Pharmacology

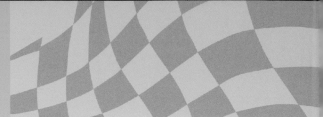

First and second edition authors:

Magali N F Taylor

Peter J W Reide

James S Dawson

Third edition author:

Gada Yassin

4th Edition
CRASH COURSE

SERIES EDITOR
Dan Horton-Szar
BSc (Hons), MBBS (Hons), MRCGP
Northgate Medical Practice Canterbury

FACULTY ADVISOR
Clive Page
BSc, PhD
Sackler Institute of Pulmonary Pharmacology
King's College London, UK

Pharmacology

Elisabetta Battista
BSc (Hons)
Fifth Year Medical Student
Guy's, King's and St Thomas'
King's College London
London, UK

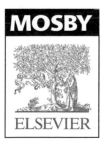

MOSBY
ELSEVIER

Edinburgh London New York Oxford Philadelphia St Louis Sydney Toronto 2015

ELSEVIER
MOSBY

Commissioning Editor: **Jeremy Bowes**
Development Editor: **Ailsa Laing**
Project Manager: **Cheryl Brant**
Designer: **Stewart Larking**
Icon Illustrations: **Geo Parkin**
Illustrations: **Marion Tasker**

First edition 2002

Second edition 2004

Third edition 2007

Fourth edition 2012

Updated Fourth edition 2015

ISBN: 978-0-7234-3851-9

British Library Cataloguing in Publication Data
A catalogue record for this book is available from the British Library

Library of Congress Cataloging in Publication Data
A catalog record for this book is available from the Library of Congress

Notices
Knowledge and best practice in this field are constantly changing. As new research and experience broaden our understanding, changes in research methods, professional practices, or medical treatment may become necessary.

Practitioners and researchers must always rely on their own experience and knowledge in evaluating and using any information, methods, compounds, or experiments described herein. In using such information or methods they should be mindful of their own safety and the safety of others, including parties for whom they have a professional responsibility.

With respect to any drug or pharmaceutical products identified, readers are advised to check the most current information provided (i) on procedures featured or (ii) by the manufacturer of each product to be administered, to verify the recommended dose or formula, the method and duration of administration, and contraindications. It is the responsibility of practitioners, relying on their own experience and knowledge of their patients, to make diagnoses, to determine dosages and the best treatment for each individual patient, and to take all appropriate safety precautions.

To the fullest extent of the law, neither the Publisher nor the authors, contributors, or editors, assume any liability for any injury and/or damage to persons or property as a matter of products liability, negligence or otherwise, or from any use or operation of any methods, products, instructions, or ideas contained in the material herein.

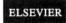

your source for books,
journals and multimedia
in the health sciences
www.elsevierhealth.com

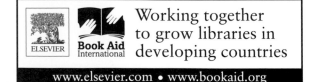

Working together
to grow libraries in
developing countries

www.elsevier.com • www.bookaid.org

The
Publisher's
policy is to use
**paper manufactured
from sustainable forests**

Printed in China

Last digit is the print line: 10 9 8 7 6 5 4 3 2 1

Series editor foreword

The *Crash Course* series first published in 1997 and now, 15 years on, we are still going strong. Medicine never stands still, and the work of keeping this series relevant for today's students is an ongoing process. These fourth editions build on the success of the previous titles and incorporate new and revised material, to keep the series up-to-date with current guidelines for best practice, and recent developments in medical research and pharmacology.

We always listen to feedback from our readers, through focus groups and student reviews of the *Crash Course* titles. For the fourth editions we have completely re-written our self-assessment material to keep up with today's 'single-best answer' and 'extended matching question' formats. The artwork and layout of the titles has also been largely re-worked to make it easier on the eye during long sessions of revision.

Despite fully revising the books with each edition, we hold fast to the principles on which we first developed the series. *Crash Course* will always bring you all the information you need to revise in compact, manageable volumes that integrate basic medical science and clinical practice. The books still maintain the balance between clarity and conciseness, and provide sufficient depth for those aiming at distinction. The authors are medical students and junior doctors who have recent experience of the exams you are now facing, and the accuracy of the material is checked by a team of faculty advisors from across the UK.

I wish you all the best for your future careers!

Dr Dan Horton-Szar

Prefaces

Author

This book aims to explain both the theory and clinical application of pharmacology. It is easily accessible and can be used to support learning and aid revision.

The introductory chapter gives a comprehensive overview of the basic concepts of pharmacology. The following chapters then elaborate on these concepts, focusing on specific systems within the body. This new edition is clear and concise, featuring clinical vignettes and illustrations throughout. New material regarding recent pharmacological advances has been included. The self-assessment section has been updated to reflect current testing strategies, now featuring a 'Best of fives' section.

I hope you find the book informative and enjoyable, and wish you luck in learning the fascinating subject of pharmacology.

Elisabetta Battista

Faculty advisor

This volume of *Crash Course: Pharmacology* has been thoroughly revised from the previous three editions. Even more than ever it provides a comprehensive and approachable text on pharmacology for medical students and others interested in the study of pharmacology. As part of the *Crash Course* series, the overall style is user friendly, consisting of concise bulleted text with informative illustrations, many of which are new, along with a useful glossary of commonly used terms. The content provides a comprehensive overview of the core material needed to pass the pharmacology component of the undergraduate medical curriculum. At the end of the book, there is a self-assessment section consisting of multiple-choice questions, short-answer questions and extended-matching questions which test the reader's understanding of the topic.

In line with the new style of curriculum recommended by the General Medical Council, the pharmacology is organized logically into body systems and the clinical relevance of the pharmacology is stressed throughout.

I have no doubt that this volume will be a useful study and revision aid for students. It provides a refreshing means of bringing the medical student up to speed in pharmacology and many congratulations go to Elisabetta Battista for the professional way she has updated this volume, significantly increasing its usefulness as a revision aid for students.

Clive Page

Acknowledgements

I would like to thank Professor Clive Page for his continual guidance and encouragement. Further thanks to everyone involved with the book at Elsevier. A massive thank you to all of my friends and family who have supported me during the writing of this book and throughout my medical course. I would like to thank everyone at Kings College London for aiding me in reading medicine and clinical pharmacology. Finally, a very special thanks to Emlyn Clay and Colette Davidson for their unwavering friendship, and my wonderful parents, who have always encouraged me.

Figure credits

Figures 1.3–1.5, 1.11B, 2.1–2.4, 5.2, 5.4, 5.11, 5.18, 5.19, 6.1–6.5, 6.7, 6.11, 6.17, 7.1–7.5, 8.1, 10.8–10.10 and 10.13 redrawn with kind permission from *Integrated Pharmacology*, 3rd edn, edited by Professor C Page, Dr M Curtis, Professor M Walker and Professor B Hoffman, Mosby, 2006.

Key to Icons

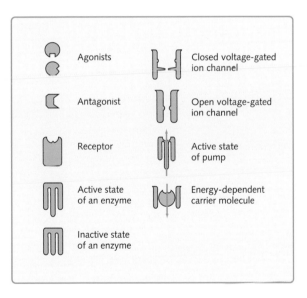

Agonists	Closed voltage-gated ion channel
Antagonist	Open voltage-gated ion channel
Receptor	Active state of pump
Active state of an enzyme	Energy-dependent carrier molecule
Inactive state of an enzyme	

Contents

Contents

Introduction to pharmacology 1

Objectives

After reading this chapter, you will:
- Understand the principles by which drugs act in the body
- Know the main mechanisms by which drugs act and the features of different receptor systems
- Understand that the pharmacodynamics and pharmacokinetics of a drug determine the drug's effect on the body and the body's response to the drug
- Know the importance of drug interactions, adverse drug effects and their monitoring
- Have a basic knowledge of the drug development process.

MOLECULAR BASIS OF PHARMACOLOGY

What is pharmacology?

Pharmacology is the study of the actions, mechanisms, uses and adverse effects of drugs.

A drug is any natural or synthetic substance that alters the physiological state of a living organism. Drugs can be divided into two groups:

- **Medicinal drugs:** substances used for the prevention, treatment and diagnosis of disease.
- **Non-medicinal (social) drugs:** substances used for recreational purposes. These drugs include illegal substances such as cannabis, heroin and cocaine as well as everyday substances such as caffeine, nicotine and alcohol.

Although drugs are intended to have a selective action, this is rarely achieved.

There is always a risk of adverse effects associated with the use of any drug and the prescriber should weigh up the effects when choosing drugs.

Drug names and classification

A single drug can have a variety of names (Fig. 1.1) and belong to many classes. Drugs are classified according to their:

- Pharmacotherapeutic actions
- Pharmacological actions
- Molecular actions
- Chemical nature.

When a drug company's patent expires, the marketing of the drug is open to other manufacturers. Although the generic name is retained the brand names can be changed.

How do drugs work?

Most drugs produce their effects by targeting specific cellular macromolecules. The majority act on receptors but they can also inhibit enzymes and transport systems. Some drugs directly target pathogens. For example, β-lactam antibiotics are bactericidal, acting by interfering with bacterial cell wall synthesis.

Certain drugs do not have conventional targets. For example, succimer is a chelating drug that is used to treat heavy metal poisoning. It binds to metals, rendering them inactive and more readily excretable. Such drugs work by means of their physicochemical properties and are said to have a non-specific mechanism of action. For this reason these drugs must be given in much higher doses (mg–g) than the more specific drugs.

Transport systems

Ion channels

Ion channels are proteins that form pores across the cell membrane and allow selective transfer of ions (charged species) in and out of the cell. Opening or closing of these channels is known as 'gating'; this occurs as a result of the ion channel undergoing a change in shape. Gating is controlled either by transmitter substances or by the membrane potential (voltage-operated channels).

Some drugs modulate ion channel function directly by blocking the pore (e.g. the blocking action of local anaesthetics on sodium channels); others bind to a part of the ion channel protein to modify its action (e.g. anxiolytics acting on the GABA channel). Other drugs interact with ion channels indirectly via a G-protein and other intermediates.

Fig. 1.1 The main methods of naming drugs

Name	Description
Chemical	Describes the atomic/molecular structure of the drug, e.g. *N*-acetyl-*p*-aminophenol
Generic	Name given to government-approved drugs sold on prescription or over the counter, e.g. paracetamol
Proprietary (brand name)	The brand a particular company assigns to the drug product, indicated by®, e.g. Calpol®

Carrier molecules

Transfer of ions and molecules against their concentration gradients is facilitated by carrier molecules located in the cell membrane. There are two types of carrier molecule:

1. **Energy-independent carriers**: These are transporters (move one type of ion/molecule in one direction), symporters (move two or more ions/molecules) or antiporters (exchange one or more ions/molecules for one or more other ions/molecules).
2. **Energy-dependent carriers**: These are termed pumps (e.g. the Na^+/K^+ ATPase pump).

Enzymes

Enzymes are protein catalysts that increase the rate of specific chemical reactions without undergoing any net change themselves during the reaction. All enzymes are potential targets for drugs. Drugs either act as a false substrate for the enzyme or inhibit the enzyme's activity directly by binding to other sites on the enzyme.

Certain drugs may require enzymatic modification. This degradation converts a drug from its inactive form (prodrug) to its active form.

Receptors

Receptors are the means through which endogenous ligands produce their effects. A receptor is a specific protein molecule that is usually located in the cell membrane, although intracellular receptors and intranuclear receptors also exist.

A ligand that binds *and* activates a receptor is an agonist. However, a ligand that binds to a receptor but *does not* activate the receptor, also prevents an agonist from doing so. Such a ligand is called an antagonist.

The following are naturally occurring ligands:

- **Neurotransmitters**: Chemicals released from nerve terminals that diffuse across the synaptic cleft, and bind to pre- or postsynaptic receptors.
- **Hormones**: Chemicals that, after being released locally, or into the bloodstream from specialized cells, can act at neighbouring or distant cells.

Each cell expresses only certain receptors, depending on the function of the cell. Receptor number and responsiveness to messengers can be modulated.

In many cases there is more than one receptor for each messenger, so that the messenger often has different pharmacological specificity and different functions according to where it binds (e.g. adrenaline is able to produce different effects in different tissues).

Using conventional molecular biology techniques it is now possible to clone receptors and express them in cultured cells, thus allowing their properties to be studied. In particular, amino acid mutations can be reproduced so that the relation between protein structure and function can be evaluated.

There are four main types of receptor (Fig. 1.2).

1. Receptors directly linked to ion channels

Receptors that are directly linked to ion channels (Fig. 1.3) are mainly involved in fast synaptic neurotransmission. A classic example of a receptor linked directly to an ion channel is the nicotinic acetylcholine receptor (nicAChR).

Fig. 1.2 The four main types of receptor and their uses

Receptor type	Time for effect	Receptor example	Function example
Ion channel linked	Milliseconds	Nicotinic acetylcholine receptor	Removing hand from hot water
G-protein linked	Seconds	β-Adrenergic receptor	Airway smooth muscle relaxation
Tyrosine kinase linked	Minutes	Insulin receptor	Glucose uptake into cells
DNA linked	Hours to days	Steroid receptor	Cellular proliferation

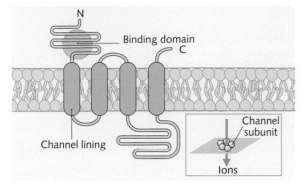

Fig. 1.3 General structure of the subunits of receptors directly linked to ion channels. (C, C-terminal; N, N-terminal.) (Redrawn from Page et al. 2006.)

The nicAChRs possess several characteristics:

- Acetylcholine (ACh) must bind to the N-terminal of both α subunits in order to activate the receptor.
- The receptor shows marked similarities with the two other receptors for fast transmission, namely the γ-aminobutyric acid (GABA$_A$) and glycine receptors.

2. G-protein linked receptors

G-protein linked receptors (Fig. 1.4) are involved in relatively fast transduction. G-protein linked receptors are the predominant receptor type in the body; muscarinic, ACh, adrenergic, dopamine, serotonin and opiate receptors are all examples of G-protein linked receptors.

Molecular structure of the receptor

Most of the G-protein linked receptors consist of a single polypeptide chain of 400–500 residues and have seven transmembrane-spanning α helices. The third

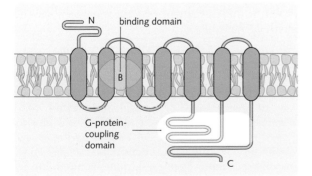

Fig. 1.4 General structure of the subunits of receptors linked to G-proteins. (C, C-terminal; N, N-terminal.) (Redrawn from Page et al. 2006.)

intracellular loop of the receptor is larger than the other loops and interacts with the G-protein.

The ligand-binding domain is buried within the membrane on one or more of the α helical segments. In contrast to the ion channel coupled receptors, the ligand binds to the extracellular N-terminal region – an area easily accessible to small hydrophobic molecules.

G-proteins

Figure 1.5 illustrates the mechanism of G-protein linked receptors:

- In resting state, the G-protein is unattached to the receptor and is a trimer consisting of α, β and γ subunits (Fig. 1.5A).
- The occupation of the receptor by an agonist produces a conformational change, causing its affinity for the trimer to increase. Subsequent association of the trimer with the receptor results in the dissociation of bound guanosine diphosphate (GDP) from the α subunit. Guanosine triphosphate (GTP) replaces GDP in the cleft thereby activating the G-protein and causing the α subunit to dissociate from the βγ dimer (Fig. 1.5B).
- α-GTP represents the active form of the G-protein (although this is not always the case: in the heart, potassium channels are activated by the βγ dimer and recent research has shown that the γ subunit alone may play a role in activation). This component diffuses in the plane of the membrane where it is free to interact with downstream effectors such as enzymes and ion channels. The βγ dimer remains associated with the membrane owing to its hydrophobicity (Fig. 1.5C).
- The cycle is completed when the α subunit, which has enzymic activity, hydrolyses the bound GTP to GDP. The GDP-bound α subunit dissociates from the effector and recombines with the βγ dimer (Fig. 1.5D).

This whole process results in an amplification effect because the binding of an agonist to the receptor can cause the activation of numerous G-proteins which in turn can each, via their association with the effector, produce many molecules of product.

Many types of G-protein exist. This is probably attributable to the variability of the α subunit. G$_s$ and G$_i$/G$_o$ cause stimulation and inhibition, respectively, of the target enzyme adenylyl cyclase. This explains why muscarinic ACh receptors (G$_i$/G$_o$ linked) and β-adrenoreceptors (G$_s$ linked) located in the heart produce opposite effects. The bacterial toxins cholera and pertussis can be used in order to determine which G-protein is involved in a particular situation. Each has enzymic action on a conjugation reaction with the α subunit, such that:

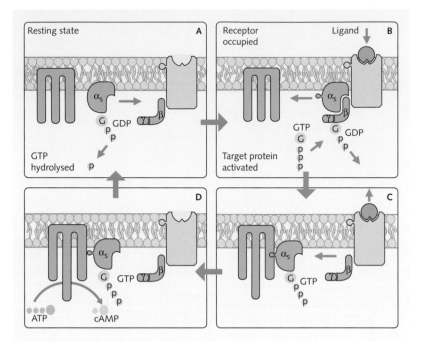

Fig. 1.5 Mechanism of action of G-protein linked receptors. (α, β, γ, subunits of G-protein; ATP, adenosine triphosphate; cAMP, cyclic adenosine monophosphate; G, guanosine; GDP, GTP, guanosine di- and triphosphate; p, phosphate.) (Redrawn from Page et al. 2006.) Integrated Pharmacology, 3rd edition, Mosby.

- Cholera affects G_s causing continued activation of adenylyl cyclase. This explains why infection with cholera toxin results in uncontrolled fluid secretion from the gastrointestinal tract.
- Pertussis affects G_i and G_o causing continued inactivation of adenylyl cyclase. This explains why infection with *Bordetella pertussis* causes a 'whooping' cough, characteristic of this infection, as the airways are constricted, and the larynx experiences muscular spasms.

Targets for G-proteins
G-proteins interact with either ion channels or secondary messengers. G-proteins may activate ion channels directly, e.g. muscarinic receptors in the heart are linked to potassium channels which open directly on interaction with the G-protein, causing a slowing down of the heart rate. Secondary messengers are a family of mediating chemicals that transduces the receptor activation in to a cellular response. These mediators can be targeted and three main secondary messenger systems exist as targets of G-proteins (Fig. 1.6).

Adenylyl cyclase/cAMP system
Adenylyl cyclase catalyses the conversion of ATP to cyclic cAMP within cells. The cAMP produced in turn causes activation of certain protein kinases, enzymes that phosphorylate serine and threonine residues in various proteins, thereby producing either activation or inactivation of these proteins. A stimulatory example of this system can be observed in the activation of β_1-adrenergic receptors found in cardiac muscle. The activation of β_1-adrenergic receptors results in the activation of cAMP-dependent protein kinase A, which phosphorylates and opens voltage-operated calcium channels. This increases calcium levels in the cells and results in an increased rate and force of contraction. An inhibitory example of this system can be observed in activation of opioid receptors. The receptor linked to the 'G_i' protein inhibits adenylyl cyclase and reduces cAMP production.

Phospholipase C/inositol phosphate system
Activation of M_1, M_3, 5-HT$_2$, peptide and α_1-adreno-receptors, via G_q, cause activation of phospholipase C, a membrane-bound enzyme, which increases the rate of degradation of phosphatidylinositol (4,5) bisphosphate into diacylglycerol (DAG) and inositol (1,4,5) triphosphate (IP$_3$). DAG and IP$_3$ act as second messengers. IP$_3$ binds to the membrane of the endoplasmic reticulum, opening calcium channels and increasing the concentration of calcium within the cell. Increased calcium levels may result in smooth muscle contraction, increased secretion from exocrine glands, increased hormone or transmitter release, or increased force and rate of contraction of the heart. DAG, which

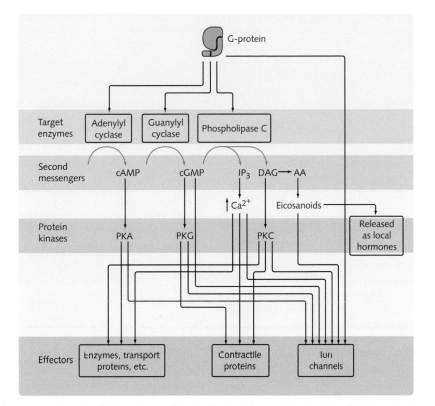

Fig. 1.6 Second-messenger targets of G-proteins and their effects. (AA, arachidonic acid ; cAMP, cyclic adenosine monophosphate; cGMP, cyclic guanosine monophosphate; DAG, diacylglycerol; IP_3, inositol (1,4,5) triphosphate; PK, protein kinase.)

remains associated with the membrane owing to its hydrophobicity, causes protein kinase C to move from the cytosol to the membrane where DAG can regulate the activity of the latter. There are at least six types of protein kinase C, with over 50 targets including:

- Release of hormones and neurotransmitters
- Smooth muscle contraction
- Inflammation
- Ion transport
- Tumour promotion.

Guanylyl cyclase system
Guanylyl cyclase catalyses the conversion of GTP to cGMP. This cGMP goes on to cause activation of protein kinase G which in turn phosphorylates contractile proteins and ion channels. Transmembrane guanylyl cyclase activity is exhibited by the atrial natriuretic peptide receptor upon the binding of atrial natriuretic peptide. Cytoplasmic guanylyl cyclase activity is exhibited when bradykinin activates receptors on the membrane of endothelial cells to generate nitric oxide, which then acts as a second messenger to activate guanylyl cyclase within the cell.

3. Tyrosine kinase linked receptors

Tyrosine kinase linked receptors are involved in the regulation of growth and differentiation, and responses to metabolic signals. The response time of enzyme-initiated transduction is slow (minutes). Examples include the receptors for insulin, platelet-derived growth factor and epidermal growth factor.

Activation of tyrosine kinase receptors results in autophosphorylation of tyrosine residues leading to the activation of pathways involving protein kinases.

4. DNA linked receptors

DNA linked receptors are located intracellularly and so agonists must pass through the cell membrane in order to reach the receptor. The agonist binds to the receptor and this receptor–agonist complex is transported to the nucleus, aided by chaperone proteins. Once in the nucleus the complex can bind to specific DNA sequences and so alter the expression of specific genes. As a result, transcription of this specific gene to mRNA is increased or decreased and thus the amount of mRNA available for translation into a protein increases or decreases.

The process is much slower than for other receptor–ligand interactions, and the effects usually last longer. Examples of molecules with DNA-linked receptors are corticosteroids, thyroid hormone, retinoic acid and vitamin D.

HINTS AND TIPS

Drugs, like naturally occurring chemical mediators, act on receptors located in the cell membrane, in the cytoplasm of the cell, or in the cell nucleus, to bring about a cellular, and eventually organ or tissue, response.

DRUG–RECEPTOR INTERACTIONS

Most drugs produce their effects by acting through specific protein molecules called receptors.

Receptors respond to endogenous chemicals in the body that are either synaptic transmitter substances (e.g. ACh, noradrenaline) or hormones (endocrine, e.g. insulin; or local mediators, e.g. histamine). These chemicals or drugs are classed as:

- **Agonists**: Activate receptors and produce a subsequent response.
- **Antagonists**: Associate with receptors but do not cause activation. Antagonists reduce the chance of transmitters or agonists binding to the receptor and thereby oppose their action by effectively diluting or removing the receptors from the system.

Electrostatic forces initially attract a drug to a receptor. If the shape of the drug corresponds to that of the binding site of the receptor, then it will be held there temporarily by weak bonds or, in the case of irreversible antagonists, permanently by stronger covalent bonds. It is the number of bonds and goodness of fit between drug and receptor that determines the affinity of the drug for that receptor, such that the greater the number of bonds and the better the goodness of fit, the higher the affinity will be.

The affinity is defined by the dissociation constant, which is given the symbol K_d. The lower the K_d, the higher the affinity. K_d values in the nanomolar range represent drugs (D) with a high affinity for their receptor (R):

$$D + R \underset{k_{-1}}{\overset{k_{+1}}{\rightleftharpoons}} DR$$

The rate at which the forward reaction occurs depends on the drug concentration [D] and the receptor concentration [R]:

$$\text{Forward rate} = K_{+1}[D][R]$$

The rate at which the backward reaction occurs mainly depends on the interaction between the drug and the receptor [DR]:

$$\text{Backward rate} = K_{-1}[DR]$$
$$K_d = K_{-1}/K_{+1}$$

K_a is the association constant and is used to quantify affinity. It can be defined as the concentration of drug that produces 50% of the maximum response at equilibrium, in the absence of receptor reserve:

$$K_a = 1/K_d$$

Drugs with a high affinity stay bound to their receptor for a relatively long time and are said to have a slow off-rate. This means that at any time the probability that any given receptor will be occupied by the drug is high.

The ability of a drug to combine with one type of receptor is termed specificity. Although no drug is truly specific, most exhibit relatively selective action on one type of receptor.

Agonists

Agonist (A) binds to the receptor (R) and the chemical energy released on binding induces a conformational change that sets off a chain of biochemical events within the cell, leading to a response (AR*). The equation for this is:

$$A + R \xrightarrow{(1)} AR \xrightarrow{(2)} AR^*$$

where: (1) affinity; (2) efficacy.

Partial agonists cannot bring about the same maximum response as full agonists, even if their affinity for the receptor is the same (Fig. 1.7).

The ability of agonists, once bound, to activate receptors is termed efficacy, such that:

- Full agonists have high efficacy and are able to produce a maximum response while occupying only a small percentage of the receptors available.
- Partial agonists have low efficacy and are unable to elicit the maximum response even if they are occupying all the available receptors.

Antagonists

Antagonists bind to receptors but do not activate them; they do not induce a conformational change and thus have no efficacy. However, because antagonists occupy the receptor, they prevent agonists from binding and therefore block their action.

Two types of antagonist exist: competitive and non-competitive.

Competitive antagonists

Competitive antagonists bind to receptors reversibly, and effectively produce a dilution of the receptors such that:

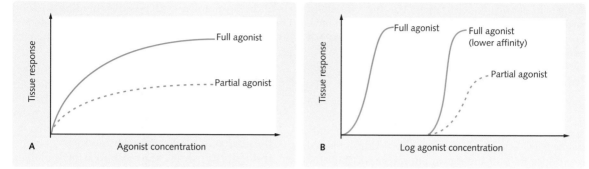

Fig. 1.7 Comparison for a partial agonist and a full agonist showing (A) the dose–response curve and (B) the log dose–response curve. (From Neal MJ 2009 *Medical Pharmacology at a Glance*, 6th edition. Wiley-Blackwell, with permission.)

- A parallel shift is produced to the right of the agonist dose–response curve (Fig. 1.8).
- The maximum response is not depressed. This reflects the fact that the antagonist's effect can be overcome by increasing the dose of agonist, i.e. the block is surmountable. Increasing the concentration of agonist increases the probability of the agonist taking the place of an antagonist leaving the receptor.
- The size of the shift in the agonist dose–response curve produced by the antagonist reflects the affinity of the antagonist for the receptor. High-affinity antagonists stay bound to the receptor for a relatively long period of time allowing the agonist little chance to take the antagonist's place.

This concept can be quantified in terms of the dose ratio. The dose ratio is the ratio of the concentration of agonist producing a given response in the presence and absence of a certain concentration of antagonist, e.g. a dose ratio of 3 tells us that three times as much agonist was required to produce a given response in the presence of the antagonist than it did in its absence.

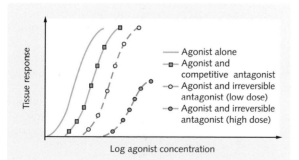

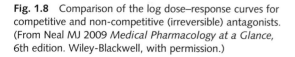

Fig. 1.8 Comparison of the log dose–response curves for competitive and non-competitive (irreversible) antagonists. (From Neal MJ 2009 *Medical Pharmacology at a Glance*, 6th edition. Wiley-Blackwell, with permission.)

> **COMMUNICATION**
>
> A 22-year-old man is admitted to hospital with signs of respiratory depression, drowsiness, bradycardia and confusion. His girlfriend tells the medical team that he uses heroin and an overdose is therefore suspected. Heroin act as an agonist, activating the opioid receptors. Naloxone is a competitive antagonist at those receptors and so is administered as treatment. Minutes later the man's condition improves and his respiratory rate rises to normal. Careful titration of the naloxone dose should allow treatment of respiratory depression without provoking acute withdrawal signs.

Non-competitive antagonists

Non-competitive antagonists are also known as irreversible antagonists. Their presence:

- Also produces a parallel shift to the right of the agonist dose–response curve (see Fig. 1.8).
- Depresses the maximum response, reflecting the fact that the antagonist's effect cannot be overcome by the addition of greater doses of agonist. At low concentrations, however, a parallel shift may occur without a reduced maximum response. This tells us that not all of the receptors need to be occupied to elicit a maximum response, because irreversible antagonists effectively remove receptors, and there must be a number of spare receptors.

Receptor reserve

Although on a log scale the relation between the concentration of agonist and the response produces a symmetrical sigmoid curve, rarely does a 50% response correspond to 50% receptor occupancy. This is because there are spare receptors.

This excess of receptors is known as receptor reserve and serves to sharpen the sensitivity of the cell to small changes in agonist concentration. The low efficacy of partial agonists can be overcome in tissues with a large receptor reserve and in these circumstances partial agonists may act as full agonists.

Potency

Potency relates to the concentration of a drug needed to elicit a response. The EC_{50}, where EC stands for effective concentration, is a number used to quantify potency. EC_{50} is the concentration of drug required to produce 50% of the maximum response. Thus, the lower the EC_{50}, the more potent the drug. For agonists, potency is related to both affinity and efficacy, but for antagonists only affinity is considered since they have no efficacy.

Pharmacokinetic variables also affect potency. For example, the acidic pH of the stomach may break down a drug that has been found to be very potent in a test tube. This means that, if given as a tablet, it would have very little potency and would be ineffective.

> **HINTS AND TIPS**
>
> The kinetic equations simply demonstrate how drugs act, and how they differ from one another. You are unlikely to be asked about them, though try to work through them as they aid in the building of a good foundation in the subject.

PHARMACOKINETICS

Pharmacology can be divided into two disciplines. These are:

- **Pharmacokinetics**: the way the body affects the drug with time, i.e. the factors that determine its absorption, distribution, metabolism and excretion.
- **Pharmacodynamics**: the biological effect of the drug on the body.

Administration

Topical

Topical drugs are applied where they are needed, giving them the advantage that they do not have to cross any barriers or membranes. Examples include skin ointments; ear, nose or eye drops; and aerosols inhaled in the treatment of asthma.

Enteral

Enteral administration means that the drug reaches its target via the gut. This is the least predictable route of administration, owing to metabolism by the liver,

chemical breakdown and possible binding to food. Drugs must cross several barriers, which may or may not be a problem according to their physicochemical properties, such as charge and size. However:

- Most drugs are administered orally unless the drug is unstable, or is rapidly inactivated in the gastrointestinal tract, or if its efficacy of absorption from the gastrointestinal tract is uncertain (owing to metabolism by the liver or the intestines, vomiting or a disease that may affect drug absorption).
- Absorption of drugs via the buccal or sublingual route avoids the portal circulation and is therefore valuable when administering drugs subject to a high degree of first-pass metabolism (which is unavoidable if taken orally). It is also useful for potent drugs with a non-disagreeable taste, such as sublingual nitroglycerin given to relieve acute attacks of angina.
- Administration of drugs rectally, such as in the form of suppositories, means that there is less first-pass metabolism by the liver because the venous return from the lower gastrointestinal tract is less than that from the upper gastrointestinal tract. It has the disadvantage, however, of being inconsistent.
- Antacids have their effect in the stomach and may be considered as being topical.

Parenteral

Parenteral administration means that the drug is administered in a manner that avoids the gut. The protein drug insulin, for example, is destroyed by the acidity of the stomach and the digestive enzymes within the gut and must therefore be injected, usually subcutaneously.

Intravenous injection of drugs has several advantages:

- It is the most direct route of administration. The drug enters the bloodstream directly and bypasses absorption barriers.
- A drug is distributed in a large volume and acts rapidly.

For drugs that must be given continuously by infusion, or for drugs that damage tissues, this is an important method of administration.

Alternative parenteral routes of administration include subcutaneous, intramuscular, epidural or intrathecal injections, and transdermal patches.

The rate of drug absorption from the site of the injection can be decreased by binding the drug to a vehicle or co-administering a vasoconstrictor, such as adrenaline, to reduce blood flow to the site.

Drug absorption

Bioavailability takes into account both absorption and metabolism and describes the proportion of the drug that passes into the systemic circulation. This will be

100% after an intravenous injection, but following oral administration it will depend on the drug, the individual and the circumstances under which the drug is given.

Drugs must cross membranes to enter cells or to transfer between body compartments; therefore, drug absorption will be affected by both chemical and physiological factors.

Cell membranes

Cell membranes are composed of lipid bi-layers and thus absorption is usually proportional to the lipid solubility of the drug. Unionized molecules (B) are far more soluble than those that are ionized (BH$^+$) and surrounded by a 'shell' of water.

$$B + H^+ \rightleftharpoons BH^+$$

Size

Small size is another factor that favours absorption. Most drugs are small molecules (molecular weight < 1000) that are able to diffuse across membranes in their uncharged state.

pH

Since most drugs are either weak bases, weak acids or amphoteric, the pH of the environment in which they dissolve, as well as the pK$_a$ value of the drug, will be important in determining the fraction in the unionized form that is in solution and able to diffuse across cell membranes. The pK$_a$ of a drug is defined as the pH at which 50% of the molecules in solution are in the ionized form, and is characterized by the Henderson–Hasselbalch equation:

For acidic molecules:

$$HA \rightleftharpoons H^+ + A$$
$$pK_a = pH + \log [HA]/[A^-]$$

For basic molecules:

$$BH^+ \rightleftharpoons B + H^+$$
$$pK_a = pH + \log [BH^+]/[B]$$

Drugs will tend to exist in the ionized form when exposed to an environment with a pH opposite to their own state. Therefore, acids become increasingly ionized with increasing pH (i.e. basic).

It is useful to consider three important body compartments in relation to plasma (pH = 7.4), stomach (pH = 2.0) and urine (pH = 8.0). For example:

- Aspirin is a weak acid (pK$_a$= 3.5) and its absorption will therefore be favoured in the stomach, where it is uncharged, and not in the plasma or the urine, where it is highly charged; aspirin in high doses may even damage the stomach.
- Morphine is a weak base (pK$_a$ = 8.0) that is highly charged in the stomach, quite charged in the plasma, and half charged in the urine. Morphine is able to cross the blood–brain barrier but is poorly and erratically absorbed from the stomach and intestines, and metabolized by the liver; it must therefore be given by injection or delayed-release capsules. Some drugs, such as quaternary ammonium compounds (e.g. suxamethonium, tubocurarine), are always charged and must therefore be injected.

Drug distribution

Once drugs have reached the circulation, they are distributed around the body. As most drugs have a very small molecular size, they are able to leave the circulation by capillary filtration to act on the tissues.

The half-life of a drug (t$_{1/2}$) is the time taken for the plasma concentration of that drug to fall to half of its original value. Bulk transfer in the blood is very quick. Drugs:

- Exist either dissolved in blood or bound to plasma proteins such as albumin. Albumin is the most important circulating protein for binding many acidic drugs.
- That are basic tend to be bound to a globulin fraction that increases with age. A drug that is bound is confined to the vascular system and is unable to exert its actions; this becomes a problem if more than 80% of the drug is bound.
- Interact and one drug may displace another. For example, aspirin can displace the benzodiazepine diazepam from albumin.

The apparent volume of distribution (V$_d$) is the calculated pharmacokinetic space in which a drug is distributed.

$$V_d = \frac{\text{dose administered}}{\text{initial apparent plasma concentration}}$$

V$_d$ values:

- That amount to less than a certain body compartment volume indicate that the drug is contained within that compartment. For example, when the volume of distribution is less than 5 L, it is likely that the drug is restricted to the vasculature.
- Less than 15 L implies that the drug is restricted to the extracellular fluid.
- Greater than 15 L suggests distribution within the total body water. Some drugs (usually basic) have a volume of distribution that exceeds body weight, in which case tissue binding is occurring. These drugs tend to be contained outside the circulation

and may accumulate in certain tissues. Very lipid-soluble substances, such as thiopental, can build up in fat. Its half-life will be much longer in obese patients than in thinner patients and this can lead to accumulations in the bone; and mepacrine, an anti-malarial drug, has a concentration in the liver 200 times that in the plasma because it binds to nucleic acids. Some drugs are even actively transported into certain organs.

Drug metabolism

Before being excreted from the body, most drugs are metabolized. A small number of drugs exist in their fully ionized form at physiological pH (7.4) and, owing to this highly polar nature, are metabolized to only a minor extent, if at all. The sequential metabolic reactions that occur have been categorized as phases 1 and 2.

Sites of metabolism

The liver is the major site of drug metabolism although most tissues are able to metabolize specific drugs. Other sites of metabolism include the kidney, the lung and the gastrointestinal tract. Diseases of these organs may affect a drug's pharmacokinetics.

Orally administered drugs, which are usually absorbed in the small intestine, reach the liver via the portal circulation. At this stage, or within the small intestine, the drugs may be extensively metabolized; this is known as first-pass metabolism and means that considerably less drug reaches the systemic circulation than enters the portal vein. This causes problems because it means that higher doses of drug must be given and, owing to individual variation in the degree of first-pass metabolism, the effects of the drug can be unpredictable. Drugs that are subject to a high degree of first-pass metabolism, such as the local anaesthetic lidocaine, cannot be given orally and must be administered by some other route.

Phase 1 metabolic reactions

Phase 1 metabolic reactions include oxidation, reduction and hydrolysis. These reactions introduce a functional group, such as OH^- or NH_2, which increases the polarity of the drug molecule and provides a site for phase 2 reactions.

Oxidation

Oxidations are the most common type of reaction and are catalysed by an enzyme system known as the microsomal mixed function oxidase system, which is located on the smooth endoplasmic reticulum. The enzyme system forms small vesicles known as microsomes when the tissue is homogenized.

Cytochrome P_{450}:

- Is the most important enzyme, although other enzymes are involved. This enzyme is a haemoprotein that requires the presence of oxygen, reduced nicotinamide adenine dinucleotide phosphate (NADPH) and NADPH cytochrome P_{450} reductase in order to function.
- Exists in several hundred isoforms, some of which are constitutive, whereas others are synthesized in response to specific signals. The substrate specificity of this enzyme depends on the isoform but tends to be low, meaning that a whole variety of drugs can be oxidized.

Although oxidative reactions usually result in inactivation of the drug, sometimes a metabolite is produced that is pharmacologically active and may have a duration of action exceeding that of the original drug. In these cases the drug is known as a prodrug, e.g. codeine which is demethylated to morphine.

Reduction

Reduction reactions also involve microsomal enzymes but are much less common than oxidation reactions. An example of a drug subject to reduction is prednisone, which is given as a prodrug and reduced to the active glucocorticoid prednisolone.

Hydrolysis

Hydrolysis is not restricted to the liver and occurs in a variety of tissues. Aspirin is spontaneously hydrolysed to salicylic acid in moisture.

Phase 2 metabolic reactions

Drug molecules that possess a suitable site that was either present before phase 1 or is the result of a phase 1 reaction, are susceptible to phase 2 reactions. Phase 2 reactions involve conjugation, the attachment of a large chemical group to a functional group on the drug molecule. Conjugation results in the drug being more hydrophilic and thus more easily excreted from the body. In conjugation:

- It is mainly the liver that is involved, although conjugation can occur in a wide variety of tissues.
- Chemical groups involved are endogenous activated moieties such as glucuronic acid, sulphate, methyl, acetyl and glutathione.
- The conjugating enzymes exist in many isoforms and show relative substrate and metabolite specificity.

Unlike the products of phase 1 reactions, the conjugate is almost invariably inactive. An important exception is morphine, which is converted to morphine 6-glucuronide, which has an analgesic effect lasting longer than that of its parent molecule.

Factors affecting metabolism

Enzyme induction is the increased synthesis or decreased degradation of enzymes and occurs as a result of the presence of an exogenous substance. For example:

- Some drugs are able to increase the activity of certain isoenzyme forms of cytochrome P_{450} and thus increase their own metabolism, as well as that of other drugs.
- Smokers can show increased metabolism of certain drugs because of the induction of cytochrome P_{448} by a constituent in tobacco smoke.
- In contrast, some drugs inhibit microsomal enzyme activity and therefore increase their own activity as well as that of other drugs.

Figure 1.9 gives some examples of enzyme-inducing agents, and the drugs whose metabolism is affected. Competition for a metabolic enzyme may occur between two drugs, in which case there is a decreased metabolism of one or both drugs. This is known as inhibition.

Enzymes that metabolize drugs are affected by many aspects of diet, such as the ratio of protein to carbohydrate, flavonoids contained in vegetables, and polycyclic aromatic hydrocarbons found in barbecued foods.

Overdose

Drugs that are taken at 2×-1000 times their therapeutic dose can cause unwanted and toxic effects. Paracetamol is a classic example of a drug that can be lethal at high doses (two to three times the maximum therapeutic dose), owing to the accumulation of its metabolites.

In phase 2 of the metabolic process, paracetamol is conjugated with glucuronic acid and sulphate. When high doses of paracetamol are ingested, these pathways become saturated and the drug is metabolized by the mixed function oxidases. This results in the formation of the toxic metabolite N-acetyl-p-benzoquinone which is inactivated by glutathione. However, when glutathione is depleted, this toxic metabolite reacts with nucleophilic constituents in the cell leading to necrosis in the liver and kidneys.

N-Acetylcysteine or methionine can be administered in cases of paracetamol overdose, because these increase liver glutathione formation and the conjugation reactions, respectively.

Drug excretion

Drugs are excreted from the body in a variety of different ways. Excretion predominately occurs via the kidneys into urine or by the gastrointestinal tract into bile and faeces. Volatile drugs are predominately exhaled by the lungs into the air. To a lesser extent, drugs may leave the body through breast milk and sweat.

Fig. 1.9 Examples of drugs that induce or inhibit drug-metabolizing enzymes

Drugs modifying enzyme action	Drugs whose metabolism is affected
Enzyme induction	
Phenobarbital and other barbiturates Rifampicin Phenytoin Ethanol Carbamazepine	Warfarin Oral contraceptives Corticosteroids Ciclosporin
Enzyme inhibition	
Allopurinol Chloramphenicol Corticosteroids Cimetidine MAO inhibitors Erythromycin Ciprofloxacin	Azathioprine Phenytoin Various drugs—TCA, cyclophosphamide Many drugs—amiodarone, phenytoin, pethidine Pethidine Ciclosporin Theophylline

MAO, monoamine oxidase; TCA, tricyclic antidepressant.

Adapted from Rang et al. 2012 Pharmacology, 7th edition, Churchill Livingstone.

The volume of plasma cleared of drug per unit time is known as the clearance.

Renal excretion

Glomerular filtration, tubular reabsorption (passive and active), and tubular secretion all determine the extent to which a drug will be excreted by the kidneys.

Glomerular capillaries allow the passage of molecules with a molecular weight $< 20\,000$. The glomerular filtrate thus contains most of the substances in plasma except proteins. In the glomerular capillaries:

- The negative charge of the corpuscular membrane also repels negatively charged molecules, including plasma proteins.
- Drugs that bind to plasma proteins such as albumin will not be filtered.

Most of the drug in the blood does not pass into the glomerular filtrate, but passes into the peritubular capillaries of the proximal tubule where, depending on its nature, it may be transported into the lumen of the tubule by either of two transport mechanisms. One transport mechanism deals with acidic molecules, the other with basic molecules. In the peritubular capillaries:

- Tubular secretion is responsible for most of the drug excretion carried out by the kidneys and, unlike glomerular filtration, allows the clearance of drugs bound to plasma proteins. Competition between drugs that share the same transport mechanism may occur, in which case the excretion of these drugs will be reduced.
- Reabsorption of a drug will depend upon the fraction of molecules in the ionized state, which is in turn dependent on the pH of the urine.
- Renal disease will affect the excretion of certain drugs. The extent to which excretion is impaired can be deduced by measuring 24-hour creatinine clearance.

Gastrointestinal excretion

Some drug conjugates are excreted into the bile and subsequently released into the intestines where they are hydrolysed back to the parent compound and reabsorbed. This 'enterohepatic circulation' prolongs the effect of the drug.

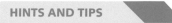

HINTS AND TIPS

The liver is the main site of drug inactivation, and the kidneys and gastrointestinal tract the main sites for drug excretion. Disease of these organs will alter a drug's pharmacokinetics.

Mathematical aspects of pharmacokinetics

Kinetic order

Two types of kinetics, related to the plasma concentration of a drug, describe the rate at which a drug leaves the body:

- **Zero-order kinetics** (Fig. 1.10A) describes a decrease in drug levels in the body that is independent of the plasma concentration, and the rate is held constant by a limiting factor, such as a co-factor of enzyme availability. When the plasma concentration is plotted against time, the decrease is a straight line. Alcohol is an example of a drug that displays zero-order kinetics.
- **First-order kinetics** (Fig. 1.10B) is displayed by most drugs. It describes a decrease in drug levels in the body that is dependent on the plasma concentration, as the concentration of the substrate (drug) is the rate limiting factor. When the plasma concentration is plotted against time, the decrease is exponential.

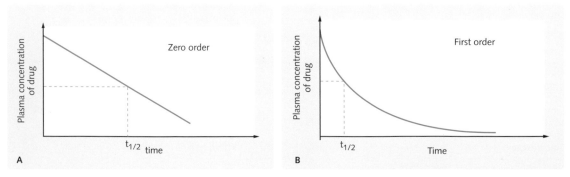

Fig. 1.10 Plasma drug concentration versus time plot. (A) For a drug displaying zero-order kinetics. (B) For a drug displaying first-order kinetics. $t_{1/2}$, half-life.

One-compartment model

The one-compartment model usually gives an adequate clinical approximation of drug concentration by considering the body to be a single compartment. Within this single compartment a drug is absorbed, immediately distributed, and subsequently eliminated by metabolism and excretion.

If the volume of the compartment is V_d and the dose administered D, then the initial drug concentration, C_o, will be:

$$C_o = D/V_d$$

The time taken for the plasma drug concentration to fall to half of its original value is the half-life of that drug. The decline in concentration may be exponential, but this situation expresses itself graphically as a straight line when the log plasma concentration is plotted against the time after intravenous dose (Fig. 1.11A).

Half-life is related to the elimination rate constant (K_{el}) by the following equation:

$$t_{1/2} \times K_{el} = \text{natural log 2 (ln 2)}$$

Half-life is related to V_d, but does not determine the ability of the body to remove the drug from the circulation, since both V_d and half-life change in the same direction. The body's ability to remove a drug from the blood is termed clearance (Cl_p) and is constant for individual drugs:

$$Cl_p = V_d \times K_{el}$$

If the drug is not administered parenterally, plotting the log plasma drug concentration against time will require the consideration of both absorption and elimination from the compartment (Fig. 1.11B).

The one-compartment model is widely used to determine the dose of drug to be administered. The two-compartment model expands on this model by considering the body as two compartments to allow some consideration of drug distribution.

Model-independent approach

For drugs displaying first-order kinetics, the level of the drug in the body increases until it is equal to the level excreted, at which point steady-state is reached (Fig. 1.12), such that:

- The time to reach steady-state is usually equal to four to five half-lives.
- The amount of drug in the body at steady-state will depend upon the frequency of drug administration: the greater the frequency, the greater the amount of drug and the less the variation between peak and trough plasma concentrations. If the frequency of administration is greater than the half-life, then accumulation of the drug will occur.

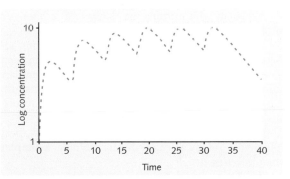

Fig. 1.12   Log plasma drug concentration versus time plot for a drug administered by mouth every 6 hours when its terminal disposition half-life is 6 hours.

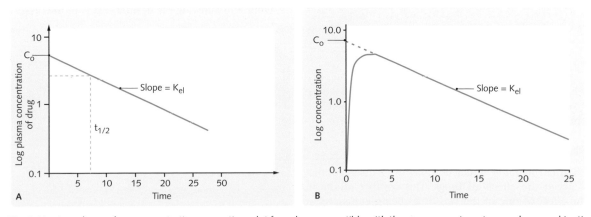

Fig. 1.11   Log plasma drug concentration versus time plot for a drug compatible with the one-compartment open pharmacokinetic model for drug disposition. (A) After a parenteral dose, assuming first-order kinetics. (B) After an oral dose. (C_o initial drug concentration; K_{el}, elimination rate constant.) (Part B redrawn from Page et al. 2006.)

The loading dose can be calculated according to the desired plasma concentration at steady-state (C_{ss}) and the volume of distribution (V_d) of the drug:

Loading dose (mg/kg) = V_d (L/kg) × C_{ss} (mg/L)

Adherence

Lastly, despite not being a pharmacological property it is important to consider adherence. For some drugs to be effective (e.g. antibiotics), they must be taken at regular intervals and for a certain period of time. For certain forms of treatment, patients may even need to come to hospital, in which case transport, work and having young children around might be a problem.

Adherence tends to be more of a problem in paediatric practice because it involves both parents and the child. The parent must remember to give the medicine and follow directions accurately; the child must cooperate and not spit out or spill the medicine. Also, elderly patients' capacity to understand and remember to take their medicines must be ascertained, as well as their physical ability to carry out the task. For example, an elderly patient with arthritis may struggle to administer medicines unaided.

Practical dosage forms are important in achieving adherence. Many tablets are now sugar coated, making them easier to take, and a large number of the drugs manufactured for children are in the form of elixirs or suspensions, which may be available in a variety of different flavours, making their administration less of a problem.

The route of administration of a drug may affect adherence. Taking a drug orally, for example, is simpler than injecting it.

The dosing schedule is also an important aspect of adherence. The easier this is to follow, and the less frequently a drug needs to be taken or administered, the more likely adherence will be achieved.

DRUG INTERACTIONS AND ADVERSE EFFECTS

Drug interactions

Drugs interact in a number of ways that may produce unwanted effects. Two types of interactions exist: pharmacodynamic and pharmacokinetic.

Pharmacodynamic interactions

Pharmacodynamic interactions involve a direct conflict between the effects of drugs. This conflict results in the effect of one of the two drugs being enhanced or reduced. For example:

- Propranolol, a β-adrenoceptor antagonist given for angina and hypertension, will reduce the effect of salbutamol, a β_2-adrenoceptor agonist given for the treatment of asthma. The administration of β-blockers to asthmatics should therefore be avoided, or undertaken with caution.
- Administration of monoamine oxidase inhibitors, which inhibit the metabolism of catecholamines, enhances the effects of drugs such as ephedrine. This enhancement causes the release of noradrenaline from stores in the nerve terminal and is known as potentiation.

Pharmacokinetic interactions

Absorption, distribution, metabolism and excretion all affect the pharmacokinetic properties of drugs. Thus any drug that interferes with these processes will be altering the effect of other drugs. For example:

- If administered with diuretics, non-steroidal anti-inflammatory drugs (NSAIDs) will reduce the anti-hypertensive action of these drugs. NSAIDs bring about this effect by reducing prostaglandin synthesis in the kidney, thus impairing renal blood flow and consequently decreasing the excretion of waste and sodium. This results in an increased blood volume and a rise in blood pressure.
- Enzyme induction, which occurs as a result of the administration of certain drugs, can affect the metabolism of other drugs served by that enzyme (see Fig. 1.9).

In some cases, however, drugs are used together so that their interaction can bring about the desired effect.

- For example, carbidopa is a drug used in conjunction with levodopa (L-dopa) in the treatment of Parkinson's disease. L-Dopa, which is converted to dopamine in the body, can cross the blood–brain barrier. Carbidopa prevents the conversion of L-dopa to dopamine; however, it cannot cross the blood–brain barrier and so acts to reduce the peripheral side-effects while still allowing the desired effects of the drug.

COMMUNICATION

Mr Abbas is a 66-year-old man who has been on metoprolol, a β-blocker, since being diagnosed with hypertension. He had a myocardial infarction (heart attack) 2 days ago and has now developed ventricular tachycardia (a type of cardiac arrhythmia). His management included receiving amiodarone, which is a class III antiarrhythmic agent.

It is vital to note that both the metoprolol and amiodarone slow the heart. This additive effect can be clinically desirable. However, as well as this dual effect, it is important the medical team is aware that amiodarone inhibits the cytochrome P_{450} enzymes responsible for breaking down metoprolol. Meaning, that in the presence of amiodarone, the plasma concentration of metoprolol is higher than would normally be expected (Fig. 1.13). This should be taken into account when deciding the drug dosage, so that excessively slow beating of the heart and conduction block of heart impulses do not occur.

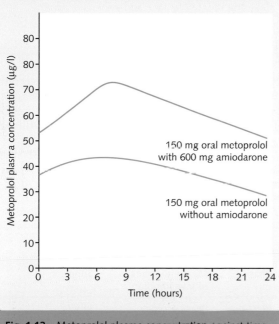

Fig. 1.13 Metoprolol plasma concentration against time, with and without amiodarone. (Adapted from Werner et al. 2004. Effect of amiodarone on the plasma levels of metoprolol. *Am J Cardiol* 94:1319–1321.)

Adverse effects

As well as interacting with one another and with their target tissue, drugs will also interact with other tissues and organs and alter their function. No drug is without side-effects, although the severity and frequency of these will vary from drug to drug and from person to person.

The liver and the kidneys are susceptible to the adverse effects of drugs, as these are the sites of drug metabolism and excretion. Some drugs cause hepatotoxicity or nephrotoxicity.

Those who are more prone to the adverse effects of drugs, include:

- Pregnant women, who must be careful about taking drugs as certain drugs are teratogenic, i.e. cause fetal malformations (e.g. thalidomide taken in the 1960s for morning sickness).
- Breastfeeding women, who must also be careful about which drugs they take, as many drugs can be passed on in the breast milk to the developing infant.
- Patients with an underlying illness other than the one being treated, such as liver or kidney disease. These illnesses will result in decreased metabolism and excretion of the drug and will produce the side-effects of an increased dose of the same drug.
- Elderly people, who tend to take a large number of drugs, greatly increasing the risk of drug interactions and the associated side-effects. In addition, elderly patients have a reduced renal clearance, and a nervous system that is more sensitive to drugs. The dose of drug initially given is usually 50% of the adult dose, and certain drugs are contraindicated.
- Children, who, like the elderly, are at an increased risk of toxicity due to immature clearance systems.
- Patients with genetic enzyme defects, such as glucose 6-phosphate dehydrogenase deficiency. The deficiency will result in haemolysis if an oxidant drug, e.g. aspirin, is taken.

Certain drugs are carcinogenic, i.e. induce cancer. Genotoxic carcinogens cause mutations, either directly (primary carcinogens) or through their metabolites (secondary carcinogens). Epigenetic carcinogens, such as phorbol esters, do not induce mutations themselves, but increase the likelihood that a mutagen will do so.

Allergic reactions to certain drugs are common, occurring in 2–25% of cases. Most of these are not serious, e.g. skin reactions; however, rarely, reactions such as anaphylactic shock (type 1 hypersensitivity) occur that may be lethal, unless treated with intravenous adrenaline. The most common allergic reaction is to penicillin, which produces anaphylactic shock in approximately 1:50 000 people.

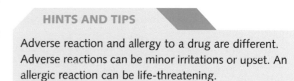

HINTS AND TIPS

Adverse reaction and allergy to a drug are different. Adverse reactions can be minor irritations or upset. An allergic reaction can be life-threatening.

Some drugs, e.g. the vasodilator hydralazine, induce autoimmune reactions similar to systemic lupus erythematosus. Stopping the drug usually puts an end to this reaction, although in some cases glucocorticoid therapy may be needed.

DRUG HISTORY AND DRUG DEVELOPMENT

Drug history

A patient's drug history is a crucial component of the clerking process, as drug effects account for a significant proportion of hospital admissions, and potential drug interactions and adverse events are crucial to foresee.

A complete list of the names and doses of prescribed drugs taken by the patient (noting the proprietary and the generic name, e.g. Viagra® and sildenafil, respectively) and any other medications or supplements they may have bought themselves over the counter at a pharmacy should be documented. Women often forget the contraceptive pill and hormone replacement therapy, and should be sensitively questioned about these. NSAIDs and paracetamol are often taken by patients with arthritis and should be specifically asked about. Make sure to note how often the drugs were taken, and at what times.

If presented with numerous bottles and packets of tablets, it is important to ensure that they all belong to the patient, and not the partner of the patient, or to someone else. Always ask the patient if they are taking all their medicines as prescribed.

Occasionally it is useful to know what drugs have been taken in the recent and distant past; for example, monoamine oxidase inhibitors should be stopped at least 3 weeks prior to starting a different antidepressant therapy.

Previous adverse reaction to drugs, and to non-drug products such as latex, is essential to ascertain. Explore what happened to the patient, and what was done about it. A simple upset stomach and loose stools just for one day after taking penicillin previously is an acceptable side-effect, and is not grounds for choosing another antibiotic when treating a penicillin-sensitive infection in the future. Widespread cutaneous rash and difficulty breathing which required adrenaline and hospital admission is a genuinely worrying adverse effect of a penicillin, and any such drug should be clearly avoided in the future as this was an allergic drug reaction. Allergy to drugs should be clearly marked in the patient's notes and drug charts.

Family history of adverse drug reactions is usually confined to the anaesthetic history, where the concern is largely in relation to the muscle relaxing drugs, particularly suxamethonium.

A history of recreational or illicit drug use is an important but sensitive issue to approach. One must use discretion when questioning the patient. A history of smoking should also be established.

Knowledge about any hepatic or renal disease and general health problems is important when it comes to management and prescribing, as are specific considerations, such as not prescribing aspirin in peptic ulcer disease, or oestrogen to patients with oestrogen-dependent cancers. These aspects are usually brought to light in the rest of the history taking.

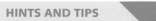

HINTS AND TIPS

The salient points of the drug history are:
- current and previous drugs and their doses
- adverse drug reactions and allergies
- family history of allergies
- recreational drug use
- existing renal or hepatic and general disease.

Drug development

Hundreds of thousands of substances have been produced by the pharmaceutical industry over the past 50 years, though very few ever get past preclinical screening, and fewer than 10% of these survive clinical assessment.

There are four clinical stages a potential drug goes through as part of the assessment of its pharmacokinetics and pharmacodynamics: efficacy, dose–response relationship and safety (Fig. 1.14).

Phase	Main aims/means of investigation	Subjects
Preclincal	Pharmacology Toxicology	*In vitro* In laboratory animals
Phase 1	Clinical pharmacology and toxicology Drug metabolism and bioavailability Evaluate safety	Healthy individuals and/or patients
Phase 2	Initial treatment studies Evaluate efficacy	Small numbers of patients
Phase 3	Large randomized controlled trials Comparing new to old treatments Evaluate safety and efficacy	Large numbers of patients
Phase 4	Post-marketing surveillance Long-term safety and rare events Yellow card scheme	All patients prescribed the drug

Fig. 1.14 The five stages of drug development and monitoring

Phase 4 can be regarded as an ongoing phase, where drugs are monitored once licensed for general use. By this stage, the efficacy and dose–response relationship are known, although the side-effect profile is often incomplete, and information is gathered on these 'adverse reactions' which are due to, or likely due to new drugs.

In the UK this is known as the yellow card scheme. The *British National Formulary (BNF)* contains detachable yellow cards, which medical staff complete, documenting adverse drug reactions in their patients, which can then be forwarded to the Medicines Control Agency. The Medicines Control Agency collates these data, and uses them for surveillance of common or severe adverse effects. The data are publicized in future copies of the *BNF,* or used in the reassessment of certain drug licences.

Cardiovascular system $\boxed{2}$

● **Objectives**

After reading this chapter, you will:
• Be able to describe the functions of the heart and blood
• Know which drugs affect heart function and circulating blood, and understand how they do so
• Be aware of any indications, contraindications and adverse drug reactions.

THE HEART

Basic concepts

The heart is a pump which together with the vascular system supplies the tissues with blood containing oxygen and nutrients, and removes waste products.

The flow of blood around the body is as follows (Fig. 2.1):

• Deoxygenated blood from body tissues reaches the right atrium through the systemic veins (the superior and inferior venae cavae).
• Blood flows into the right ventricle, which then pumps the deoxygenated blood via the pulmonary artery to the lungs, where the blood becomes oxygenated before reaching the left atrium via the pulmonary vein.
• Blood flows from the left atrium into the left ventricle. From here it is pumped into the systemic circulation via the aorta, to supply the tissues of the body.

Cardiac rate and rhythm

The sinoatrial node (SAN) and the atrioventricular node (AVN) govern the rate and timing of the cardiac action potential. The SAN is located in the superior part of the right atrium near the entrance of the superior vena cava; the AVN is located at the base of the right atrium. The SAN discharges at a frequency of 80 impulses/min; it is the pacemaker for the heart and as such determines the heart rate. The action potential generated by the SAN spreads throughout both atria, reaching the AVN. The AVN delays the action potential arising from the SAN to encourage the complete emptying of the atria before the ventricles contract.

The secondary action potential generated by the AVN descends into the interventricular septum via the bundle of His. The bundle of His splits into left and right branches making contact with the Purkinje fibres,

which conduct the impulse throughout the ventricles, causing them to contract (Fig. 2.2).

Cardiac action potential
The shape of the action potential is characteristic of the location of its origin (i.e. whether from nodal tissue, the atria or the ventricles) (Fig. 2.2).

Non-nodal cells
The resting membrane potential across the ventricular cell membrane is approximately -85 mV; this is because the resting membrane is more permeable to potassium than to other ions. Four phases occurring at the ventricular cell membrane are (Fig. 2.3):

• **Phase 0 or depolarization:** Occurs when the membrane potential reaches a critical value of -60 mV. The upstroke of the action potential is due to the transient opening of voltage-gated sodium channels, allowing sodium ions into the cell. In addition, potassium conductance falls to very low levels.
• **Phase 1 (partial repolarization):** Occurs as a result of the inactivation of the sodium current, and a transient outward potassium current.
• **Phase 2 (plateau phase):** The membrane remains depolarized at a plateau of approximately 0 mV. This is due to the activation of a voltage-dependent slow inward calcium current (conducting positive charge into the cell) and a delayed rectifier potassium current conducting positive charge out of the cell.
• **Phase 3 (repolarization):** Repolarization is due to the inactivation of the calcium current and an increase in potassium conductance.

Nodal cells
The resting membrane potential of nodal cells is approximately -60 mV.

In nodal cells, there is no fast sodium current. Instead, the action potential is initiated by an inward calcium current, and, because calcium spikes conduct slowly, there is a delay of approximately 0.1 s between atrial and ventricular contraction.

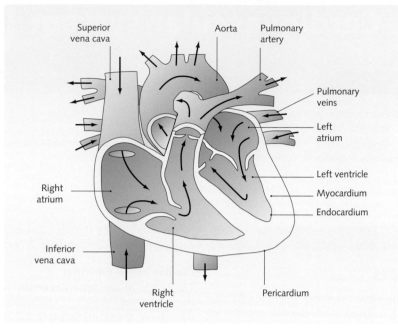

Fig. 2.1 Blood flow through the heart chambers. (Redrawn from Page et al. 2006.)

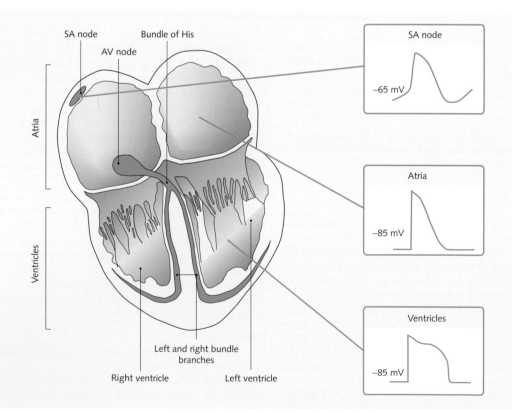

Fig. 2.2 Regional variation in action potential configuration throughout the heart. (AV, atrioventricular; SA, sinoatrial.) (Redrawn from Page et al. 2006.)

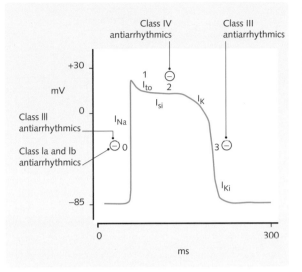

Fig. 2.3 Configuration of a typical ventricular action potential showing the ionic currents, the phases and where class I, III and IV antiarrhythmic drugs act. (0, 1, 2 and 3, phases of the action potential; I_{Na}, fast inward Na^+ current; I_{si}, slow inward Ca^{2+} current; I_{to}, transient outward K^+ current; I_K, delayed rectifier K^+ current; I_{Ki}, inward rectifier K^+ current.) (Redrawn from Page et al. 2006.)

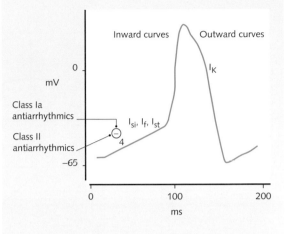

Fig. 2.4 Configuration of a typical sinoatrial node action potential showing the ionic currents, the phases and where class Ia and II antiarrhythmic drugs act. (4, phase of the action potential; I_{si}, an inward current carried by Ca^{2+} ions; I_f, a 'funny' current carried by Na^+ and Ca^{2+} ions; I_{st}, the sustained inward Na^+ current; I_K, the delayed rectifier current which is an outward K^+ current.) (Redrawn from Page et al. 2006.)

Nodal cells have a phase known as phase 4 (the pacemaker potential). This phase involves a gradual depolarization that occurs during diastole and is known as the f current (I_f funny). The f current is activated by hyperpolarization at $-45\,mV$, and consists of sodium and calcium ions entering the cell (Fig. 2.4).

Autonomic control of the heart

Both the parasympathetic and sympathetic nervous systems influence the heart, though parasympathetic activity predominates. This explains why the heart rate is lower than the inherent firing frequency of the sinoatrial node (SAN).

The sympathetic nervous system mediates its effects through the cardiac nerve, and activation of β_1-adrenoceptors. These are linked to adenylyl cyclase and their activation causes increased levels of cyclic adenosine monophosphate (cAMP), and a subsequent increase in intracellular calcium levels.

The parasympathetic nervous system mediates its effects through the vagus nerve, and activation of M_2 receptors. These are also linked to adenylyl cyclase, but their activation causes decreased levels of cAMP, and a subsequent decrease in intracellular calcium levels.

The effects of the sympathetic and parasympathetic nervous systems on the heart are summarized in Figure 2.5.

Fig. 2.5 Effects of the sympathetic and parasympathetic nervous systems on the heart

	Sympathetic	Parasympathetic
Heart rate	Increased	Decreased
Force of contraction	Increased	Decreased
Automaticity	Increased	Reduced
AV node conduction	Facilitated	Inhibited
Cardiac efficiency	Reduced	Increased
AV, atrioventricular.		

Cardiac contractility

Myocardial contraction is the result of calcium entry through L-type channels, giving rise to an increase in cytosolic calcium in the myocytes (Fig. 2.6).

The calcium is derived from two sources:

- The sarcoplasmic reticulum within the cell
- The extracellular medium.

Extracellular calcium enters the cell, triggering larger amounts of calcium to be released from the sarcoplasmic reticulum, a process known as calcium-induced calcium release.

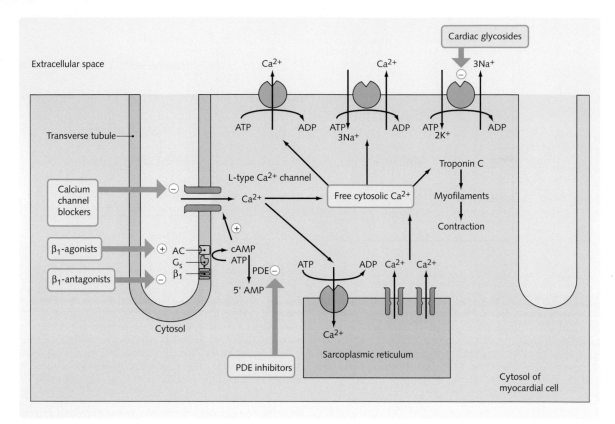

Fig. 2.6 Effects of drugs on cardiac contractility. (AC, adenylyl cyclase; β_1, β_1-adrenoceptor; G_s, stimulatory G-protein; PDE, phosphodiesterase.)

During contraction, the intracellular levels of calcium increase to levels 10 000 times greater than those at rest. Calcium binds to troponin C, thereby modifying the position of actin and myosin filaments, and allowing the cell to contract. Contraction ceases only once calcium has been removed from the cytoplasm. This occurs through two mechanisms:

- Calcium is pumped out of the cell via the electrogenic Na^+/Ca^{2+} exchanger, which pumps one calcium ion out for every three sodium ions in.
- Calcium is re-sequestered into sarcoplasmic reticulum stores by a Ca^{2+} ATPase pump.

Cardiac dysfunction and treatment

Congestive cardiac failure

Congestive cardiac failure (CCF) is the combined failure of both the left and right sides of the heart. The incidence of cardiac failure in the UK is between 1 and 5 per 1000 per year, and doubles for each decade of life after the age of 45.

CCF occurs when the cardiac output does not meet the needs of the tissues. This is thought to be due to defective excitation–contraction coupling, with progressive systolic and diastolic ventricular dysfunction. Some of the causes, symptoms and signs of acute and chronic cardiac failure are given in Figure 2.7. The characteristics of left and right ventricular failure are listed in Figure 2.8.

The body attempts to compensate for the effects of CCF by two processes: extrinsic and intrinsic.

Extrinsic cardiac compensation

Extrinsic cardiac compensation mechanisms aim to maintain cardiac output and blood pressure. The reflex pathway is as follows: hypotension → activation of baroreceptors (receptors responding to changes in pressure) → increased sympathetic activity → increased heart rate and vasoconstriction → increased cardiac contractility and vascular tone → increased arterial pressure.

However, the greater the resistance (arterial pressure) against which the heart must pump, the greater the

Fig. 2.7 Causes and symptoms/signs of acute and chronic cardiac failure (CF)

Causes		Symptoms/signs	
Acute CF	Chronic CF	Acute CF	Chronic CF
Myocardial infarction Acute valvular lesion	Systemic hypertension Myocardial infarction Valvular lesions Cardiomyopathies	Tachycardia Hypotension Dyspnoea Pulmonary oedema Systemic oedema	Exertional dyspnoea Systemic oedema Cardiomegaly Fatigue Orthopnoea

Fig. 2.8 Characteristics of right and left ventricular failure

Right ventricular failure	Left ventricular failure
Reduced cardiac output	Reduced cardiac output
Hypotension	**Hypotension**
Peripheral oedema	Pulmonary oedema
Raised jugular venous pressure	Dyspnoea
Hepatomegaly Ascites	Fatigue

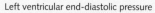

Positive inotropes and congestive cardiac failure (CCF)

— Left ventricular end-diastolic pressure vs CO
Low output symptoms: fatigue (forward failure)
Congestive symptoms: dyspnoea, oedema (backward failure)
Forward and backward failure
○ Normal set point
◉ New set point

Fig. 2.9 Normal cardiac output is determined by the pressure in the left ventricle at end-diastole. In CCF, the set point for cardiac output is reduced and cardiac output falls (1). Compensatory neurohumoral responses become activated which increase end-diastolic pressure and improve cardiac output; however, this can give rise to backward failure (2). Positive inotropic agents increase cardiac output (3). The improved cardiac output reduces the drive for a high end-diastolic pressure, and decompensation occurs to a new set point (4).

reduction in both the ejection fraction and the perfusion of the tissues.

The reduced perfusion of the kidneys activates the renin–angiotensin system (RAS), leading to renin secretion and subsequent elevation of plasma angiotensin II and aldosterone levels (see Fig. 2.13). Angiotensin II causes peripheral vasoconstriction and aldosterone increases sodium retention, leading to increased water retention, oedema and an increased preload.

Intrinsic cardiac compensation
The increased cardiac preload leads to incomplete emptying of the ventricles and an increase in end-diastolic pressure. The heart eventually fails, owing to the massive increase in myocardial energy requirements.

Drugs used in heart failure

Cardiac glycosides
Prototypical cardiac glycosides are digoxin and digitoxin. The drugs in this class shift the Frank–Starling ventricular function curve to a more favourable position (Fig. 2.9).

Chemically, cardiac glycosides have an aglycone steroid nucleus (the pharmacophore) that causes positive inotropic. An unsaturated lactone ring is responsible for cardiotonic activity and by adding additional sugar moieties the potency and pharmacokinetic distribution can be modulated.

Positive inotropic actions of cardiac glycosides improve the symptoms of CCF but there is no evidence they have a beneficial effect on the long-term prognosis of patients with CCF.

Mechanism of action—Cardiac glycosides act by inhibiting the membrane Na^+/K^+ ATPase pump (see Fig. 2.6). This increases intracellular Na^+ concentration, thus reducing the sodium gradient across the membrane and decreasing the amount of calcium pumped out of the cell by the Na^+/Ca^{2+} exchanger during diastole. Consequently, the intracellular calcium concentration rises, thus increasing the force of cardiac contraction and maintaining normal blood pressure.

In addition, cardiac glycosides alter the electrical activity of the heart, both directly and indirectly. At therapeutic doses they indirectly decrease the heart rate, slow atrioventricular (AV) conductance and shorten the atrial action potential by stimulating vagal activity. This is useful in atrial fibrillation. At toxic doses they indirectly increase the sympathetic activity of the heart, and cause arrhythmias, including heart block. The direct effects are mainly due to loss of intracellular potassium, and are most pronounced at high doses. The resting membrane potential is reduced, causing enhanced automaticity slowed cardiac conduction, and increased atrioventricular node (AVN) refractory period.

The increased cytosolic calcium concentration may reach toxic levels thereby saturating the sarcoplasmic reticulum sequestration mechanism and causing oscillations in calcium owing to calcium-induced calcium release. This results in oscillatory after-potentials and subsequent arrhythmias.

In addition, cardiac glycosides have a direct effect on α-adrenoceptors, causing vasoconstriction and a consequent increase in peripheral vascular resistance, which is further enhanced by a centrally mediated increase in sympathetic tone.

Route of administration—Oral.

Indications—Heart failure, supraventricular arrhythmias.

Contraindications—Heart block, hypokalaemia associated with the use of diuretics (the lack of competition from potassium potentiates the effects of cardiac glycosides on the Na^+/K^+ ATPase pump).

Adverse effects—Arrhythmias, anorexia, nausea and vomiting, visual disturbances, abdominal pain and diarrhoea.

Therapeutic notes—The cardiac glycosides have a very narrow therapeutic window, and toxicity is therefore relatively common. If this occurs, the drug should be withdrawn and, if necessary, potassium supplements and antiarrhythmic drugs administered. For severe intoxication, antibodies specific to cardiac glycosides are available.

☠ **Dangerous drug interaction**

Cardiac glycosides + loop diuretics = potassium loss, arrhythmias

---

Phosphodiesterase inhibitors

Examples of phosphodiesterase (PDE) inhibitors include enoximone and milrinone. These have been developed as a result of the many adverse effects and problems associated with cardiac glycosides. There is no evidence that these improve the mortality rate.

Mechanism of action—The type III PDE isoenzyme is found in myocardial and vascular smooth muscle.

Phosphodiesterase is responsible for the degradation of cAMP; thus, inhibiting this enzyme raises cAMP levels and causes an increase in myocardial contractility and vasodilatation (Fig. 2.6). Cardiac output is increased, and pulmonary wedge pressure and total peripheral resistance are reduced, without much change in heart rate or blood pressure.

Route of administration—Intravenous.

Indications—PDE inhibitors are given for severe acute heart failure that is resistant to other drugs.

Adverse effects—Nausea and vomiting, arrhythmias, liver dysfunction, abdominal pain, hypersensitivity.

β-Adrenoceptor agonists

Examples of β-adrenoceptor agonists (p. 35) include dobutamine and dopamine. They are used intravenously in CCF emergencies (see Fig. 2.6).

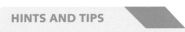

HINTS AND TIPS

Drugs with proven mortality benefits in cardiac failure should be remembered. They are β-adrenoceptor antagonists, angiotensin-converting enzyme (ACE) inhibitors, nitrates with hydralazine and spironolactone.

Diuretics

The main diuretic drug classes are:

- Thiazides
- Loop diuretics
- Spironolactone.

Diuretics inhibit sodium and water retention by the kidneys, and so reduce oedema due to heart failure. Venous pressure and thus cardiac preload are reduced, increasing the efficiency of the heart as a pump (see Ch. 7). Spironolactone appears to have a beneficial effect in cardiac failure at doses lower than it would be expected to function as a diuretic.

Angiotensin-converting-enzyme inhibitors

For details of angiotensin converting enzyme (ACE) inhibitors see p. 32.

Nitrates

See antianginal drugs (p. 28).

Vasodilating drugs

Hydralazine is discussed on page 33.

Arrhythmias

The most common cause of sudden death in developed countries is arrhythmia and it usually results from underlying cardiovascular pathology such as atherosclerosis.

Myocardial ischaemia is one of the most important causes of arrhythmias, and occurs when a coronary artery becomes occluded, thus preventing sufficient blood from reaching the myocardium. Accumulation of endogenous biological mediators, including potassium, cAMP, thromboxane A_2 and free radicals, is believed to initiate arrhythmias.

Reperfusion after coronary occlusion is necessary for tissue recovery and prevention of myocardial necrosis, but spontaneous resumption of coronary flow is often itself a cause of arrhythmia.

Arrhythmias have been defined according to their appearance on the electrocardiogram (ECG) by the Lambeth Conventions. These include:

- **Ventricular:** premature beats, tachycardia, fibrillation and torsades de pointes.
- **Atrial:** premature beats, tachycardia, flutter and fibrillation.

The two main mechanisms by which cardiac rhythm becomes dysfunctional are:

- Abnormal impulse generation (automatic or triggered).
- Abnormal impulse conduction.

Abnormal impulse generation

Automatic—Automatic abnormal impulse generation is likely to cause sinus and atrial tachycardia, and ventricular premature beats. It can be:

- **Enhanced:** pathological conditions, such as ischaemia, may effect nodal and conducting tissue so their inherent pacemaker frequency is greater than that of the SAN. Ischaemia causes partial depolarization of tissues (owing to a decrease in the activity of the electrogenic sodium pump) and catecholamine release, thus enhancing the automaticity of the slow pacemakers (AVN, Purkinje fibres, bundle of His) and often giving rise to an ectopic focus triggering the development of a premature beat.
- **Abnormal:** A premature beat may also develop in atrial or ventricular tissue, which are not normally automatic.

Triggered—Forms of triggered abnormal impulse generation are:

- **Early after-depolarizations (EADs):** These are likely to cause torsade de pointes and reperfusion-induced arrhythmias. EADs are triggered during repolarization, i.e. phase 2 or 3, of a previously normal impulse. They may result from a decrease in the delayed rectifier K^+ current and are associated with abnormally long action potentials. They are therefore more likely to occur during bradycardia and class III antiarrhythmic drug treatment.
- **Delayed after-depolarizations (DADs):** DADs are triggered once the action potential has ended, i.e. during phase 4, of a previously normal impulse. DADs usually result from cellular calcium overload, associated with ischaemia, reperfusion and cardiac glycoside intoxication.

Abnormal impulse conduction

Heart block—Heart block is likely to cause ventricular premature beats and results from damage to nodal tissue (most commonly the AVN) caused by conditions such as infarction. AV block may be first, second or third degree, manifesting itself from slowed conduction to complete block of conduction, where the atria and ventricles beat independently.

Re-entry—Re-entry is likely to cause ventricular and atrial tachycardia and fibrillation, atrial flutter and Wolff–Parkinson–White syndrome. Re-entry is of two types, circus movement and reflection:

- **Circus movement:** An impulse re-excites an area of the myocardium recently excited and after the refractory period has ended. This usually occurs in a ring of tissue in which a unidirectional block is present, preventing anterograde conduction of the impulse, but allowing retrograde conduction of the same impulse. This results in its continuous circulation, termed circus movement. The time taken for the impulse to propagate around the ring must exceed the refractory period; thus, administration of drugs that prolong the refractory period will interrupt the circuit and terminate re-entry.
- **Reflection:** Occurs in non-branching bundles within which electrical dissociation has taken place. Owing to this electrical dissociation, an impulse can return over the same bundle.

COMMUNICATION

Mrs Fibbs, a 70-year-old retired financier with a history of mitral stenosis, presented with palpitations and dyspnoea. On examination, she had an irregularly irregular pulse, diagnostic of atrial fibrillation.

This was confirmed on ECG by absent P waves and irregular QRS complexes. Digoxin was given to slow the heart rate. Her management also included anticoagulation by warfarin, since she is over 65 and her atrial fibrillation puts her at increased risk of embolic stroke.

Fig. 2.10 Effects of antiarrhythmic drugs

Class	Example	Myocardial contractility	AV conduction	AP duration	Effective refractory period
Ia	Procainamide	↓	↓	↑	↑
Ib	Lidocaine	–	–	↓	↑↑
Ic	Flecainide	↓↓	↓↓	–	–
II	Propranolol	↓↓	–/↓	–	–
III	Amiodarone	–	↑	↑↑↑	↑↑↑
IV	Verapamil	↓↓↓	↓↓	↓↓	–

AP, action potential; AV, atrioventricular.
The number of arrows indicates the degree of the effect caused.

Antiarrhythmic drugs

Antiarrhythmic drugs are classified according to a system devised by Vaughan Williams in 1970, and later modified by Harrison. A summary of the effects of the different classes of drug is given in Figure 2.10.

Class I

All class I drugs block the voltage-dependent sodium channels in a dose-dependent manner. Their action resembles that of local anaesthetics (Ch. 9).

All class I drugs have the following effects:

- They prolong the effective refractory period (terminate re-entry).
- They convert unidirectional block to bidirectional block (prevent re-entry).

Class Ia

Examples of class Ia drugs include quinidine, procainamide and disopyramide.

Class Ia drugs affect atrial muscle, ventricular muscle, the bundle of His, the Purkinje fibres and the AVN.

Mechanism of action—Class Ia drugs block voltage-dependent sodium channels in their open (activated) or refractory (inactivated) state (see Figs. 2.3 and 2.4). Their effects are to slow phase 0 (increasing the effective refractory period) and phase 4 (reducing automaticity), and to prolong action potential duration.

Route of administration—Oral, intravenous. Consult the *British National Formulary (BNF)*.

Indications—Ventricular, supraventricular arrhythmias.

Contraindications—Heart block, sinus node dysfunction, cardiogenic shock, severe uncompensated heart failure. Procainamide should not be given to patients with systemic lupus erythematosus.

Adverse effects—Arrhythmias, nausea and vomiting, hypersensitivity, thrombocytopenia and agranulocytosis. Procainamide can cause a lupus-like syndrome, and disopyramide causes hypotension.

Class Ib

Examples of class Ib drugs include lidocaine, mexiletine and phenytoin.

Mechanism of action—Class Ib drugs exert their effects in several ways (see Fig. 2.3). These include:

- Blocking voltage-dependent sodium channels in their refractory (inactivated) state, i.e. when depolarized, as occurs in ischaemia.
- Binding to open channels during phase 0, and dissociating by the next beat, if the rhythm is normal, but abolishing premature beats.
- Decreasing action potential duration.
- Increasing the effective refractory period.

Route of administration—Lidocaine is administered intravenously, and mexiletine and phenytoin either orally or intravenously.

Indications—Ventricular arrhythmias following myocardial infarction. Phenytoin is used in epilepsy (Ch. 5).

Contraindications—Class Ib drugs should not be given to patients with SA disorders, AV block and porphyria.

Adverse effects—Hypotension, bradycardia, drowsiness and confusion, convulsions and paraesthesia (pins and needles).

Lidocaine may cause dizziness and respiratory depression; mexiletine may cause nausea and vomiting, constipation, arrhythmias and hepatitis; and phenytoin may cause nausea and vomiting and peripheral neuropathy.

Class Ic

Flecainide is the only drug used from class Ic.

Mechanism of action—Flecainide blocks sodium channels in a fashion similar to the class Ia and Ib drugs, but shows no preference for refractory channels. This results in a general reduction in the excitability of the myocardium.

Route of administration—Oral, intravenous.

Indications—Ventricular tachyarrhythmias.

Contraindications—Heart failure, history of myocardial infarction.

Adverse effects—Dizziness, visual disturbances, arrhythmias.

Class II

Examples of class II drugs include propranolol, atenolol and pindolol (see Figs. 2.4 and 2.6).

Class II drugs are β-adrenoceptor antagonists (atenolol is β$_1$ selective). They have been shown to prevent sudden death after myocardial infarction by 50% (although this is believed to be due to prevention of cardiac rupture as opposed to prevention of ventricular fibrillation).

Class III

Examples of class III drugs include bretylium, amiodarone, sotalol and ibutilide.

Mechanism of action—All class III drugs used clinically are potassium-channel blockers. They prolong cardiac action potential duration (increased QT interval on the ECG), and prolong the effective refractory period (see Fig. 2.3).

Amiodarone also blocks sodium and calcium channels, i.e. slows phases 0 and 3, and blocks α- and β-adrenoceptors. Sotalol is a β-adrenoceptor antagonist with class III activity.

Route of administration—Bretylium is administered intravenously whereas amiodarone and sotalol are administered orally or intravenously.

Indications—Class III drugs are given for ventricular and supraventricular arrhythmias.

Contraindications—Bretylium should not be given to patients with phaeochromocytoma; amiodarone should not be given to those with AV block, sinus bradycardia or thyroid dysfunction.

For contraindications regarding sotalol, see under β-blockers (p. 28).

Adverse effects—Class III drugs can cause arrhythmias, especially torsades de pointes. Bretylium may cause hypotension, nausea and vomiting, whereas amiodarone may cause thyroid dysfunction, liver damage, pulmonary disorders, photosensitivity and neuropathy.

For adverse effects regarding sotalol see under β-blockers (p. 28).

Class IV

Examples of class IV drugs include verapamil and diltiazem (see Fig. 2.3 and Fig. 2.6).

Class IV drugs are calcium antagonists that shorten phase 2 of the action potential, thus decreasing action potential duration. They are particularly effective in nodal cells, where calcium spikes initiate conduction.

Details of the drugs are given in the section on antianginal drugs (p. 28).

Other antiarrhythmics

The cardiac glycosides and adenosine are agents used in arrhythmias, but which do not fit into the four classes described.

Adenosine

Adenosine is produced endogenously, and acts upon many tissues, including the lungs, afferent nerves and platelets.

Mechanism of action—Adenosine acts at A$_1$ receptors in cardiac conducting tissue and causes myocyte hyperpolarization. This acts to slow the rate of rise of an action potential, and brings about delay in conduction.

Route of administration—Intravenous.

Indications—Paroxysmal supraventricular tachycardia. Aids diagnosis of broad and narrow complex supraventricular tachycardia.

Contraindications—Second- or third-degree heart block, sick sinus syndrome.

Adverse effects—Transient facial flushing, chest pain, dyspnoea, bronchospasm. Side-effects are very short lived, often lasting less than 30 seconds.

Angina pectoris

Angina is associated with acute myocardial ischaemia, and results from underlying cardiovascular pathology. When coronary flow does not meet the metabolic needs of the heart, a radiating chest pain results. This is angina pectoris.

Stable or classic angina is due to fixed stenosis of the coronary arteries, and is brought on by exercise and stress. Unstable angina (crescendo angina) can occur suddenly at rest, and becomes progressively worse, with an increase in the number and severity of attacks. The following conditions can all cause unstable angina:

- Coronary atherosclerosis
- Coronary artery spasm
- Transient platelet aggregation and coronary thrombosis
- Endothelial injury causing the accumulation of vasoconstrictor substances
- Coronary vasoconstriction following adrenergic stimulation.

Variant angina (Prinzmetal's angina) occurs at rest, at the same time each day and is usually due to coronary artery spasm. It is characterized by an elevated ST segment on the ECG during chest pain, and may be accompanied by ventricular arrhythmias.

> **HINTS AND TIPS**
>
> The drugs used in stable angina pectoris are β-adrenoceptor antagonists, nitrates, calcium antagonists, antiplatelets and potassium-channel activators.

Antianginal drugs

Treatment of angina aims to dilate coronary arteries to allow maximal myocardial perfusion, decrease the heart rate to minimize oxygen demands of the myocardium, lengthen diastole when cardiac perfusion occurs and to prevent platelets from aggregating and forming platelet plugs.

Acute attacks of angina are treated with:

• Sublingual nitrates.

In the hospital setting, acute anginal pain is treated with an opiate (Ch. 9).

Stable angina is treated with:

• Long-acting nitrates
• Antiplatelet agents
• β-Adrenoceptor antagonists
• Calcium antagonists
• Potassium-channel activators.

Unstable angina is a medical emergency, and requires hospital admission. Unstable angina is treated with:

• Antiplatelets: aspirin, clopidogrel, dipyridamole and the glycoprotein IIb/IIIa inhibitors, (p. 41).
• Heparin/low-molecular-weight heparin (p. 41).
• Standard antianginal drug regimen.

Organic nitrates

The organic nitrates, glyceryl trinitrate (GTN), isosorbide mononitrate (ISMN) and isosorbide dinitrate (ISDN), can relieve angina within minutes.

Mechanism of action—Most nitrates are prodrugs, decomposing to form nitric oxide (NO), which activates guanylyl cyclase, thereby increasing the levels of cyclic guanosine monophosphate (cGMP). Protein kinase G is activated and contractile proteins are phosphorylated. Dilatation of the systemic veins decreases preload and thus the oxygen demand of the heart, while dilatation of the coronary arteries increases blood flow and oxygen delivery to the myocardium.

Route of administration—Sublingual, oral (modified release), transcutaneous patches. GTN can be given by intravenous infusion.

Indications—Organic nitrates are given for the prophylaxis and treatment of angina, and in left ventricular failure.

Contraindications—Organic nitrates should not be given to patients with hypersensitivity to nitrates, or those with hypotension and hypovolaemia.

Adverse effects—Postural hypotension, tachycardia, headache, flushing and dizziness.

Therapeutic notes—To avoid nitrate tolerance, a drug-free period of approximately 8 hours is needed.

β-Adrenoceptor antagonists (β-blockers)

Examples of β-blockers include propranolol, atenolol, bisoprolol and metoprolol.

β-Adrenoceptors are found in many tissues, though the β_1-adrenoceptor is found predominantly in the heart, and the β_2-adrenoceptor is found mainly in the smooth muscle of the vasculature. Some overlap does exist.

Different β-blockers have different affinity for the two types of adrenoceptor. Propranolol is non-selective, having equal affinity for both the β_1- and β_2-adrenoceptors. Atenolol, bisoprolol and metoprolol have greater affinity for the β_1-adrenoceptor and are therefore more 'cardiac-specific'. Some β-blockers even appear to have partial agonistic effects at β-adrenoceptors, as well as antagonistic effects.

Mechanism of action—The aim of using β-adrenoceptor antagonists in cardiac disease is to block β-adrenoceptors in the heart. This has the effect of causing a fall in heart rate (slowing of phase 4; Fig. 2.4), in systolic blood pressure, in cardiac contractile activity and in myocardial oxygen demand.

Route of administration—Oral, intravenous.

Indications—Angina, post-myocardial infarction, arrhythmias, hypertension, thyrotoxicosis, glaucoma, anxiety.

Contraindications—Non-selective β-blockers (e.g. propranolol) must not be given to asthmatic patients. At high doses β_1-adrenoceptor antagonists lose their selectivity, and should be used with caution in those with asthma. Other contraindications for β-blockers include bradycardia, hypotension, AV block and CCF.

Adverse effects—Bronchospasm, fatigue and insomnia, dizziness, cold extremities (β_2-adrenoceptor effect), bradycardia, heart block, hypotension and decreased glucose tolerance in diabetic patients.

Calcium-channel blockers

There are two types of calcium-channel blocker (CCBs):

• Rate-limiting CCBs (verapamil).
• Dihydropyridine CCBs (short acting nifedipine or long acting felodipine).

Mechanism of action—Rate-limiting CCBs block L-type calcium channels found in the heart and in the vascular smooth muscle, thereby reducing calcium entry into cardiac and vascular cells (Figs. 2.3, 2.6 and 2.12). This decrease in intracellular calcium reduces cardiac contractility and causes vasodilatation, which results in several effects: reduced preload due to the reduced venous pressure; reduced afterload due to the reduced arteriolar pressure; increased coronary blood flow; reduced cardiac contractility and thus reduced myocardial oxygen consumption; and a decreased heart rate. High doses of these drugs affect AVN conduction.

Dihydropyridines block L-type calcium channels in vascular cells. They do not affect cardiac contractility or AVN conduction, and the beneficial effects are due to increased coronary flow and peripheral vasodilatation.

Route of administration—Oral.

Indications—Prophylaxis and treatment of angina and hypertension. Dihydropyridines are especially useful in angina associated with coronary vasospasm, with the long-acting dihydropyridines being particularly useful for hypertension management. Verapamil and diltiazem are given for supraventricular arrhythmias, and nifedipine for Raynaud's syndrome (peripheral vasoconstriction).

Contraindications—CCBs should not be given to patients in cardiogenic shock.

Dihydropyridines are contraindicated in advanced aortic stenosis. Verapamil and diltiazem should not be given to patients in severe heart failure (owing to their negative inotropic action), to those taking β-blockers (risk of AV block and impaired cardiac output), and those with severe bradycardia.

Adverse effects—Verapamil and diltiazem may cause hypotension, rash, bradycardia, CCF, heart block and constipation.

Dihydropyridines may cause hypotension, rash, tachycardia, peripheral oedema, and flushing and dizziness.

> **HINTS AND TIPS**
>
> There are three classes of calcium-channel blockers. Two of them act mostly on the heart (verapamil and diltiazem) and the other acts mostly on peripheral vascular tone (nifedipine). Concurrent use of a β-adrenoceptor antagonist and a calcium-channel blocker could result in profound bradycardia.

Potassium-channel activators

Nicorandil is the only licensed drug in this class.

Mechanism of action—Nicorandil acts to activate the potassium channels of the vascular smooth muscle. Once activated, potassium flows out of the cells, causing hyperpolarization of the cell membrane. The hyperpolarized membrane inhibits the influx of calcium, and therefore inhibits contraction; the overall effect is relaxation of the smooth muscle and vasodilatation (see Fig. 2.12).

Route of administration—Oral.

Indications—Angina prophylaxis.

Contraindications—Cardiogenic shock, left ventricular failure, hypotension.

Adverse effects—Headache, cutaneous vasodilatation, nausea and vomiting.

See Figure 2.11 for a summary of the drug classes used in cardiac dysfunction.

> **HINTS AND TIPS**
>
> The overall aim of symptom management in angina: dilate coronary arteries to allow maximal myocardial perfusion; to decrease the heart rate to minimize oxygen demands of the myocardium, and lengthen diastole when cardiac perfusion occurs; and to prevent platelets from aggregating and forming platelet plugs. In addition to this, reversible risk factors need to be addressed to limit the progression of the disease.

THE CIRCULATION

Control of vascular tone

α-Adrenoceptor activation

α-Adrenoceptor activation (Fig. 2.12) causes contraction of vascular smooth muscle through the activation of phospholipase C (PLC). The resulting increased levels of inositol triphosphate cause the release of calcium from the endoplasmic reticulum, thus increasing calcium levels. Calcium then binds to calmodulin, thus activating myosin light-chain kinase (MLCK) and allowing contraction.

$β_2$-Adrenoceptor activation

$β_2$-Adrenoceptor activation (Fig. 2.12) causes relaxation of vascular smooth muscle through the activation of adenylyl cyclase. The resulting increased levels of cAMP activate protein kinase A, which phosphorylates and inactivates MLCK.

Fig. 2.11 Classes of drugs used to treat angina, cardiac failure and arrhythmias

Angina	Heart failure	Arrhythmias
Organic nitrates	Cardiac glycosides	Na^+-channel blockers (Class I)
$β_1$-Adrenoceptor antagonists	Phosphodiesterase inhibitors	$β_1$-Adrenoceptor antagonists (Class II)
Ca^{2+} antagonists	$β_1$-Adrenoceptor agonists	K^+-channel blockers (Class III)
Antiplatelets	Diuretics	Ca^{2+} antagonists (Class IV)
Potassium-channel activators	ACE inhibitors	Cardiac glycosides
	Nitrates	Adenosine
	Vasodilating drugs	

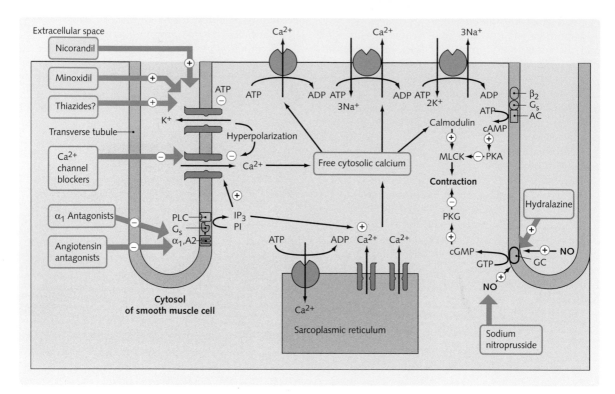

Fig. 2.12 Drugs affecting vascular tone. (AC, adenylyl cyclase; α_1, α_1-adrenoceptor; A2, angiotensin II; β_2, β_2-adrenoceptor; GC, guanylyl cyclase; G_S, stimulatory G-protein; IP$_3$, inositol triphosphate; MLCK, myosin light-chain kinase; NO, nitric oxide; PLC, phospholipase C; PI, phosphatidylinositol; PKA, protein kinase A; PKG, protein kinase G.)

M$_3$-receptor activation

M$_3$-receptor activation causes relaxation of vascular smooth muscle through the release of endothelium-derived relaxing factor (EDRF), which is believed to be NO (Fig. 2.12). Guanylyl cyclase is activated by NO, thus increasing the levels of cGMP and activating protein kinase G. Protein kinase G inhibits contraction by phosphorylating contractile proteins.

Renin–angiotensin system

A decrease in plasma volume results in the activation of the RAS (Ch. 7), which is summarized in Figure 2.13.

Angiotensin-converting enzyme (ACE) catalyses the production of angiotensin II. The effects of angiotensin II are:

- Potent direct vasoconstriction
- Indirect vasoconstriction by releasing noradrenaline
- Stimulates the secretion of aldosterone.

ACE also catalyses the inactivation of bradykinin, which is an endogenous vasodilator.

Aldosterone is a steroid that induces the synthesis of sodium channels and Na$^+$/K$^+$ ATPase pumps in the luminal membrane of the cortical collecting ducts. This results in a greater amount of sodium and consequently water being reabsorbed, thus increasing the blood volume and pressure.

Certain renal diseases and renal artery occlusion will cause activation of the RAS and result in the development of hypertension.

Hypertension

Normal blood pressure is generally regarded as 120/ 80 mmHg (systolic pressure/diastolic pressure). Hypertension is defined as a diastolic arterial pressure greater than 90 mmHg, or a systolic arterial pressure greater than 140 mmHg. The condition can be fatal if left untreated, as it greatly increases the risk of thrombosis, stroke and renal failure.

Three factors determine blood pressure:

- Blood volume
- Cardiac output
- Peripheral vascular resistance.

'Primary' or 'essential' hypertension accounts for 90–95% of all cases of hypertension. This has no known cause, but is associated with:

- Age (40+)
- Obesity

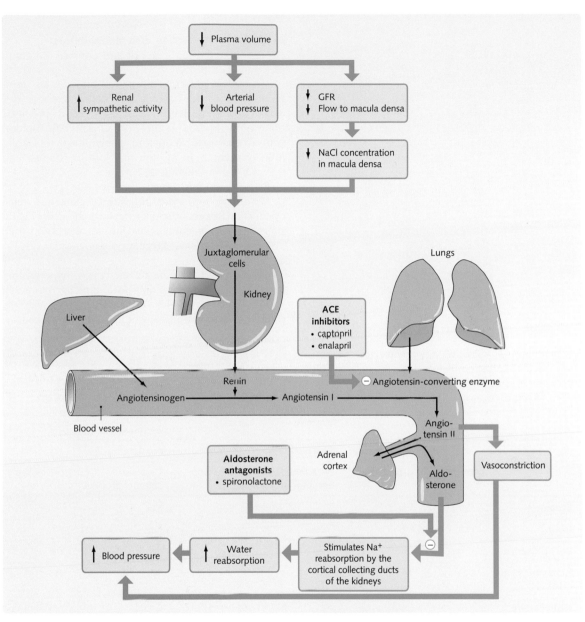

Fig. 2.13   Renin–angiotensin system and ACE inhibitors. (GFR, glomerular filtration rate.)

- Physical inactivity
- Smoking and alcohol consumption
- Genetic predisposition.

'Secondary hypertension' accounts for the remaining 5–10% of cases of hypertension. The cause is usually one of the following:

- Renal disease, which activates the RAS
- Endocrine disease, e.g. phaeochromocytoma, steroid-secreting tumour of the adrenal cortex, adrenaline-secreting tumour of the adrenal medulla.

COMMUNICATION

Mr Gill is a 41-year-old African Caribbean, who presents to his GP with increasing frequency of headaches. He has noticed recent visual disturbances as well. His GP notes he smokes about 15 cigarettes per day, undertakes very little exercise and mainly eats fast foods. Urine dipstick was immediately carried out and revealed significant proteinuria. On questioning, Mr Gill denies any family history of diabetes and a random blood glucose test gave a score of 4.7, within the normal range. However, his resting blood pressure was found to be 210/140, which is severely elevated and indicative of malignant hypertension. Fundoscopy also revealed hypertensive changes (silver wiring and cotton wool spots). He is admitted for immediate treatment.

He was given the long-acting calcium-channel blocker, amlodipine. Two days later, bendroflumethiazide (a thiazide diuretic) was also added to his management. These two drug classes have been shown to be particularly effective in African Caribbeans with hypertension because of their effect on salt sensitivity and volume expansion. He is also advised to stop smoking, eat a healthier salt-restricted diet and do more exercise.

Treatment of hypertension

The treatment of hypertension is aimed at various targets; these are summarized in Figure 2.14. When prescribing, the choice of drug is usually influenced by age (over or under 55) and ethnicity. This is called the A/CD rule (see British Hypertension Society recommendations).

Vasodilators

Angiotensin-converting enzyme inhibitors

Captopril, enalapril, lisinopril and ramipril are examples of ACE inhibitors.

Mechanism of action—ACE inhibitors cause inhibition of ACE with consequent reduced angiotensin II and aldosterone levels (Fig. 2.13), and increased bradykinin levels. This therefore causes vasodilatation with a consequent reduction in peripheral resistance, little change in heart rate and cardiac output and reduced sodium retention.

Route of administration—Oral.

Indications—Hypertension, heart failure and renal dysfunction (especially in diabetic patients to slow progression of diabetic or reduced renal functional nephropathy).

Contraindications—Pregnancy, renovascular disease, aortic stenosis.

Adverse effects—Characteristic cough, hypotension, dizziness and headache, diarrhoea, muscle cramps.

Therapeutic notes—First-dose hypotension is relatively common, and should ideally be given just before bed.

☠ **Dangerous drug interaction**

Angiotensin-converting enzyme inhibitors + NSAIDs = hypotension

Fig. 2.14 Advantages and disadvantages of drugs used in hypertension with respect to associated conditions

	Diuretics	β-Blocker	ACE inhibitor/angiotensin II receptor antagonist	Calcium-channel blockers	α-Blocker
Diabetes	Care[a]	Care[a]	Yes	Yes	Yes
Gout	No	Yes	Yes	Yes	Yes
Dyslipidaemia	Care[b]	Care[b]	Yes	Yes	Yes
Ischaemic heart disease	Yes	Yes	Yes	Yes	Yes
Heart failure	Yes	Care[c]	Yes	Care[d]	Yes
Asthma	Yes	No	Yes	Yes	Yes
Peripheral vascular disease	Yes	Care	Care[e]	Yes	Yes
Renal artery stenosis	Yes	Care	No	Yes	Yes
Pregnancy	Caution	Not in late pregnancy	No	No	Caution

[a]*Diuretics may aggravate diabetes; β-blockers worsen glucose intolerance and mask symptoms of hypoglycaemia.*
[b]*Both diuretics and β-blockers disturb the lipid profile.*
[c]*There is some evidence for beneficial effects of some β-blockers when used cautiously in heart failure.*
[d]*Verapamil and diltiazem may exacerbate heart failure, although amlodipine appears to be safe.*
[e]*Patients with peripheral vascular disease may also have renal artery stenosis; therefore ACE inhibitors should be used cautiously.*
Reproduced from Kumar and Clark, Clinical Medicine, *4th edn. WB Saunders 1998.*

Angiotensin-II receptor antagonists

Losartan and valsartan are examples of angiotensin-II receptor antagonists.

Mechanism of action—Angiotensin-II receptor antagonists cause inhibition at the angiotensin-II receptor (see Fig. 2.12), resulting in vasodilatation with a consequent reduction in peripheral resistance.

Route of administration—Oral.

Indications—Hypertension.

Contraindications—Pregnancy, breastfeeding. Caution in renal artery stenosis and aortic stenosis.

Adverse effects—Cough (less common than with ACE inhibitors), orthostatic hypotension, dizziness, head ache and fatigue, hyperkalaemia and rash.

Calcium antagonists

Nifedipine has more effect upon vascular tone than diltiazem or verapamil, which are more cardioselective (see Fig. 2.12).

α₁-Adrenoceptor antagonists

Prazosin and doxazosin are examples of α_1-adrenoceptor antagonists.

Mechanism of action—α_1-Adrenoceptor antagonists cause inhibition of α_1 adrenoceptor-mediated vasoconstriction, thus reducing peripheral resistance and venous pressure (see Fig. 2.12). They also lower plasma low-density lipoprotein (LDL) cholesterol levels, very-low-density lipoprotein (VLDL) levels and triglyceride levels, and increase high-density lipoprotein (HDL) cholesterol levels, thus reducing the risk of coronary artery disease.

Route of administration—Oral.

Indications—Hypertension (especially in patients with CCF), prostate hyperplasia (reduced bladder and prostate resistance), coronary artery disease.

Contraindications—Prazosin should not be given to people with CCF due to aortic stenosis.

Adverse effects—Postural hypotension, dizziness, headache and fatigue, weakness, palpitations, nausea.

Hydralazine

Hydralazine is a second- or third-line drug for the treatment of mild to moderate hypertension.

Mechanism of action—Hydralazine effects are unclear, though it appears to interfere with the action of inositol triphosphate in vascular smooth muscle, thereby reducing peripheral resistance and blood pressure (Fig. 2.12).

Route of administration—Oral, intravenous.

Indications—Moderate to severe hypertension. Also used in conjunction with β-blockers and thiazides in hypertensive emergencies, and in hypertensive pregnant women.

Contraindications—Idiopathic systemic lupus erythematosus, severe tachycardia.

Adverse effects—Tachycardia, fluid retention, nausea and vomiting, headache.

Minoxidil

Owing to its adverse effects, minoxidil is the drug of last resort in the long-term treatment of hypertension.

Mechanism of action—Minoxidil activates vascular smooth muscle ATP-sensitive potassium channels, resulting in hyperpolarization of the cell membrane and consequent reduced calcium entry through L-type channels (see Fig. 2.12). The overall effect is inhibition of smooth muscle contraction, and subsequent vasodilatation.

Route of administration—Oral for hypertension; topical cream for baldness.

Indications—Severe hypertension, baldness.

Contraindications—Phaeochromocytoma, porphyria.

Adverse effects—Hirsutism (limits use in women), sodium and water retention, tachycardia, cardiotoxicity.

Therapeutic notes—Though unrelated chemically, the drug diazoxide acts in a similar fashion to minoxidil, and activates potassium channels, resulting in vasodilatation.

Sodium nitroprusside

Mechanism of action—Sodium nitroprusside is a prodrug that spontaneously decomposes into NO inside smooth muscle cells. NO activates guanylyl cyclase, thus increasing intracellular cGMP levels, and causing vasodilatation (see Fig. 2.12).

Route of administration—Intravenous.

Indications—Sodium nitroprusside is given in hypertensive crises, and for controlled hypotension in surgery, and in heart failure.

Contraindications—Sodium nitroprusside should not be given to patients with severe hepatic impairment, vitamin B_{12} deficiency or Leber's optic atrophy.

Adverse effects—Headache and dizziness, nausea, abdominal pain, palpitations, retrosternal discomfort.

Therapeutic notes—Sodium nitroprusside is broken down in the body to thiocyanate, which has a half-life of only a few minutes, though prolonged exposure to nitroprusside and thiocyanate can result in thiocyanate toxicity (weakness, nausea and inhibition of thyroid function).

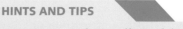

HINTS AND TIPS

The more common adverse effects of the vasodilating drugs are hypotension and headache, both of which result directly from reducing peripheral vascular resistance.

Diuretic drugs

The main diuretics drug classes used in hypertension are:

- Thiazides
- Loop diuretics
- Potassium-sparing diuretics.

See Chapter 7 for details of each of these drugs.

Mechanism of action—The antihypertensive action of diuretic drugs does not seem to correlate with their diuretic activity: loop diuretics are powerful diuretics but only moderate antihypertensives while thiazides are moderate diuretics but powerful antihypertensives.

It has recently been suggested that the antihypertensive effects of diuretics (especially the thiazides) are not necessarily due to their diuretic effect, but rather may be due to activation of ATP-regulated potassium channels in resistance arterioles, with a mechanism of action similar to that of nicorandil (p. 29) and minoxidil. This causes hyperpolarization, and thus inhibition of calcium entry into vascular smooth muscle cells with consequent vasodilatation and reduced peripheral vascular resistance (see Fig. 2.12).

Centrally acting antihypertensive drugs

Clonidine, methyldopa and moxonidine are examples of centrally acting antihypertensive drugs. These agents are second- or third-line drugs in the treatment of hypertension.

Mechanism of action—Centrally acting antihypertensive drugs are α_2-adrenoceptor agonists. The activation of presynaptic α_2-adrenoceptors causes inhibition of noradrenaline release and consequent vasodilatation. The activation of postsynaptic α_2-adrenoceptors causes vasoconstriction, although presynaptic effects dominate.

Centrally acting antihypertensive drugs reduce the activity of the vasomotor centre in the brain, causing reduced sympathetic activity and subsequent vasodilatation. They also reduce heart rate and cardiac output.

Route of administration—Oral. Clonidine can be given by intravenous infusion.

Indications—Hypertensive patients when first-line antihypertensive agents are ineffective or contraindicated. Methyldopa is safe for hypertension in pregnancy, asthmatic patients and those with heart failure.

Contraindications—Methyldopa should not be given to people with depression, liver disease or phaeochromocytoma.

Adverse effects—Dry mouth, sedation, orthostatic hypotension, male sexual dysfunction, galactorrhoea. Methyldopa can cause diffuse parenchymal liver injury, fever and, rarely, haemolytic anaemia. Clonidine can cause a withdrawal hypertensive crisis on stopping treatment.

Phaeochromocytoma

Phaeochromocytoma is a rare endocrine tumour, most commonly of the adrenal gland. These tumours can secrete adrenaline and various intermediates in its biosynthesis. These vasoactive compounds result in the clinical signs and symptoms of phaeochromocytomas, which include facial flushing, sweating, breathlessness, anxiety, tachycardia and paroxysmal hypertension.

Medical management of phaeochromocytoma-induced hypertension relies on the powerful α-Adrenoceptor antagonist phenoxybenzamine. α-adrenoceptor blockade reduces peripheral vascular resistance and lowers blood pressure. The use of β-adrenoceptor antagonists is dangerous, as tumour-secreted sympathomimetics act unopposed on α-adrenoceptors, increasing both peripheral vascular resistance and blood pressure.

Phenoxybenzamine

Mechanism of action—Phenoxybenzamine antagonises α-adrenoceptors in the vascular smooth muscles, resulting in vasodilatation.

Route of administration—Oral, intravenous.

Indications—Hypertensive episodes in phaeochromocytoma.

Contraindications—History of cerebrovascular events, post-myocardial infarction.

Adverse effects—Postural hypotension, tachycardia, nasal congestion.

Therapeutic notes—Phentolamine is another powerful α-adrenoceptor antagonist which can be used in phaeochromocytoma, though it has a much shorter half-life, and is commonly used prior to, and during, surgery to excise the tumour.

Vasoconstrictors and the management of shock

Shock

Shock is a state of circulatory collapse, characterized by an arterial blood pressure unable to maintain adequate tissue perfusion. Shock is a life-threatening condition.

The body responds inappropriately to shock, releasing mediators such as histamine, prostaglandins, bradykinin and serotonin, which cause capillary dilatation and increased capillary permeability. This further reduces blood pressure and cardiac output.

Signs of shock include:

- Very low arterial blood pressure
- A weak, rapid pulse
- Cold, pale, sweaty skin
- Rapid breathing
- Dry mouth
- Reduced urine output
- Anxiousness.

Causes of shock include:

- Haemorrhage
- Burns
- Dehydration
- Severe vomiting or diarrhoea
- Bacterial septicaemia
- Myocardial infarction
- Pulmonary embolism.

Types of shock include:

- **Hypovolemic:** caused by a reduction in the circulating blood volume.
- **Cardiogenic:** reduced cardiac output due to 'pump failure'.
- **Septic:** caused by massive vasodilatation.
- **Anaphylactic:** a severe allergic reaction, in which there is a massive generalized release of vasodilating mediators.
- **Spinal:** disruption of neuronal control on vascular tone and cardiac output.

Management of shock

The medical management of shock ultimately depends upon its underlying cause, e.g. if a child is shocked due to chronic diarrhoea and vomiting, fluid and electrolyte replacement is the most appropriate management.

The following drugs are useful in restoring blood pressure and tissue perfusion, but on the whole do not address the underlying cause of the different types of shock.

Sympathomimetic amines

Examples of sympathomimetic amines include adrenaline, noradrenaline, phenylephrine and ephedrine.

Sympathomimetic amines raise blood pressure at the expense of vital organs such as the kidneys, and raise peripheral resistance, which is already high in patients with shock.

Mechanism of action—Adrenaline and noradrenaline are agonists at both α- and β-adrenoceptors, and phenylephrine is an α_1-adrenoceptor agonist. Ephedrine is a β-adrenoceptor agonist and causes noradrenaline release. These drugs work either by activating α-adrenoceptors which then activate phospholipase C, causing vasoconstriction and a consequent increase in arterial blood pressure, or by activating β-adrenoceptors which then activate adenylyl cyclase, causing an increased heart rate, increased cardiac contractility and vasodilatation.

Route of administration—Parenterally, commonly intravenously.

Indications—Shock, acute hypotension and reversal of hypotension caused by spinal or epidural anaesthesia. Adrenaline is used in cardiac arrest and anaphylaxis.

Contraindications—Sympathomimetic amines should not be given in pregnancy or in people who have hypertension.

Adverse effects—Tachycardia, anxiety, insomnia, arrhythmias, dry mouth, cold extremities.

Therapeutic notes—In a cardiac arrest, adrenaline is used at a concentration of 1 mg/10 mL (1:10 000) intravenously, whereas in anaphylaxis, adrenaline is used at a concentration of 1 mg/1 mL (1:1000) intramuscularly.

Dopamine and dobutamine

Mechanism of action—Dopamine is a precursor of noradrenaline. It activates dopamine receptors and α- and β-adrenoceptors. When administered by intravenous infusion, dopamine acts on:

- Dopamine receptors, causing vasodilatation in the kidneys at low doses
- α_1-Adrenoceptors, causing vasoconstriction in other vasculature
- β_1-Adrenoceptors, causing positive inotropic and chronotropic effects.

Dobutamine has no effect on dopaminergic receptors, but does activate β_1-adrenoceptors.

If renal perfusion is not impaired, dobutamine and dopamine are a more appropriate means of treating shock than α-adrenoceptor agonists. This form of treatment maintains renal perfusion, and inhibits the activation of the RAS.

Route of administration—Intravenous.

Indications—CCF (emergencies only), cardiogenic shock, septic shock, hypovolaemic shock, cardiomyopathy, cardiac surgery.

Contraindications—Tachyarrhythmias. Dopamine is contraindicated in people with phaeochromocytoma.

Adverse effects—Tachycardia and hypertension; dopamine causes nausea and vomiting and hypotension.

Therapeutic notes—Although low doses of dopamine cause vasodilatation, high doses cause vasoconstriction and may exacerbate heart failure.

Vasopressin and desmopressin

Vasopressin (antidiuretic hormone; ADH), and desmopressin are examples of antidiuretic peptides.

Vasopressin is short acting ($t_{1/2} = 10$ minutes) whereas desmopressin is longer acting ($t_{1/2} = 75$ minutes).

Mechanism of action—Antidiuretic peptides activate V_1 receptors on smooth muscle cells, which stimulate phospholipase C, causing contraction. They also activate V_2 receptors on the tubular cells of the kidneys, which stimulate adenylyl cyclase and thereby increase the permeability of these cells to water, and reduce sodium and water excretion. Vasopressin has a much greater affinity for V_2 receptors than V_1 receptors whereas desmopressin is selective for V_1 receptors.

Route of administration—Oral, intravenous, intranasal.

Indications—Pituitary diabetes insipidus. The antidiuretic peptides are no longer used in the management of shock, though their pharmacology is both academically interesting and a potential target for future drugs.

Contraindications—Vascular disease, chronic nephritis.

Adverse effects—Fluid retention, nausea, pallor, abdominal cramps, belching. They may induce anginal attacks (due to coronary vasoconstriction).

Corticosteroids

The use of corticosteroids in septic shock remains controversial, though they are also given by intravenous injection in the treatment of anaphylactic shock as an adjunct to adrenaline (Ch. 6).

HINTS AND TIPS

It is possible to distinguish between the types of shock clinically:

- Hypovolaemic – low jugular venous pressure (JVP), cool, clammy peripheries, confusion/restlessness.
- Cardiogenic – raised JVP, cool, clammy peripheries, anxiousness/agitation.
- Septic – warm, sweaty peripheries, pyrexia, nausea.
- Anaphylactic – warm peripheries, ureterica, nausea.
- Spinal – history of trauma or spinal anaesthesia.
- Tachycardia, hypotension and tachypnoea will feature in all types of shock.

Lipoprotein circulation and atherosclerosis

Lipoproteins provide a means of transporting lipids (cholesterol, triglycerides and phospholipids), which are insoluble in the blood, around the body.

Four classes of lipoproteins exist. These differ in size, density, constituent lipids and type of surface protein (apoprotein). These lipoproteins are:

- High-density lipoproteins (HDL)
- Low-density lipoproteins (LDL)
- Very-low-density lipoproteins (VLDL)
- Chylomicrons.

Lipid transport in the blood is via two pathways, exogenous and endogenous, which are summarized in Figure 2.15.

In the exogenous pathway (numbers refer to those in Fig. 2.15):

1. Diet-derived lipid breakdown leads to the formation of chylomicrons.
2. Lipoprotein lipase (LPL), found in the endothelium of extrahepatic tissues, hydrolyses the triglycerides in chylomicrons to glycerol and free fatty acids (FFAs), for use by the tissues.
3. The chylomicron remnant is taken up by the liver.
4. The liver secretes cholesterol and bile acids into the gut, creating an enterohepatic circulation.

In the endogenous pathway (numbers refer to those in Fig. 2.15):

1. The liver secretes VLDLs, the components of which may be derived either endogenously or from the diet.
2. Lipoprotein lipase (LPL), found in the endothelium of extrahepatic tissues, hydrolyses triglycerides in the VLDLs to glycerol and FFAs, for use by the tissues, and leaves LDL.
3. LDL is then taken up by the liver and extrahepatic tissues.
4. HDL is secreted by the liver into the plasma, where it is modified by lecithin cholesterol acyltransferase (LCAT) and uptake of cholesterol from the tissues. LCAT transfers cholesterol esters to LDLs and VLDLs.

Hyperlipidaemias

Hyperlipidaemias are characterized by markedly elevated plasma triglycerides, cholesterol and lipoprotein concentrations.

Cholesterol is deposited in various tissues:

- Deposition in arterial plaques results in atherosclerosis, which leads to heart attacks, strokes and peripheral vascular disease.
- Deposition in tendons and skin results in xanthomas.

Primary

Primary hyperlipidaemias are genetic, and numerous types exist.

Secondary

Secondary hyperlipidaemias are the consequences of other conditions such as:

- Diabetes
- Liver disease
- Nephrotic syndrome
- Renal failure
- Alcoholism
- Hypothyroidism
- Oestrogen administration.

Treatment (lipid-lowering drugs)

Changing a patient's diet alone can lower serum cholesterol, and should be the first-line treatment option in mild to moderate hyperlipidaemia. The following drug classes, however, provide pharmacological control of a patient's cholesterol level, inhibiting its synthesis and its uptake from the intestine.

HMG CoA reductase inhibitors ('statins')

Atorvastatin, pravastatin and simvastatin are examples of 3-hydroxy-3-methylglutaryl co-enzyme A (HMG CoA) reductase inhibitors. These drugs have been shown to reduce blood cholesterol by up to 35% in some patients.

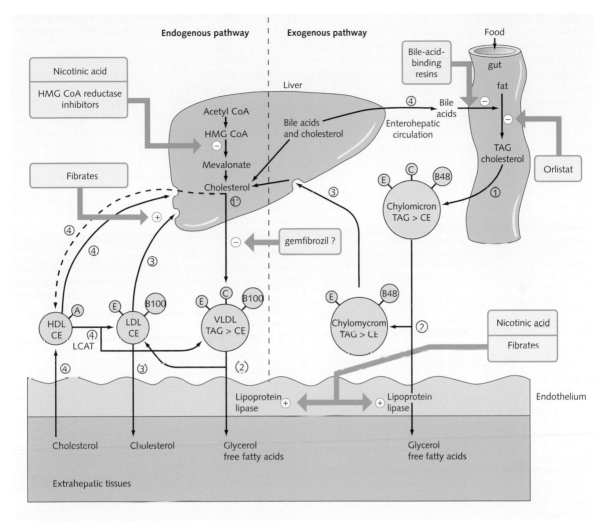

Fig. 2.15 Endogenous and exogenous pathways of lipid transport. (CE, cholesterol ester; HDL, high density lipoprotein; LCAT, lecithin cholesterol acyltransferase; TAG, triacylglycerol; VLDL, very-low-density lipoproteins; numbers refer to steps in pathways, see p. 36.)

HMG CoA reductase inhibitors can reduce the risk of dying from a coronary event by up to nearly half.

Mechanism of action—Statins reversibly inhibit the enzyme HMG CoA reductase, which catalyses the rate-limiting step in the synthesis of cholesterol. The decrease in cholesterol synthesis also increases the number of LDL receptors, thus decreasing LDL levels.

Route of administration—Oral.

Indications—Hyperlipidaemia resistant to dietary control, as part of secondary prevention in patients with serum cholesterol greater than 5.5 mmol/L (this value will vary depending upon local policy).

Contraindications—Pregnancy, breastfeeding, liver disease.

Adverse effects—Reversible myositis (rare), constipation or diarrhoea, abdominal pain and flatulence, nausea and headache, fatigue, insomnia, rash.

Fibrates

Fibrates include bezafibrate, ciprofibrate and gemfibrozil. These are broad-spectrum lipid-modulating agents that are ineffective in patients with elevated cholesterol but normal triglyceride concentrations.

Mechanism of action—Fibrates work in several ways (Fig. 2.15):

- Stimulation of lipoprotein lipase, thus reducing the triglyceride content of VLDLs and chylomicrons
- Stimulation of hepatic LDL clearance, by increasing hepatic LDL uptake (Fig. 2.15).
- Reduction of plasma triglyceride, LDL and VLDL concentrations.

Increase of HDL-cholesterol concentration (except bezafibrate). Gemfibrozil decreases lipolysis and may decrease VLDL secretion.

Route of administration—Oral.

Indications—Hyperlipidaemia unresponsive to dietary control.

Contraindications—Gallbladder disease, severe renal or hepatic impairment, hypoalbuminaemia, pregnancy, breastfeeding.

Adverse effects—Myositis-like syndrome (especially if renal function is impaired), gastrointestinal disturbances, dermatitis, pruritus, rash and urticaria, impotence, headache, dizziness, blurred vision.

HINTS AND TIPS

Changing a patient's diet alone can lower serum cholesterol, and should be the first-line treatment option in mild to moderate hyperlipidaemia.

Nicotinic acid

The side-effects of nicotinic acid limit its use in the treatment of hyperlipidaemias. Nicotinic acid has been shown to reduce the incidence of coronary artery disease.

Mechanism of action—Nicotinic acid has the following effects (Fig. 2.15):

- Inhibits cholesterol synthesis thereby decreasing VLDL and thus LDL production.
- It stimulates lipoprotein lipase thus reducing the triglyceride content of VLDLs and chylomicrons.
- It increases HDL-cholesterol.
- It increases the levels of tissue plasminogen activator (p. 39).
- It decreases the levels of plasma fibrinogen.

Route of administration—Oral.

Indications—Hyperlipidaemias unresponsive to other measures.

Contraindications—Pregnancy, breastfeeding.

Adverse effects—Flushing, dizziness, headache, palpitations, nausea and vomiting, pruritus.

Bile acid binding resins

Colestyramine and colestipol have been shown to decrease the rate of mortality from coronary artery disease.

Mechanism of action—Basic anion exchange resins act by binding bile acids in the intestine (Fig. 2.15), thus preventing their reabsorption and promoting hepatic conversion of cholesterol into bile acids. This increases hepatic LDL receptor activity, thus increasing the breakdown of LDL-cholesterol. Plasma LDL-cholesterol is therefore lowered.

Route of administration—Oral.

Indications—When elevated cholesterol is due to a high LDL concentration.

Colestyramine is used in the primary prevention of coronary heart disease in men aged 35–59 years with primary hypercholesterolaemia. It also relieves pruritus associated with partial biliary obstruction and primary biliary cirrhosis.

Contraindications—Complete biliary obstruction.

Adverse effects—Bile acid binding resins are not absorbed, and therefore have very few systemic side-effects. Side-effects include nausea and vomiting, constipation, heartburn, abdominal pain and flatulence, and aggravation of hypertriglyceridaemia. They may interfere with the absorption of fat-soluble vitamins and certain drugs.

Therapeutic regimen—To avoid interference with their absorption, other drugs should not be taken within 1 hour before or 3–4 hours after colestyramine or colestipol administration.

Other lipid-lowering drugs

Fish oils rich in omega-3 marine triglycerides can be useful in the treatment of severe hypertriglyceridaemia, though may sometimes worsen hypercholesteraemia. Their role in clinical practice remains to be thoroughly ascertained.

Ispaghula husk is taken orally, and is presumed to act by binding bile acids, preventing their reabsorption, and is potentially useful in patients with hypercholesterolaemia but not hypertriglyceridaemia.

HAEMOSTASIS AND THROMBOSIS

Haemostasis

Haemostasis is the cessation of bleeding from damaged blood vessels. If haemostasis is defective or unable to cope with blood loss from larger vessels, blood may accumulate in the tissues. This accumulated blood is called a haematoma.

Three stages are involved in haemostasis:

- Blood vessel constriction
- Formation of a platelet plug
- Formation of a clot.

Blood vessel constriction

The first response to a severed blood vessel is contraction of the smooth muscle of the vessel. This is mediated by the release of thromboxane A_2 and other substances from platelets.

Blood vessel constriction slows the flow of blood through the vessel, thus reducing the pressure, and pushes opposing surfaces of the vessel together. In very small vessels this results in permanent closure of the vessel, but in most cases blood vessel constriction is insufficient for this to occur.

Platelet plug formation

Exposure to the collagen underlying the vessel endothelium, as occurs during vessel injury, allows platelets to adhere to the collagen by binding to von Willebrand's factor. This factor, secreted by the platelets and endothelium, binds to the exposed collagen; platelets then bind to this complex.

Release of ADP, serotonin, thromboxane A_2 and other substances by the platelets causes the platelets to aggregate. Fibrin binds them together. The synthesis and release of prostacyclin by the intact endothelium inhibits platelet aggregation limiting the extent of the platelet plug.

Intact endothelial cells also produce NO, a potent vasodilator and inhibitor of platelet aggregation.

Clot formation

Blood coagulation is the conversion of liquid blood into a solid gel, known as a clot. A clot:

- Consists of a meshwork of fibrin within which blood cells are trapped
- Functions to reinforce the platelet plug.

Fibrin is formed from its precursor fibrinogen, through the action of an enzyme called thrombin. The formation of thrombin occurs via two distinct pathways, the intrinsic and the extrinsic pathways, which together are known as the coagulation cascade. Both pathways involve the conversion of inactive factors into active enzymes, which then go on to catalyse the conversion of other factors into enzymes (Fig. 2.15). The liver is important in coagulation as it is the site at which many of the clotting factors are produced. It also produces bile salts necessary for the absorption of vitamin K, which is needed by the liver to produce prothrombin and clotting factors VII, IX and X.

The extrinsic pathway is thus termed because the component needed for its initiation is contained outside the blood. Tissue factor binds factor VII on exposure of blood to subendothelial cells, and converts it to its active form, VIIa. This enzyme then catalyses the activation of factors X and IX.

The intrinsic pathway is thus termed because its components are contained in the blood. It merges with the extrinsic pathway at the step prior to thrombin activation.

The thrombin formed stimulates the activation of factors XI, VIII and V, and thus acts as a form of positive feedback.

Three naturally occurring anticoagulants limit the extent of clot formation. These are:

- Tissue factor pathway inhibitor, which binds to the tissue factor–VIIa complex, and inhibits its actions.

- Protein C, which is activated by thrombin, and inactivates factors VII and V.
- Antithrombin III, which is activated by heparin, and inactivates thrombin and other factors.

Fibrinolysis

The fibrinolytic or thrombolytic system functions to dissolve a clot once repair of the vessel is under way.

Plasmin digests fibrin. It is formed from plasminogen through the action of plasminogen activators, the best example of which is tissue plasminogen activator (tPA).

Thrombosis

Thrombosis is the pathological formation of a clot known as a thrombus, which may cause occlusion within blood vessels or the heart, and result in death. Thrombosis causes:

- Arterial occlusion – which may lead to myocardial infarction, stroke and peripheral ischaemia.
- Venous occlusion – which may lead to deep venous thrombosis and pulmonary embolism.

COMMUNICATION

Mr Patel is 50 years old with a body mass index of 31, who presented to casualty with central crushing chest pain, shortness of breath and sweating. He is a longstanding smoker with a 60-pack a year history and his younger brother recently died from a stroke associated with significant vascular disease. ECG showed ST segment elevation (a recognized ECG pattern), which combined with the history is highly suggestive of myocardial infarction.

He was given oxygen, aspirin (antithrombotic agent) to prevent further platelet aggregation, morphine for pain relief and the anti-ischaemic vasodilating spray (glyceryl trinitrate). To decrease ischaemia, he was then given atenolol intravenously, which acts by decreasing cardiac workload and therefore oxygen demand as well as causing vasodilatation. He was also given the thrombolytic streptokinase to dissolve any clots that may have caused the myocardial infarction.

Arterial thrombi form because of endothelial injury which is in turn the result of underlying arterial wall pathology such as atherosclerosis.

Venous and atrial thrombi tend to form as a result of blood stasis, allowing the build-up of platelets and fibrin. People with hypercoagulability, due to a lack of one or more of the naturally occurring anticoagulants, are particularly susceptible.

Arterial thrombi consist mainly of platelets, whereas venous thrombi consist mainly of fibrin.

Treatment of thrombosis

Anticoagulants

Vitamin K antagonists
Warfarin, nicoumalone and phenindione are examples of vitamin K antagonists.

Mechanism of action—Vitamin K antagonists block the reduction of vitamin K epoxide, which is necessary for its action as a co-factor in the synthesis of factors II, VII, IX and X (see Figs. 2.16 and 2.17).

Route of administration—Oral.

Indications—Prophylaxis and treatment of deep vein thrombosis and pulmonary embolism, the prophylaxis of embolization in atrial fibrillation and rheumatic disease, and in patients with prosthetic heart valves.

Contraindications—Cerebral thrombosis, peripheral arterial occlusion, peptic ulcers, hypertension, pregnancy.

Adverse effects—Haemorrhage.

Therapeutic notes—The onset of action of vitamin K antagonists takes several hours, owing to the time needed for the degradation of factors that have already been carboxylated ($t_{1/2}$: VII = 6 hours, IX = 24 hours, X = 40 hours, II = 60 hours).

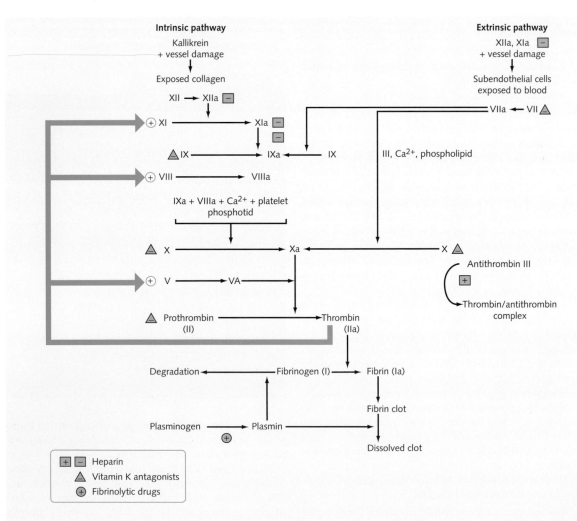

Fig. 2.16 Effects of heparin, vitamin K and fibrinolytic drugs on the coagulation cascade. Factor III, factor/tissue thromboplastin.

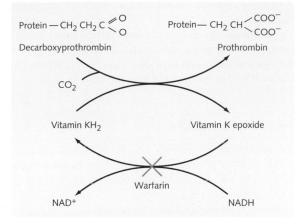

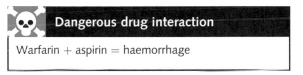

Fig. 2.17 Role of vitamin K in prothrombin formation. Warfarin inhibits the reduction of vitamin K epoxide.

☠ **Dangerous drug interaction**

Warfarin + aspirin = haemorrhage

Heparin and the low-molecular-weight heparins

Mechanism of action—Heparin activates antithrombin III, which limits blood clotting by inactivating thrombin and factor X. Heparin also inhibits platelet aggregation, possibly as a result of inhibiting thrombin. Low-molecular-weight heparins (LMWHs) are simply fragments of heparin which exhibit very similar activity to heparin. LMWHs are used more frequently because their dosing is more predictable and less frequent.

Route of administration—Intravenous, subcutaneous.

Indications—Treatment of deep vein thrombosis and pulmonary embolism; prophylaxis against postoperative deep vein thrombosis and pulmonary embolism in high-risk patients; myocardial infarction.

Contraindications—Heparin should not be given to patients with haemophilia, thrombocytopenia or peptic ulcers.

Adverse effects—Haemorrhage (treated by stopping therapy or administering a heparin antagonist such as protamine sulphate), skin necrosis, thrombocytopenia, hypersensitivity reactions.

Therapeutic regimen—Heparin is given intravenously by intravenous infusion, or 12-hourly by the subcutaneous route. LMWHs are given as a once-daily subcutaneous injection.

Therapeutic notes—Heparin has an immediate onset and can therefore be used in emergencies.

Hirudins

Mechanism of action—Derived from the medical leech. Hirudin or rather its recombinant derivatives, desirudin and lepirudin, inactivate thrombin.

Route of administration—Subcutaneous, intravenous.

Indications—Desirudin is used in patients with type II (immune) heparin-induced thrombocytopenia. Desirudin is used for prophylaxis of deep-vein thrombosis in patients undergoing hip and knee replacement.

Contraindications—Active bleeding, renal or hepatic impairment.

Adverse effects—Haemorrhage, hypersensitivity reactions.

Antiplatelet agents

Aspirin

Aspirin is acetylsalicylic acid, originally derived from the willow tree.

Mechanism of action—Aspirin blocks the synthesis of thromboxane A_2 from arachidonic acid in platelets, by acetylating and thus inhibiting the enzyme cyclooxygenase. Thromboxane A_2 stimulates phospholipase C, thus increasing calcium levels and causing platelet aggregation. Aspirin also blocks the synthesis of prostacyclin from endothelial cells, which inhibits platelet aggregation. However, this effect is short lived because endothelial cells, unlike platelets, can synthesize new cyclooxygenase (Fig. 2.18).

Route of administration—Oral.

Indications—Prevention and treatment of myocardial infarction and ischaemic stroke. Aspirin is also used as an analgesic and an anti-inflammatory agent (Ch. 10).

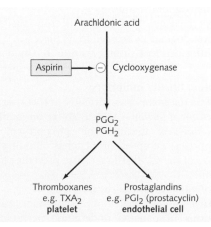

Fig. 2.18 Inhibition of cyclooxygenase by aspirin, leading to a reduction in the formation of thromboxane and prostacyclin. (PG, prostaglandin; PGI_2, prostacyclin; TXA_2, thromboxane A_2.)

Contraindications—Children under 12 years of age (risk of Reye's syndrome), during breastfeeding, haemophilia, peptic ulcers or known hypersensitivity reactions.

Adverse effects—Bronchospasm, gastrointestinal haemorrhage.

Therapeutic regimen—Aspirin at 150 mg daily after myocardial infarction has been shown to decrease mortality significantly. Given on alternate days, aspirin may reduce the incidence of primary myocardial infarction.

Dangerous drug interaction

Aspirin + warfarin = haemorrhage

Dipyridamole

Mechanism of action—Dipyridamole causes inhibition of the phosphodiesterase enzyme that hydrolyses cAMP. Increased cAMP levels result in decreased calcium levels and inhibition of platelet aggregation.

Route of administration—Oral.

Indications—Dipyridamole is used in conjunction with warfarin and other oral anticoagulants in the prophylaxis against thrombosis associated with prosthetic heart valves.

Adverse effects—Hypotension, nausea, diarrhoea, headache.

Clopidogrel

Mechanism of action—Clopidogrel inhibits activation of the glycoprotein IIb/IIIa receptor on the surface of platelets, which is required for aggregation to occur.

Route of administration—Oral.

Indications—Secondary prevention of cardiovascular and cerebrovascular events.

Adverse effects—Haemorrhage, abdominal discomfort, nausea and vomiting.

Therapeutic notes—If a patient is truly allergic to aspirin, clopidogrel can be used in its place.

Ticlopidine acts in a similar fashion to clopidogrel.

Glycoprotein IIb/IIIa inhibitors

Abciximab is the main drug currently in this class.

Mechanism of action—Abciximab is an antibody fragment directed towards the glycoprotein IIb/IIIa (GPIIb/IIIa) receptor of platelets. Binding and inactivation of the GPIIb/IIIa receptor prevents platelet aggregation.

Route of administration—Intravenous.

Indications—Prevention of ischaemic cardiac complications in patients undergoing percutaneous coronary intervention; short-term prevention of myocardial infarction in patients with unstable angina.

Contraindications—Active bleeding.

Adverse effects—Haemorrhage, nausea, vomiting, hypotension.

Therapeutic notes—Tirofiban and eptifibatide also act by inhibiting the GPIIb/IIIa receptor, though are peptide fragments. As peptides, these agents are potentially antigenic, and should only be used once.

Fibrinolytic agents

Streptokinase

Mechanism of action—Streptokinase forms a complex with, and activates, plasminogen into plasmin, a fibrinolytic enzyme.

Route of administration—Intravenous.

Indications—Life-threatening venous thrombosis, pulmonary embolism, arterial thromboembolism, acute myocardial infarction.

Contraindications—Recent haemorrhage, trauma, surgery, bleeding diathesis, aortic dissection, coma, history of cerebrovascular disease. Consult the *BNF* for a comprehensive list of contraindications.

Adverse effects—Nausea and vomiting, bleeding.

Therapeutic regimen—Streptokinase is often used in conjunction with antiplatelet and anticoagulant drugs. The clinical preference is to use fibrinolytics with a faster onset of action, such as tissue plasminogen activators. Furthermore, streptokinase is derived from haemolytic streptococci, and is thus antigenic. Repeated administration of streptokinase could result in an anaphylaxis-like reaction. If repeated fibrinolytic therapy is needed, the non-antigenic tissue-type plasminogen activators should be employed.

Tissue-type plasminogen activators (tPAs)

Alteplase and reteplase are examples of tPAs.

Mechanism of action—tPAs are tissue-type plasminogen activators.

Route of administration—Intravenous.

Indications—Myocardial infarction, pulmonary embolism.

Contraindications—As for streptokinase.

Adverse effects—Nausea and vomiting, bleeding.

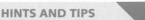
HINTS AND TIPS

While the administration of a fibrinolytic drug could improve the life expectancy of someone suffering from an acute myocardial infarction, it could also have disastrous effects. There are stringent criteria for administering or not administering fibrinolytic drugs. You should learn these.

Bleeding disorders

Hereditary bleeding disorders are rare. Haemophilia is a genetic disorder in which excessive bleeding occurs, owing to the absence of factor VIII (haemophilia A) or IX (haemophilia B). Von Willebrand's disease is characterized by abnormal bruising and mucosal bleeding.

Acquired bleeding disorders may be due to liver disease, vitamin K deficiency or anticoagulant drugs. Caution should be taken when using the aforementioned drugs in patients with thromboembolic disease.

Treatment of bleeding disorders

Vitamin K

Mechanism of action—Vitamin K is needed for the post-transcriptional γ-carboxylation of glutamic acid residues of prothrombin (factor II) and clotting factors VII, IX and X by the liver (Fig. 2.17). Vitamin K is also necessary for normal calcification of bone.

Route of administration—Oral, intramuscular, intravenous.

Indications—Vitamin K is used as an antidote to the effects of oral anticoagulants, and in patients with biliary obstruction or liver disease, where Vitamin K deficiency may be a problem. It is also used after prolonged treatment with antibiotics that inhibit the formation of vitamin K by intestinal bacteria, and as prophylaxis against hypoprothrombinaemia in the newborn.

Adverse effects—Side-effects of vitamin K include haemolytic anaemia and hyperbilirubinaemia in the newborn.

Protamine

Mechanism of action—Protamine is a strongly basic protein, which forms an inactive complex with heparin, and as such is used in patients in whom heparin treatment has resulted in haemorrhage. High doses of protamine appear to have anticoagulant effects through an unknown mechanism.

Route of administration—Intravenous.

Indications—Haemorrhage secondary to heparinization.

Adverse effects—Nausea, vomiting, flushing, hypotension.

Clotting factors

Deficiencies of clotting factors can be replaced by the administration of fresh plasma. Factors VIII and IX are available as freeze-dried concentrates.

Mechanism of action—All clotting factors are necessary for normal blood coagulation.

Route of administration—Intravenous.

Indications—Haemophilia; antidote to the effects of oral anticoagulants.

Adverse effects—Allergic reactions, including fevers and chills.

Desmopressin

Desmopressin is a synthetic analogue of vasopressin.

Mechanism of action—Desmopressin causes the release of factor VIII. It is also used in diabetes insipidus, as it has antidiuretic effects.

Route of administration—Parenteral.

Indications—Desmopressin is given for mild factor VIII deficiency, and in the treatment of diabetes insipidus.

Adverse effects—Fluid retention, hyponatraemia, and headache, nausea and vomiting.

Tranexamic acid

Mechanism of action—Tranexamic acid is antifibrinolytic, inhibiting plasminogen activation and therefore preventing fibrinolysis.

Route of administration—Oral, intravenous.

Indications—Tranexamic acid agents are used for gastrointestinal haemorrhage and conditions in which there is haemorrhage or risk of haemorrhage, e.g. haemophilia, menorrhagia and dental extraction.

Contraindications—Thromboembolic disease.

Adverse effects—Nausea and vomiting, diarrhoea. Thromboembolic events are rare.

Aprotinin

Mechanism of action—Aprotinin inhibits the proteolytic enzymes plasmin and kallikrein, thus inhibiting fibrinolysis.

Route of administration—Intravenous.

Indications—Aprotinin is used when there is a risk of blood loss after open heart surgery, and in hyperplasminaemia.

Adverse effects—Allergy, localized thrombophlebitis.

Etamsylate

Mechanism of action—Etamsylate corrects abnormal platelet adhesion.

Route of administration—Oral, intravenous.

Indications—Etamsylate is used to reduce capillary bleeding and periventricular haemorrhage in premature infants.

Contraindications—Porphyria.

Adverse effects—Nausea, headache, rashes.

THE BLOOD AND FLUID REPLACEMENT

Anaemia

Anaemia is a common problem worldwide. In the young it is commonly due to nutritional deficiencies (vitamin B_{12}, folate and iron), in fertile women menstrual loss accounts for most cases, and in the elderly malignancy and renal failure are the commoner causes.

Iron

Ferrous sulphate, ferrous fumarate and ferrous gluconate are the commoner iron salt preparations.

Mechanism of action—Dietary supplementation of iron increases serum iron and stored iron in the liver and bone. Adequate iron is necessary for normal erythropoiesis, as well as for numerous iron-containing proteins.

Route of administration—Oral. Parenteral preparations of iron exist, but are seldom used.

Indications—Iron-deficiency anaemia.

Contraindications—Caution in pregnancy.

Adverse effects—Gastrointestinal irritation, nausea, epigastric pain, altered bowel habits.

Therapeutic notes—Iron overdose or chronic iron overload can be harmful, and either acquired or inherited in the form of haemochromatosis. The iron-chelating agent desferrioxamine can be given parenterally, which allows iron to be excreted in the urine.

Vitamin B$_{12}$

Hydroxocobalamin and cyanocobalamin are vitamin B$_{12}$ drug preparations.

Mechanism of action—Vitamin B$_{12}$ is required for DNA synthesis and effective erythropoiesis.

Route of administration—Intramuscular, oral.

Indications—Pernicious anaemia, other macrocytic megaloblastic anaemias.

Contraindications—None.

Adverse effects—Itching, fever, chills, flushing, nausea.

Therapeutic notes—Initial treatment requires regular weekly injections, but once serum vitamin B$_{12}$ is normalized, injections should be given at 3-monthly intervals.

Folate

Folic acid in the form folate is administered.

Mechanism of action—Folate is required for DNA synthesis and effective erythropoiesis.

Route of administration—Oral.

Indications—Macrocytic megaloblastic anaemia, prevention of neural tube defects in pregnancy.

Contraindications—None.

Adverse effects—None.

Therapeutic notes—Since the introduction of folate acid supplements for pregnant women, the rate of neural tube defects in newborn babies has fallen markedly.

Erythropoietin

Epoetin is a recombinant erythropoietin. Erythropoietin is synthesized in the kidney in response to a fall in the oxygen tension of the blood passing through it.

Mechanism of action—Erythropoietin acts upon the bone marrow to stimulate stem cells to divide, to produce cells of the red cell lineage.

Route of administration—Parenteral.

Indications—Anaemia of chronic renal failure, anaemia following cancer chemotherapy, prior to autologous blood donation.

Contraindications—Uncontrolled hypertension.

Adverse effects—Dose-dependant increase in blood pressure and platelet count, influenza-like symptoms.

Therapeutic notes—Erythropoietin often features in the news, as an increased haemoglobin concentration most probably improves an athlete's performance, making this drug a potential drug of 'misuse' in sport.

Myeloproliferative disorders

The pharmacological management of the myeloproliferative disorders is outside the scope of this text, although it relies on cytotoxic drugs. Information on these agents should be learnt from a haematology or general medical textbook.

Fluid replacement

Fluid replacement should ideally be achieved orally, though this is often not practical. Intravenous administration of fluids is commonplace in hospital.

- Intravenous fluids are given for many reasons. In trauma they are used to replace blood loss, in septicaemia they are used to raise blood pressure and tissue perfusion, in the unconscious they are used to replace water and electrolytes lost in the urine and via insensible routes.
- There are many types of intravenous fluid. The commoner fluids given intravenously are blood, the crystalloids (sodium chloride and dextrose saline) and the colloids (dextrans and gelatin). Supplements can be added to intravenous fluids.
- The art of fluid replacement and fluid management is best learnt from an anaesthetics or general medical textbook. The names and compositions of the various intravenous fluids can be obtained from the *BNF*.

Respiratory system

After reading this chapter, you will:
- Be able to describe the characteristics of the main diseases of the respiratory system and their pharmacological management
- Know the main drug categories, their mechanism of action, when they are and are not used, and their adverse effects.

BASIC CONCEPTS

Respiration is the process of exchange of oxygen and carbon dioxide between an organism and its external environment. This principally involves the lungs, which possess the largest surface area in the body in contact with the external environment. The respiratory system (Fig. 3.1) has defence mechanisms which can be divided into physical (such as coughing or the mucociliary escalator, to remove foreign agents) and immunological (such as enzymes, pulmonary macrophages and lymphoid tissue, to 'disarm' foreign agents). These defence mechanisms can be launched inappropriately or may be insufficient to deal with the triggering agent, and thus disease may occur.

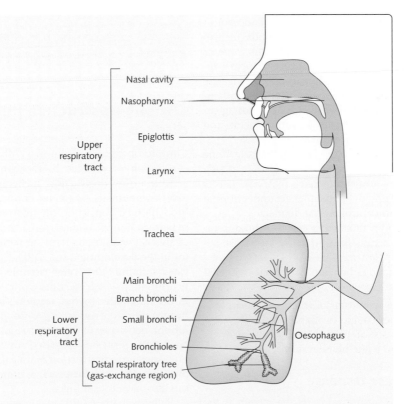

Fig. 3.1 A schematic diagram of the respiratory tract. (From McGowan et al. *Respiratory System*, 2nd edition. Mosby, London, 2003.)

OBSTRUCTIVE AIRWAYS DISEASES

Asthma

Asthma is a chronic inflammatory disease of the bronchiolar airways. It is characterized by recurrent reversible obstruction to airflow causing airflow limitation, airway hyperresponsiveness and inflammation of the bronchi. Asthma may be allergic (extrinsic) or non-allergic (intrinsic).

In asthma, smooth muscle that surrounds the bronchi is hyperresponsive to stimuli, and underlying inflammatory changes are present in the airways. Asthmatic stimuli include inhaled allergens (e.g. pollen, animal dander), occupational allergens, and drugs or non-specific stimuli such as cold air, exercise, stress and pollution.

The stimuli cause asthmatic changes through several complex pathways (Fig. 3.2). The possible mechanisms of these pathways include the following:

- Immune reactions (type 1 hypersensitivity) and release of inflammatory mediators: the cross-linking of IgE by allergens causes mast cell degranulation which releases histamine, eosinophilic and neutrophilic chemotactic factors. The eosinophils, neutrophils and other inflammatory cells release inflammatory mediators that cause a bronchial inflammatory reaction, tissue damage and an increase in bronchial hyperresponsiveness. Bronchial inflammatory mediators include leukotrienes, prostaglandins, thromboxane, platelet-activating factor and eosinophilic major basic protein.
- An imbalance in airway smooth muscle tone involving the parasympathetic nerves (vagus), non-adrenergic non-cholinergic (NANC) nerves and circulating noradrenaline that act under normal circumstances to control airway diameter.
- Abnormal calcium flux across cell membranes, increasing smooth muscle contraction and mast cell degranulation.
- Leaky tight junctions between bronchial epithelial cells allowing allergen access.

The above result in symptoms of wheezing, breathlessness and sometimes cough. In many people the asthmatic attack consists of two phases: an immediate-phase response and a late-phase response.

Immediate-phase response

An immediate-phase response occurs on exposure to the eliciting stimulus. The response consists mainly of bronchospasm. Bronchodilators are effective in this early phase.

Late-phase response

Several hours later, the late-phase response occurs. This consists of bronchospasm, vasodilatation, oedema and mucus secretion caused by inflammatory mediators released from eosinophils, platelets and other cells, and neuropeptides released by axon reflexes. Anti-inflammatory drug action is necessary for the prevention and/or treatment of this phase (Fig. 3.2).

COMMUNICATION

Children with asthma who are very young can have difficulty using inhalers or nebulizers, and it is therefore more effective to give them theophylline, as this can be given in tablet form. Zara is a 4-year-old girl who is on theophylline for this reason. Zara presents to accident and emergency (with her mother) in pain, distress and with pyrexia (a high temperature). She is found to have an infection. Should she be given erythromycin as normal? No! Theophylline plasma concentrations would increase because enzymes involved in its breakdown would be occupied with erythromycin as well. Theophylline has a very narrow therapeutic range and so small increases above the therapeutic dose can be toxic and even fatal.

Chronic obstructive pulmonary disease

Chronic obstructive pulmonary disease (COPD) is a chronic and progressive disease with fixed or poorly reversible airflow obstruction. It encompasses several disease components, namely chronic bronchitis and bronchiolitis, consisting of inflammation and mucus hypersecretion and emphysema, involving destruction of alveolar walls. Long-term smoking is the leading factor in the development of COPD. Cigarette smoke activates inflammatory cells (mainly macrophages and neutrophils), which can cause connective tissue damage in the lung parenchyma, resulting in emphysema and hypersecretion of mucus. α_1-Antitrypsin is a protease inhibitor, deficiency of which can result in decreased inhibition of proteases released by neutrophils, thus predisposing to destruction of lung tissue leading to emphysema. Other factors, such as atmospheric pollution, can also have causal links.

Patients with COPD experience cough with the production of sputum, wheeze and breathlessness. Infective exacerbations can occur, giving purulent sputum.

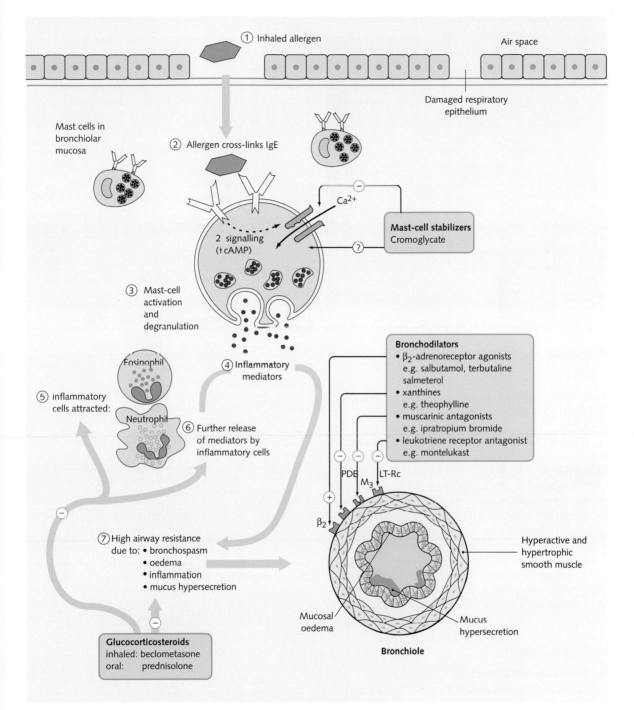

Fig. 3.2 Pathogenesis and drug action in asthma. Allergens interact with respiratory mucosa (1), and trigger IgE-mediated mast cell response (2). Activation of mast cells causes them to degranulate (3) and release various proinflammatory mediators (4) which attract and recruit further inflammatory response cells (5). These cells also secrete mediators which amplifies the inflammatory response (6). The overall effect is narrowing of small airways (7) by bronchospasm, oedema and increased secretions. (PDE, phosphodiesterase; LT-Rc, leukotriene receptor.)

Mrs Connors is a 62-year-old woman who has been smoking approximately 15 cigarettes a day for the past 40 years. She presents with breathlessness and a 3-month history of cough, which is productive of sputum. After examination a diagnosis of COPD is made, concurrent with her presenting history. She is given Combivent® – a mixture of salbutamol (a β-agonist) and ipratropium bromide (an anticholinergic) – to relax the airways and increase the flow of air. In her case, she was not given a corticosteroid (such as fluticasone propionate) because her condition is currently mild, and it stabilized with the Combivent® treatment. In the future, as the disease progresses, a corticosteroid may be added and she may also be put on long-term oxygen therapy. She is advised to have regular flu and pneumonia vaccinations to prevent exacerbation of her COPD.

Fig. 3.3 Management of asthma in adults and children over the age of 5 years. Therapy should be started at step 1 and worked upwards until control of symptoms is achieved. Once symptoms have been controlled it may be possible to step down

Step 1	Inhaled short-acting β_2-agonist as required
Step 2	Inhaled short-acting β_2-agonist as required *Plus* *Either* regular standard-dose inhaled corticosteroid *Or* regular cromoglycate or nedocromil
Step 3	Inhaled short-acting β_2-agonist as required *Plus* *Either* regular high-dose inhaled corticosteroid *Or* regular standard-dose inhaled corticosteroid *Plus* regular inhaled long-acting β_2-agonist
Step 4	Inhaled short-acting β_2-agonist as required *With* Regular high-dose inhaled corticosteroid *Plus sequential therapeutic trial of one or more of:* Inhaled long-acting β_2-agonist Modified-release oral theophyllines Inhaled ipratropium or, in adults, oxitropium Modified-release oral β_2-agonist High-dose inhaled bronchodilators Cromoglycate or nedocromil
Step 5	Inhaled short-acting β_2-agonist as required *With* Regular high-dose inhaled corticosteroid *And* one or more long-acting bronchodilators *Plus* Regular prednisolone tablets
Stepping down	If control is achieved, stepwise reduction may be possible

Adapted from the British National Formulary, 41, March 2001.

Management of obstructive airways disease

Anti-asthmatic drugs include symptomatic bronchodilators (these are most effective in the immediate-phase response), and prophylactic or anti-inflammatory agents, which prevent and/or resolve the late-phase response. The step-wise management of asthma is summarized in Figure 3.3; the stage-dependent treatment of COPD is shown in Figure 3.4. Most patients with COPD get some symptom relief from bronchodilators and anti-inflammatory agents in a fashion similar to people with asthma, yet the response of their airways to these drugs is much less marked, and there are no proved benefits for life expectancy. Long-term oxygen therapy does prolong survival in patients with COPD; however, this must be undertaken with care in patients with carbon dioxide retention because it will reduce their hypoxic drive to breathe.

Bronchodilators

β₂-Adrenoceptor agonists
Examples of β_2-adrenoceptor agonists include salbutamol (short acting) and salmeterol (long acting).

Mechanism of action—Airway smooth muscle does not have a sympathetic nervous supply, but it does contain β_2-adrenoceptors that respond to circulating adrenaline. The stimulation of β_2-adrenoceptors leads to a rise in intracellular cAMP levels and subsequent smooth muscle relaxation and bronchodilation.

- β_2-Adrenoceptor agonists may also help prevent the activation of mast cells, as a minor effect.

- Modern selective β_2-adrenoceptor agonists are potent bronchodilators and have very few β_1-stimulating properties (i.e. they do not affect the heart).

Route of administration—Inhaled.

Oral administration is reserved for children and people unable to use inhalers; intravenous administration for status asthmaticus.

Indications—β_2-Adrenoceptor agonists are used to relieve bronchospasm. They may be used alone in mild, occasional asthma, but are more commonly used in conjunction with other drugs, e.g. corticosteroids.

Fig. 3.4 Stage-dependent COPD treatment

Stage	0 (at risk)	1 (mild)	II (moderate)	III (severe)	IV (very severe)
Characteristics	Normal spirometry; exposure to risk factors; chronic symptoms (cough, sputum production)	$FEV_1/FVC < 0.7$ $FEV_1 \geq 80\%$ predicted $\pm$ chronic symptoms	$FEV_1/FVC < 0.7$ $50\% \leq FEV1$ $<80\%$ predicted $\pm$ chronic symptoms	$FEV_1/FVC < 0.7$ $30\% \leq FEV_1$ $\leq 50\% \pm$ chronic symptoms	$FEV_1/FVC < 0.7$ $FEV_1 < 30\%$ or $FEV_1 < 50\% +$ chronic respiratory failure
Treatment	Avoidance of risk factor(s); influenza vaccination				
		Add short-acting bronchodilator when needed			
			Add regular treatment with one or more long-acting bronchodilators Add rehabilitation		
				Add inhaled glucocorticosteroids if repeated exacerbations	
					Add long-term oxygen therapy if chronic respiratory failure

FEV_1, forced expiratory volume in one second; FVC, forced vital capacity.

Adapted from the GOLD Executive Summary (2005 update).

Contraindications—Caution in hyperthyroidism, cardiovascular disease, arrhythmias.

Adverse effects—Fine tremor, tachycardia, hypokalaemia after high doses.

Therapeutic notes—β_2-Adrenoceptor agonists treat the symptoms of asthma but not the underlying disease process. Salmeterol is a long-acting drug that can be administered twice daily. It is not suitable for relief of an acute attack.

Anticholinergics

Ipratropium bromide (short acting) and tiotropium (long acting) are examples of anticholinergic (antimuscarinic) drugs.

Mechanism of action—Parasympathetic vagal fibres provide a bronchoconstrictor tone to the smooth muscle of the airways. They are activated by reflex on stimulation of sensory (irritant) receptors in the airway walls.

Muscarinic antagonists act by blocking muscarinic receptors, especially the M_3 subtype, which responds to this parasympathetic bronchoconstrictor tone.

Route of administration—Inhaled.

Indications—Anticholinergics are used as adjuncts to β_2-adrenoceptor agonists in the treatment of asthma.

Contraindications—Glaucoma, prostatic hypertrophy, pregnancy.

Adverse effects—Dry mouth may occur. Systemic anticholinergic effects are rare.

Therapeutic notes—Anticholinergics have a synergistic effect when administered with β_2-adrenoreceptor agonists in asthma.

Xanthines

Theophylline is an example of a xanthine.

Mechanism of action—The xanthines appear to increase cAMP levels in the bronchial smooth muscle cells by inhibiting phosphodiesterase, an enzyme which catalyses the hydrolysis of cAMP to AMP. Increased cAMP relaxes smooth muscle, causing bronchodilation.

Route of administration—Oral.

Aminophylline is the intravenous xanthine used in severe asthma attacks.

Indications—Xanthines are used in asthmatic children unable to use inhalers, and adults with predominantly nocturnal symptoms. They are administered intravenously in status asthmaticus.

Contraindications—Cardiac disease, hypertension, hepatic impairment.

Adverse effects—Nausea, vomiting, tremor, insomnia, tachycardia.

Therapeutic notes—Oral xanthines are formulated as sustained-release preparations. Xanthines often cause adverse effects, having a narrow therapeutic window, but are useful as oral drugs in preventing attacks for up to 12 hours. Infants with asthma who are very young can have difficulty using inhalers or nebulizers, and it is therefore more effective to give them theophylline, as this can be given in tablet form. Theophylline has a very narrow therapeutic range and so small increases above the therapeutic dose can be toxic and even fatal.

Leukotriene receptor antagonists

Montelukast and zafirlukast are examples of leukotriene receptor antagonists.

Mechanism of action—The leukotriene receptor antagonists are believed to act at leukotriene receptors in the bronchiolar muscle, antagonising endogenous leukotrienes, thus causing bronchodilation.

Leukotrienes are thought to be partly responsible for airway narrowing which is sometimes observed with the use of non-steroidal anti-inflammatory drugs (NSAIDs; see Ch. 9) in asthmatic people. The NSAIDs inhibit cyclooxygenase, and divert arachidonic acid breakdown via the lipoxygenase pathway, liberating leukotrienes among other mediators.

Route of administration—Oral.

Indications—Prophylaxis of asthma.

Contraindications—Elderly, pregnancy, Churg–Strauss syndrome.

Adverse effects—Gastrointestinal disturbance, dry mouth, headache.

Therapeutic notes—The leukotriene receptor antagonists are not yet widely used, though their potential as an agent in the combination therapy of asthma is becoming more widely accepted.

HINTS AND TIPS

In an asthmatic emergency, when thinking what drugs to use, don't forget oxygen.

Prophylactic and anti-inflammatory drugs

Mast-cell stabilizers

Sodium cromoglycate and nedocromil sodium are examples of mast-cell stabilizers.

Mechanism of action—The exact modes of action of mast-cell stabilizers are unclear. These drugs appear to stabilize antigen-sensitized mast cells by reducing calcium influx and subsequent release of inflammatory mediators.

Route of administration—Inhaled.

Indications—Mast-cell stabilizers are useful in young patients (<20 years old) with marked allergic disease and moderate asthma.

Adverse effects—Cough, transient bronchospasm, throat irritation.

Therapeutic notes—Mast-cell stabilizers have a prophylactic action; they must be taken regularly for several weeks before any beneficial effects are noted. These drugs are therefore not of use in acute asthma attacks.

Glucocorticoids

Anti-inflammatory glucocorticoids include beclometasone, fluticasone, budesonide and prednisolone.

Mechanism of action—Corticosteroids depress the inflammatory response in bronchial mucosa and so diminish bronchial hyperresponsiveness. The specific effects include:

- Reduced mucosal oedema and mucus production
- Decreased local generation of prostaglandins and leukotrienes, with less inflammatory-cell activation
- Adrenoceptor up-regulation
- Long-term reduced T-cell cytokine production, and reduced eosinophil and mast-cell infiltration of bronchial mucosa.

For the intracellular events involved in corticosteroid action see Chapter 6.

Route of administration—Corticosteroids are usually delivered by metered-dose inhaler. Oral and intravenous administration is reserved for severe asthma and status asthmaticus.

Indications—Corticosteroids are used in patients with more than minimal symptoms, often in combination with β_2-agonists or drugs that block allergies (Fig. 3.3).

Contraindications—Caution in growing children and in those with systemic and local respiratory/ear, nose and throat (ENT) infections.

Adverse effects—Dysphonia, oral thrush and systemic distribution in high dosage. If given orally, cushingoid effects may occur (Ch. 6).

Therapeutic notes—The initial treatment of severe or refractory asthma may require oral corticosteroids. If possible, maintenance should be achieved with inhaled corticosteroids via a metered dose, to minimize side-effects. Inhaled corticosteroids are usually effective in 3–7 days, but must be taken regularly.

Use of inhalers, nebulizers and oxygen

In the treatment of asthma, inhalers and nebulizers are used to deliver drugs directly to the airways. This allows higher drug concentrations to be achieved locally, while minimizing systemic effects. Whatever device is used, less than 15% of the dose is deposited on the bronchial mucosa.

Inhalers

There are several types of inhaler: metered dose, breath-activated spray, breath-activated powder. They vary in cost, delivery efficiency and ease of use.

Spacer devices, used in conjunction with inhalers, improve drug delivery and are easy to use. Spacers are particularly effective in children.

Nebulizers
Nebulizers convert a solution of drug into an aerosol for inhalation. They are more efficient than inhalers and are used to deliver higher doses of drug. They are useful in status asthmaticus and for the acute hospital treatment of severe asthma.

The long-term use of nebulizers is limited by cost, convenience and the danger of patient over-reliance.

Oxygen
High-flow oxygen should be given to any patient in respiratory distress unless they have COPD and a 'hypoxic drive'. In this situation, oxygen can be administered, but at a lower concentration.

Oxygen increases alveolar oxygen tension and decreases the work of breathing necessary to maintain arterial oxygen tension.

Allergic rhinitis

'Rhinitis' means an inflammatory response of the membrane lining the nose. 'Allergic rhinitis' means that the inflammatory response is due to specific allergens causing a type 1 hypersensitivity reaction. Based on symptoms, it may be further classified as seasonal or perennial (throughout the year). The inflammation can cause swelling, blockages to airflow and overactivity of the mucous membrane glands, causing excessive mucus production. Allergic rhinitis is treated with antihistamine drugs or local steroid sprays (see Ch. 10). Decongestants can sometimes be helpful.

Decongestants

Nasal decongestion can occur acutely, or be a chronic disorder.

Decongestion relies on administration of agents which ultimately have sympathomimetic effects. This results in vasoconstriction of the mucosal blood vessels of the nose, and a reduction in oedema and secretions.

Ephedrine
This drug is the most commonly used decongestant.

Mechanism of action—Ephedrine's sympathomimetic activity results in vasoconstriction of nasal blood vessels, limiting oedema and nasal secretions.

Route of administration—Topical or oral.

Indications—Nasal congestion.

Contraindications—Caution in children.

Adverse effects—Local irritation, nausea, headache. Re-bound nasal congestion on withdrawal.

Therapeutic notes—Oral preparations are less effective than topical, and are contraindicated in diabetes, hypertension and hyperthyroidism.

RESPIRATORY STIMULANTS AND PULMONARY SURFACTANTS

Respiratory stimulants

Respiratory stimulants, or analeptic drugs, have a very limited place in the treatment of ventilatory failure in patients with chronic obstructive airways disease. They have largely been replaced by the use of ventilatory support. Example drugs are naloxone, flumazil and Doxapram.

Doxapram
Mechanism of action—Doxapram is used to improve both rate and depth of breathing. Doxapram is a central stimulant drug that acts on both carotid chemoreceptors and the respiratory centre in the brainstem to increase respiration.

Route of administration—Intravenous.

Indications—Acute respiratory failure.

Adverse effects—Perineal warmth, dizziness, sweating, increase in blood pressure and heart rate.

Pulmonary surfactants

Pulmonary surfactants are used in the management of respiratory distress syndrome, which is most common amongst premature babies. Pulmonary surfactants act to decrease the surface tension of the alveoli, and allow ventilation to occur more easily. They are usually administered via endotracheal tubes directly into the pulmonary tree.

ANTITUSSIVES AND MUCOLYTICS

Antitussives

Antitussives are drugs that inhibit the cough reflex.

Cough is usually a valuable protective reflex mechanism for clearing foreign material and secretions from the airways. In some conditions, however, such as inflammation or neoplasia, the cough reflex may become inappropriately stimulated and in such cases antitussive drugs may be used.

Antitussives either reduce sensory receptor activation or work by an ill-defined mechanism, depressing a 'cough centre' in the brainstem.

Drugs that reduce receptor activation

Menthol vapour and topical local anaesthetics
Benzocaine is an example of a topical local anaesthetic.

Mechanism of action—Menthol vapour and topical local anaesthetics reduce the sensitivity of peripheral sensory 'cough receptors' in the pharynx and larynx to irritation.

Route of administration—Topical as a spray, lozenge or vapour.

Indications—Menthol vapour and topical local anaesthetics are used for unwanted cough.

Drugs that reduce the sensitivity of the 'cough centre'

Opioids

Opioids (See ch. 9) reduce the sensitivity of the 'cough centre'. Examples of these drugs include codeine and pholcodine.

Mechanism of action—Although not clearly understood, opioids seem to work via agonist action on opiate receptors, depressing a 'cough centre' in the brainstem.

Route of administration—Oral.

Indications—Opioids are used for inappropriate coughing.

Adverse effects—There are generally few side-effects of opioids at antitussive doses. Unlike pholcodine, codeine can cause constipation and inhibition of mucociliary clearance.

Mucolytics

Mucolytics are drugs that reduce the viscosity of bronchial secretions. They are sometimes used when excess bronchial secretions need to be cleared.

Carbocisteine and mecysteine hydrochloride

These drugs act as mucolytics.

Mechanism of action—Carbocisteine and mecysteine hydrochloride reduce the viscosity of bronchial secretions by cleaving disulphide bonds cross-linking mucus glycoprotein molecules.

Route of administration—Oral.

Indications—Carbocisteine and mecysteine hydrochloride may be of benefit in some chronic obstructive airways disease, although there is no evidence supporting their use.

Therapeutic notes—A novel drug with 'mucolytic' properties is dornase alfa, a genetically engineered enzyme which cleaves extracellular DNA, and is used in cystic fibrosis, being administered by inhalation.

After reading this chapter, you will:
- Have a good understanding of the peripheral nervous system and neurotransmitter action
- Know the different classes of drugs that are used in disorders of the peripheral nervous system and how their mechanisms of action result in beneficial and adverse effects.

NERVE CONDUCTION

Conduction of impulses through nerves occurs as an all-or-none event called the action potential. The action potential is caused by voltage-dependent opening of sodium and potassium channels in the cell membrane.

The sodium equilibrium potential (Eq Na^+) is $+60$ mV and the potassium equilibrium potential (Eq K^+) is -90 mV. Since a resting nerve has 50–75 more potassium channels open than sodium channels, the resting membrane potential is -70 mV.

Figure 4.1 shows the concentrations of sodium and potassium inside and outside a resting nerve. The Na^+/K^+ pump (Na^+/K^+ ATPase) is an energy-dependent pump that functions to maintain the concentration gradient of these two ionic species across the membrane. Three sodium ions are pumped out of the cell for every two potassium ions pumped in, and thus the excitability of the cell is retained. Figures 4.2 and 4.3 summarize the events that occur during a nerve action potential. During a nerve action potential:

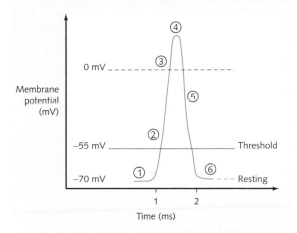

Fig. 4.2 Nerve action potential. For explanation of points 1–6, see Figure 4.3.

- The rate of sodium entry into the nerve axon becomes greater than the rate of potassium out of the axon, at which point the membrane becomes depolarized (the loss of an electrical gradient across the membrane).
- Depolarization sets off a sodium-positive feedback whereby more voltage-gated sodium channels open and the membrane becomes more depolarized.
- A threshold, which is usually 15 mV greater than the resting membrane potential, must be reached if an action potential is to be generated.
- The membrane repolarizes when the sodium channels become inactivated; a special set of potassium channels open and potassium leaves the axon.
- The sodium channels; eventually regain their resting excitable state and the Na^+/K^+ ATPase restores the membrane potential back to -70 mV.

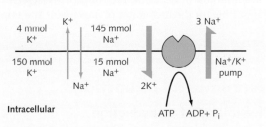

Fig. 4.1 Intracellular and extracellular sodium and potassium concentrations. The Na^+/K^+ pump maintains these concentration gradients across the cell membrane.

Figure 4.4 shows the voltage-operated sodium channels in their inactivated, activated and resting states. Two types of gate exist within the channel; the m-gates and

Fig. 4.3 State of sodium and potassium channels and membrane potential at different stages of the neuronal action potential

	Sodium channels	Potassium channels	Membrane potential
1	Closed resting	Closed resting	Resting (-70 mV)
2	Open	Closed resting	Depolarization (action potential upstroke)
3	More channels open	Closed resting	More depolarization
4	Channels close (inactive)	Special set of channels start opening	Peak of action potential reached
5	All inactivated	More channels open	Re-polarization
6	Closed resting	Channels close	Resting membrane potential re-established

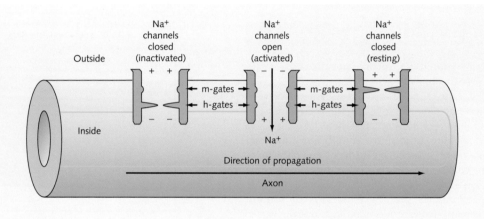

Fig. 4.4 Voltage-operated sodium channels in their inactivated, activated and resting states. The m-gates and h-gates open or close according to the state of the channel.

the h-gates. These gates are open or closed according to the state of the channel.

In the resting sodium channel, the m-gates are held closed by the strongly negative (-70 mV) electrical gradient across the membrane. Once an action potential begins to propagate, the loss of the membrane potential causes the m-gates to open, allowing sodium into the cell, further propagating the action potential. After a very short time, a further conformational change causes the h-gates to close, inactivating the sodium channel. The membrane then re-polarizes, and once at -70 mV the m-gates again close, and the h-gates open so the sodium channel is back in its resting state.

Sodium channel

The voltage-operated sodium channel is present in all excitable tissues. It is a transmembrane protein made up of four domains, each with six transmembrane regions. It is sensitive to membrane potential and selectively passes sodium ions.

Local anaesthetics block the sodium channel, and thus nerve conduction, by binding to the sixth transmembrane region of the fourth domain.

Size of the nerve fibre

Small nerve fibres are preferentially blocked because of their high surface-area to volume ratio. This results in a differential block whereby the small nociceptive (pain) and autonomic fibres are blocked but not the larger fibres responsible for the mediation of movement and touch.

SOMATIC NERVOUS SYSTEM

Neuromuscular junction

Physiology of transduction

Skeletal (voluntary) muscle is innervated by motor neurons, the axons of which are able to propagate action potentials at high velocities. The area of muscle that lies below the axon terminal is known as the motor end-plate, and the chemical synapse between the two is known as the neuromuscular junction (NMJ).

The axon terminal incorporates membrane-bound vesicles containing the neurotransmitter acetylcholine (ACh). Depolarization of the presynaptic terminal of the nerve by an action potential (generated by sodium influx) causes voltage-sensitive calcium channels to open, allowing calcium ions into the terminal. Normally, the level of calcium ions inside the nerves is very low, much lower relative to the external concentration. This calcium influx results in the release of ACh by exocytosis from vesicles. ACh diffuses across to the muscle membrane where it binds to the nicotinic acetylcholine receptor (nicAChR) and/or is inactivated by acetylcholinesterase (Fig. 4.5). Several events then occur:

- During association, ACh binds to the nicAChR, which is an ion channel that allows cations into the muscle (mainly sodium but also potassium to a lesser extent).

- During the conformational change, the pore of the ion channel is open for 1 ms, during which approximately 20 000 sodium ions enter the cell. The resulting depolarization, called an end-plate potential (EPP), depolarizes the adjacent muscle fibre.
- If the cellular response is large enough, an action potential is generated in the rest of the muscle fibre (sodium influx), resulting in the opening of voltage-operated calcium channels, but this time the calcium influx mediates contraction.
- ACh is rapidly inactivated by an enzyme called acetylcholinesterase (AChE) which hydrolyses ACh into the inactive metabolites choline and acetic acid.
- In the synthesis of ACh, the choline generated is taken up by the nerve terminal where another enzyme, choline acetyl transferase (ChAT), converts it back to ACh to be reused.

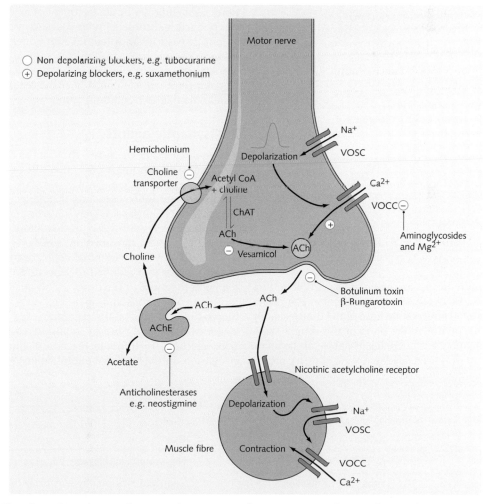

Fig. 4.5 Physiology of impulse transduction at the neuromuscular junction (NMJ) showing the site of action of drugs used in conjunction with the NMJ. (ChAT, choline acetyltransferase; vesamicol, an experimental drug; VOCC, voltage-operated calcium channel; AChE, acetylcholinesterase; VOSC, voltage-operated sodium channel.)

Nicotinic acetylcholine receptor

The nicAChR is made up of five subunits (two α, one β, one γ and one γ) that traverse the membrane and surround a central pore. All the subunits show high sequence identity. The binding site for ACh lies on the α subunits, therefore ACh must bind to both α subunits to open the channel.

Each subunit has four membrane-spanning regions (helices), i.e. each receptor has a total of 20 regions. One of the transmembrane helices (M_2) from each subunit forms the lining of the channel pore.

Pharmacological targets

There are three major targets within the NMJ for clinically useful drugs (Fig. 4.6):

- Presynaptic release
- Nicotinic acetylcholine receptor
- Acetylcholinesterase.

Drugs affecting the neuromuscular junction

Presynaptic agents

Drugs inhibiting ACh synthesis—The rate-limiting step in the synthesis of ACh is the uptake of choline into the nerve terminal.

Hemicholinium is an analogue of choline that competitively blocks the choline transporter and causes a depletion of ACh stores. Because of the time taken for the stores to run down, the onset of this drug is slow. This, and the frequency-dependent nature of the block (depletion of stores is related to release of ACh), means

that it is not useful clinically. The block is reversed by the addition of choline.

Drugs inhibiting vesicular packaging of ACh—Vesamicol inhibits the active transport of ACh into storage vesicles and results in neuromuscular block.

Drugs inhibiting ACh release—Calcium entry into the nerve terminal is necessary for the release of ACh; thus, agents such as aminoglycoside antibiotics (e.g. streptomycin) that prevent this step will cause neuromuscular blockade. Muscle paralysis is occasionally a side-effect of aminoglycoside antibiotics, but it can be reversed by the administration of calcium salts.

Botulinum toxin is a neurotoxin produced by the anaerobic bacillus *Clostridium botulinum*. The toxin is very potent and it is believed to inhibit ACh release by inactivating actin, which is necessary for exocytosis. In botulism, a serious type of food poisoning caused by this toxin, victims experience progressive parasympathetic and motor paralysis. Botulinum toxin type A is sometimes used clinically in the treatment of excessive muscle contraction disorders (dystonias) such as strabismus (squint), spasticity and tremors. More often, however, it is used cosmetically to diminish the appearance of wrinkles.

β-Bungarotoxin contained in snake venom acts in a similar manner to botulinum toxin.

Postsynaptic agents

Non-depolarizing blockers—These act as competitive antagonists by binding to the nicAChR but not activating it, and producing motor paralysis. Details of the most commonly used non-depolarizing blockers are given in Figure 4.7

Approximately 80–90% of receptors must be blocked to prevent transmission, since the amount of ACh released by nerve terminal depolarization usually greatly exceeds that required to generate an action potential in the muscle. The drugs are all quaternary ammonium compounds and, therefore, do not cross the blood–brain barrier or the placenta. They are poorly absorbed orally and must be administered by intravenous injection. 'Tetanic fade' (i.e. non-maintained muscle tension during brief nerve stimulation) is seen with

Fig. 4.6 Targets for clinically useful drugs at the neuromuscular junction

Site	Action	Use
nicAChR	Block transmission	Neuromuscular blockers for surgery
AChE	Enhance transmission	Peripheral neuropathy, e.g. myasthenia gravis
Release	Block transmission	Spasms, e.g. squints, tics, tremors, etc.

AChE, acetylcholine esterase; nicAChR, nicotinic acetylcholine receptor.

Fig. 4.7 Non-depolarizing blockers of postsynaptic receptors at the neuromuscular junction

Drug	Approximate duration (mins)	Side effects		Other	Elimination
		Ganglion block	Histamine release		
Pancuronium	40–60	X	Minimal	Block of muscarinic receptors in the heart → tachycardia	Mainly renal
Gallamine	15	X	X	Block of muscarinic receptors in the heart → tachycardia	Mainly renal: avoid in patients with renal disease
Alcuronium	20	X	X	Dose dependency	Mainly hepatic
Vecuronium	20–30	X	X		Mainly hepatic
Atracurium	15–30	X	Sometimes		Degradation in plasma at body pH (Hofmann elimination)

some of these drugs. This is due to the blocking of presynaptic autoreceptors which usually maintain the release of ACh during repeated stimulation.

The block can be reversed by anticholinesterases and depolarizing drugs. It is also enhanced in patients with myasthenia gravis. The main side-effect from these drugs is hypotension caused by the blocking of ganglionic transmission. Histamine release from mast cells, resulting in bronchospasm, may be a problem in certain individuals.

Depolarizing (non-competitive) blockers—Depolarizing blockers initially activate receptors, causing depolarization, but in doing so block further activation.

Depolarizing blockers act on the motor end-plate in the same manner as ACh, i.e. they are agonists and increase the cation permeability of the end-plate. However, unlike ACh, which is released in brief spurts and rapidly hydrolysed, depolarizing blockers remain associated with the receptors long enough to cause a sustained depolarization and a resulting loss of electrical excitability (phase I).

Repeated or continuous administration of depolarizing blockers leads to the block becoming more characteristic of non-depolarizing drugs. This is known as phase II and is probably due to receptor desensitization, whereby the end-plate becomes less sensitive to ACh. The block starts to show and it is partly reversed by anticholinesterase drugs.

Suxamethonium is the only depolarizing blocker used clinically because of its rapid onset time and short duration of action (approximately 4 mins). It must be given by intravenous injection. It is rapidly hydrolysed by plasma cholinesterase, although certain people with a genetic variant of this enzyme may experience a neuromuscular block that may last for hours.

Depolarizing blockers have no effect in patients with myasthenia gravis, since these patients have a decreased number of receptors at the end-plate. In this instance, the blocking potency of depolarizing blockers is reduced.

The side-effects of depolarizing blockers include:

- Initial spasms, which occur prior to paralysis, often resulting in postoperative muscle pain.
- Muscarinic receptor activation resulting in bradycardia. Bradycardia can be prevented by the administration of atropine.
- Potassium release from muscle resulting in elevated plasma potassium levels. This is usually a problem only in the case of trauma.

Anticholinesterases

Anticholinesterases inhibit AChE and thus increase the amount of ACh in the synaptic cleft and enhance cholinergic transmission. Most of the anticholinesterases used are quaternary ammonium compounds and, therefore, they do not penetrate the blood–brain barrier.

Short-acting anticholinesterases include edrophonium. This is selective for the NMJ and clinically relevant in the diagnosis of myasthenia gravis. Edrophonium's duration of action is only 2–10 mins because it binds by electrostatic forces (no covalent bonds) to the active site of the enzyme. It is therefore not used therapeutically but rather as a diagnostic test in myasthenia gravis.

Intermediate-acting anticholinesterases include neostigmine, pyridostigmine and physostigmine.

Neostigmine is used intravenously to reverse the effects of non-depolarizing blockers. Its duration of action is 2–4 hours, and it is used orally in the treatment of myasthenia gravis. Although neostigmine shows some selectivity for the NMJ, atropine is sometimes co-administered to block the muscarinic effects of the drug.

Pyridostigmine has a duration of action of 3–6 hours, and it is also used orally in the treatment of myasthenia gravis. It has few parasympathetic actions.

Physostigmine shows selectivity for the postganglionic parasympathetic junction. It is associated with central effects such as initial excitation followed by depression, and possibly respiratory depression and unconsciousness. The central cerebral side-effects can be antagonized by atropine. Physostigmine is used in the form of eye drops to constrict the pupil and contract the ciliary muscle in the treatment of glaucoma.

Most of the long-lasting or irreversible anticholinesterases are organophosphorus compounds. For example, sarin and tabun were developed as nerve gases, and parathion was developed as an insecticide, as well as for clinical use. These drugs have many adverse effects, such as bradycardia, hypotension, breathing problems, depolarizing neuromuscular block, central effects and possible death from peripheral nerve demyelination. Echothiophate shows selectivity for the postganglionic parasympathetic junction, and it is used in the treatment of glaucoma.

HINTS AND TIPS

In the treatment of myasthenia gravis, prednisolone can be added to help manage symptoms, usually with azathioprine to allow a lower dose of the steroid.

COMMUNICATION

Mrs Thumma, 34 years old, presented to her doctors with a 3-month history of early fatigue and muscle weakness. She finds it difficult to finish meals as she gets tired chewing and has now lost 2 kg. She is otherwise a healthy non-smoker, who rarely drinks alcohol. Her husband has noticed her voice becoming quieter, especially towards the end of the day.

On examination, she looks well. Power in all muscle groups is grossly normal but weakens after repeated testing. Tone, coordination, reflexes and sensation are normal. She is referred to a neurologist, who orders more investigations. Serum acetylcholine receptor antibodies test positive. A CT scan of her thymus reveals an enlarged thymus gland.

She therefore has a thymectomy, histopathological examination of which revealed benign hyperplasia. She is also given the anticholinesterase pyridostigmine and an appointment for review.

AUTONOMIC NERVOUS SYSTEM

The autonomic nervous system comprises the sympathetic and parasympathetic systems, which generally have opposite effects on the body. It innervates all tissues, except skeletal muscle (Fig. 4.8). The axons of the autonomic nervous system arise from their cell body, located in the central nervous system (CNS), as preganglionic fibres. These synapse in the appropriate ganglion, and leave as postganglionic fibres, which reach the effector cells.

The neurotransmitter released by preganglionic fibres at autonomic ganglia is ACh. The ACh receptors located on postganglionic nicotinic fibres.

Autonomic ganglia

Figure 4.9 summarizes the differences between ganglionic nicAChR and those found on skeletal muscle at the NMJ.

Ganglion-stimulating drugs

Nicotinic agonists

There are few agonists that act selectively on the nicAChR without affecting muscarinic receptors. Carbachol is the best example of a drug that shows preference for the nicotinic receptor, but still its action is not selective. Nicotine and lobeline both show preference for ganglionic nicotinic receptors (meaning slightly higher concentrations are needed when they stimulate the NMJ).

These drugs have no clinical use, since their range of effects is vast, affecting both sympathetic and parasympathetic transmission:

- Sympathetic effects include tachycardia and vasoconstriction leading to hypertension.
- Parasympathetic effects include increased gastrointestinal motility and glandular secretions.

Ganglion-blocking drugs

Autonomic ganglia can be blocked presynaptically by inhibiting ACh synthesis, vesicular packaging or release (p. 64), or postsynaptically by blocking the nicotinic receptors.

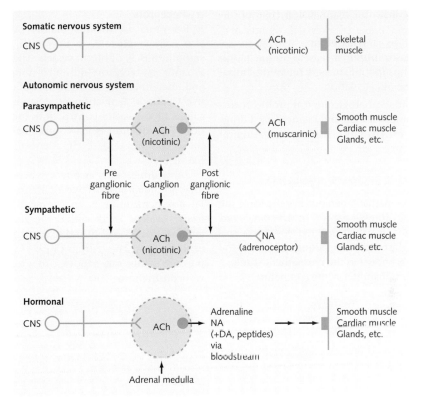

Fig. 4.8 Somatic and autonomic nervous systems: organization and neurotransmitters. (ACh, acetylcholine; CNS, central nervous sytem; DA,dopamine; NA, noradrenaline.)

Non-depolarizing ganglion blockers

A few of these drugs act solely as competitive antagonists, blocking receptors without depolarizing the ganglion. Most block the ion channel, as well as the associated receptor, and they produce their action through this former mechanism.

Ganglion-blocking drugs have a wide range of complex effects, although the sympathetic and parasympathetic systems tend to oppose one another. The effects of ganglion-blocking drugs include:

- Arteriolar vasodilatation leading to a marked reduction in blood pressure (block of sympathetic ganglia).

Fig. 4.9 Distinguishing features of the ganglionic nicotinic acetylcholine receptors and those found on skeletal muscle at the neuromuscular junction

	Skeletal muscle	Neurons
Structure	2α 1β 1γ or ε 1δ	2α 3β
Specific agonists	Suxamethonium	DMPP
Specific antagonists	Gallamine Tubocurarine α-Bungarotoxin	Hexamethonium Mecamylamine κ-Bungarotoxin
Function	End-plate region depolarization at NMJ	Neuronal depolarization in ganglia and CNS
(DMPP, dimethylphenylpiperazinium.)		

- Postural and postexercise hypotension (loss of cardiac reflexes).
- Slight reduction in cardiac output.
- Inhibition of gastrointestinal secretions and motility, leading to constipation, urinary retention, impotence and failure of ejaculation.

Despite having a broad pharmacological profile, rocuronium and vecuronium are the only widely used drugs of this class; they are used as muscle relaxants in surgical intubuation.

Sympathetic nervous system

The fibres of the sympathetic nervous system leave the CNS from the thoracolumbar regions of the spinal cord (T1–L3). They synapse in ganglia located close to the spinal cord. These ganglia form a chain along each side of the spinal cord, which is known as the sympathetic trunk.

The major neurotransmitter is noradrenaline.

HINTS AND TIPS

Sympathetic transmission is enhanced under conditions of stress, known as the 'fight-or-flight response'.

Adrenal medulla

Some postganglionic neurons in the sympathetic division do not have axons, but instead they release their transmitters directly into the bloodstream. These neurons are located in the adrenal medulla.

On stimulation by preganglionic fibres, the adrenal medulla acts as an endocrine gland, releasing its hormones/transmitters into the systemic circulation and consist of $\sim 80\%$ adrenaline, $\sim 20\%$ noradrenaline, as well as small amounts of dopamine, neuropeptides and ATP.

Adrenoceptors

The two receptor subtypes are α and β. Potency at:

- α receptors is noradrenaline > adrenaline > isoprenaline
- β receptors is isoprenaline > adrenaline > noradrenaline.

Effects mediated by α-adrenoreceptors

α_1-Receptors

α_1-Receptors are located postsynaptically. Their activation causes smooth muscle contraction (except for the non-sphincter part of the gastrointestinal tract, where activation causes relaxation), glycogenolysis in the liver, and potassium release from the liver and salivary glands. Transduction is via G-proteins and an increase in the second messengers inositol (1,4,5) triphosphate (IP_3) and diacylglycerol (DAG).

α_2-Receptors

α_2-Receptors are located mainly presynaptically, but also postsynaptically on liver cells, platelets and the smooth muscle of blood vessels. The activation of presynaptic α_2-receptors inhibits noradrenaline release and, therefore, provides a means of end-product negative feedback. Activation of postsynaptic α_2-receptors causes blood vessel constriction and platelet aggregation. Transduction is via G-proteins and a decrease in the second messenger cyclic adenosine monophosphate (cAMP).

Some drugs, such as phenoxybenzamine and phentolamine, are non-selective α-adrenoceptor antagonists. Phenoxybenzamine is an irreversible antagonist as it forms covalent bonds with the receptor, while phentolamine binds reversibly and so has a much shorter duration of action. These drugs cause a fall in arterial blood pressure, due to block of α-receptor-mediated vasoconstriction.

COMMUNICATION

Mrs Pharasha, a 26-year-old librarian, presents to her doctor with episodes of anxiety, sweating, tremor and palpitations. These attacks had been increasing in frequency and are now occurring almost daily. The only change Mrs Pharasha can think of is the increased stress at work, which she now feels she is not handling well. She is a non-smoker and seldom drinks alcohol. She is on no medication.

On examination, her heart rate is 106 beats per minute and her blood pressure is elevated. To treat her hypertension she is prescribed propranolol, a β-blocker, which causes her blood pressure to increase by 30 mmHg and her heart rate to reach 145 beats per minute. So her condition worsens markedly. She is rushed to accident and emergency where the doctor suspects phaeochromocytoma.

Resting plasma catecholamines and urinary metanephrines (catecholamine metabolites) are raised, supporting the diagnosis. Imaging reveals a tumour in the adrenal medulla, which is resectable. Intravenous phentolamine is given to safely reduce her blood pressure. Following stabilization of her blood pressure, she is put on phenoxybenzamine to achieve α-blockade, with propranolol added later to achieve β-blockade as well. She is maintained on this until complete α- and β-blockade is established and plasma volume has re-expanded. Surgery to remove the secreting tumour can then be performed, with an expert anaesthetist and surgeon, and readily available nitroprusside.

Effects mediated by β-adrenoceptors

β₁-Receptors

β₁-Receptors are mainly postsynaptic and located in the heart, platelets and non-sphincter part of the gastrointestinal tract. They can, however, be found presynaptically. Activation causes an increase in the rate and force of contraction of the heart, relaxation of the non-sphincter part of the gastrointestinal tract, aggregation of platelets, an increase in the release of noradrenaline, lipolysis in fat, and amylase secretion from the salivary glands. Presynaptically, their activation causes an increase in noradrenaline release. Transduction is via G-proteins and an increase in the second messenger cAMP.

β₂-Receptors

β₂-Receptors are located postsynaptically. Their activation causes smooth muscle relaxation, glycogenolysis in the liver, inhibition of histamine release from mast cells, and tremor in skeletal muscle. Transduction is via G-proteins and an increase in the second messenger cAMP.

Drugs acting on the sympathetic system

Figure 4.10 summarizes the drugs acting on the sympathetic system.

Presynaptic agents

Noradrenaline synthesis—The precursor to noradrenaline is L-tyrosine, which is taken up by adrenergic neurons.

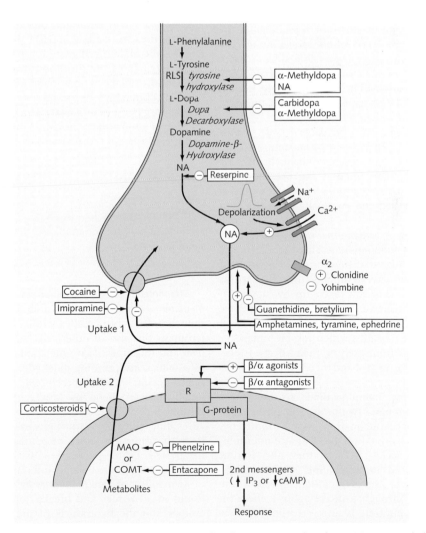

Fig. 4.10 Drugs affecting adrenergic transmission. (cAMP, cyclic adenosine monophosphate; COMT, catechol-O-methyltransferase; IP₃, inositol triphosphate; MAO, monoamine oxidase; NA, noradrenaline; RLS, rate-limiting step.)

Drugs decreasing noradrenaline synthesis—The rate-limiting step (RLS) is the conversion of tyrosine to dihydroxyphenylalanine (dopa), which is catalysed by tyrosine hydroxylase and inhibited by metyrosine. Noradrenaline provides a negative feedback upon this step. Carbidopa inhibits dopa decarboxylase and is used in Parkinson's disease to increase dopamine levels. Because this is not the RLS, drugs that inhibit dopa decarboxylase do not greatly affect noradrenaline synthesis. Administering α-methyldopa (used in hypertension) results in the formation of a false transmitter, α-methylnoradrenaline.

Drugs increasing noradrenaline synthesis—Levodopa (L-dopa) administration bypasses the RLS and is used in Parkinson's disease. Noradrenaline is stored in vesicles as a complex with ATP and a protein called chromogranin A.

Drugs inhibiting noradrenaline storage—Reserpine is a drug used in the treatment of hypertension and schizophrenia. It reduces stores of noradrenaline by preventing the accumulation of noradrenaline in vesicles. Its action is effectively irreversible since it has a very high affinity for the noradrenaline storage site. The displaced noradrenaline is immediately broken down by monoamine oxidase (MAO) and is therefore unable to exert sympathetic effects.

Drugs inhibiting the breakdown of leaked noradrenaline stores—They include monoamine oxidase inhibitors (MAOIs) and catechol-O-methyltransferase (COMT) inhibitors. They prevent the breakdown of leaked catecholamines so that noradrenaline that leaves the vesicles is protected and eventually leaks out from the nerve ending.

Drugs inhibiting noradrenaline release—These include guanethidine and bretylium. These are adrenergic neuron-blocking drugs that prevent the exocytosis of noradrenaline from nerve terminals; they are used as hypotensive drugs. They are taken up by 'uptake 1' and concentrated in nerve terminals where they have a local anaesthetic effect on impulse conduction. The tricyclic antidepressants, which inhibit 'uptake 1', prevent these drugs from exerting their effects. Clonidine is an α_2-receptor agonist and therefore inhibits noradrenaline release.

Drugs promoting noradrenaline release—These include amphetamines, tyramine and ephedrine, which are sympathomimetic drugs that act indirectly. They are taken up by uptake 1 and displace noradrenaline from the vesicles. Because they also inhibit MAO, the displaced noradrenaline is not broken down, and is able to exert sympathetic effects. These drugs act in part through a direct agonist effect on adrenoceptors. Yohimbine is an α_2-receptor antagonist and it therefore prevents noradrenaline from exerting a negative feedback effect on noradrenaline release.

Postsynaptic agents

Adrenoceptor agonists—These are termed 'sympathomimetics'. They activate postsynaptic receptors, eliciting a response (Fig. 4.11).

Adrenoceptor antagonists—These are termed 'sympatholytics'. They block postsynaptic receptors (Fig. 4.12).

Inactivation

Uptake 1—This is located on neuronal terminals, and it is the main mechanism for noradrenaline inactivation. Uptake 1 has a high affinity for the uptake of noradrenaline (K = 0.3 mmol/L in the rat), but the maximum rate of uptake is low (V_{max} = 1.2 nmol/g per min in the rat). It has a specificity rank of noradrenaline > adrenaline > isoprenaline; it is blocked by cocaine, amphetamines and tricyclic antidepressants (e.g. imipramine), which therefore potentiate the actions of noradrenaline.

Uptake 2—This is located outside neurons (e.g. in smooth muscle, cardiac muscle and endothelium), and it is the main mechanism for the removal of circulating adrenaline from the bloodstream. It has a low affinity for the uptake of noradrenaline (K = 250 mmol/L in the rat) but a high maximum rate of uptake (V_{max} = 100 nmol/g per min in the rat). Uptake 2 has a specificity rank of adrenaline > noradrenaline > isoprenaline, and it is blocked by corticosteroids.

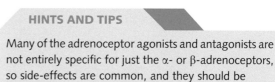

HINTS AND TIPS

Many of the adrenoceptor agonists and antagonists are not entirely specific for just the α- or β-adrenoceptors, so side-effects are common, and they should be remembered.

Metabolism of catecholamines by the enzyme monoamine oxidase—MAO is found on the surface of mitochondria, principally within adrenergic nerve terminals but also in other cells, such as those of the liver and intestines. MAO metabolizes catecholamines into their corresponding aldehydes. It comprises two major forms: MAO_A and MAO_B. Noradrenaline is mainly broken down by MAO_A in nerve terminals. Inhibitors of MAO increase the releasable store of noradrenaline, but they do not greatly potentiate sympathetic transmission, since catecholamines are mainly inactivated by reuptake. MAOIs include the antidepressant drugs phenelzine and tranylcypromine.

Metabolism of catecholamines by COMT—COMT is found in all tissues and breaks down most catecholamines and the byproducts of the actions of MAO. COMT metabolizes catecholamines to give a methoxy derivative. Entacapone, a COMT inhibitor, is a drug used clinically for parkinsonism.

Fig. 4.11 Adrenoceptor agonists and their clinical uses

Drug	Receptor	Uses	Side effects	Pharmacokinetics
Noradrenaline	α/β	No use clinically	Hypertension, tachycardia, ventricular arrhythmias	Poor oral absorption, metabolized by MAO and COMT $t_{1/2} \sim 2$ min
Adrenaline	α/β	Anaphylactic shock Cardiac resuscitation with local anaesthetics	Hypertension, tachycardia, ventricular arrhythmias	Poor oral absorption, metabolized by MAO and COMT $t_{1/2} \sim 2$ min given intravenously or intramuscularly
Oxymetazoline	α	Nasal decongestant	Rebound congestion	Given intranasally
Phenylephrine	α_1	Hypotension Nasal decongestant	Hypertension Reflex bradycardia	Metabolized by MAO $t_{1/2} < 1$ min, given intramuscularly or intranasally
Clonidine	α_2	Hypertension Migraine	Drowsiness, hypotension	Good oral absorption $t_{1/2} \sim 12$ h
Isoprenaline	β	Asthma Cardiac resuscitation	Arrhythmias, tachycardia	Metabolized by COMT, given sublingually or as aerosol $t_{1/2} \sim 2$ h
Dobutamine	β_1	Heart failure	Tachycardia	
Salbutamol	β_2	Asthma Premature labour	Arrhythmias, tachycardia, vasodilatation	Given by aerosol $t_{1/2} \sim 4$ h

COMT, catechol-O-methyltransferase; MAO, monoamine oxidase.

Fig. 4.12 Adrenoceptor antagonists and their clinical uses

Drug	Receptor	Uses	Side effects	Pharmacokinetics
Labetalol	α/β	Hypertension	Postural hypotension	Oral absorption $t_{1/2} \sim 4$ h
Phentolamine	α	No clinical use	Hypotension Tachycardia Nasal congestion	Metabolized by the liver, given intravenously $t_{1/2} \sim 4$ h
Prazosin	α_1	Hypertension	Hypotension Tachycardia Nasal congestion Drowsiness	Oral absorption, metabolized by the liver $t_{1/2} \sim 2$ h
Yohimbine	α_2	No clinical use	Hypertension Excitement	Oral absorption, metabolized by the liver $t_{1/2} \sim 4$ h
Propranolol	β	Hypertension Angina Arrhythmias	Bronchoconstriction Heart failure	Oral absorption, first-pass metabolism, 90% plasma-protein bound $t_{1/2} \sim 4$ h
Practolol	β_1	Hypertension Angina Arrhythmias	Bronchoconstriction Heart failure	Oral absorptison $t_{1/2} \sim 4$ h

Parasympathetic nervous system

The fibres of the parasympathetic nervous system leave the CNS from the sacral region (S3 and S4) of the spinal cord and via cranial nerves III, VII, IX and X. The fibres synapse in ganglia, which, unlike the sympathetic system, are located within the innervated organs themselves.

The major transmitter released by the postganglionic fibres at the junction with effector cells is ACh (Fig. 4.13).

Parasympathetic receptors

The ACh released by postganglionic nerve fibres acts on muscarinic (M) receptors, of which between three and five subtypes exist.

'Neuroparietal' M_1 receptors

M1 'neuroparietal' receptors are principally found in the CNS, peripheral neurons and gastric parietal cells. Their effects tend to be excitatory, depolarizing membranes through a decrease in potassium conductance. Activation causes central excitation and gastric acid secretion, while transduction is via G-proteins and an increase in the second messengers IP_3 and DAG through stimulation of phospholipase C.

'Neurocardiac' M_2 receptors

M_2 'neurocardiac' receptors are found in the heart and on peripheral neurons. Their effects are inhibitory, increasing potassium conductance and inhibiting calcium channels. In the heart, their activation causes a decrease in the rate (via potassium) and force of contraction (via calcium). Transduction is via G-proteins and a decrease in the second messenger cAMP through inhibition of adenylyl cyclase.

'Smooth muscle-glandular' M_3 receptors

M_3 'smooth muscle-glandular' receptors are found in smooth muscle and glands. Their effects tend to be excitatory, increasing sodium conductance. Activation causes glandular secretions such as saliva and sweat, and smooth muscle contraction. Transduction is via G-proteins and an increase in the second messengers IP_3 and DAG. M_3 receptors are also located on vascular endothelium, activation of which causes vasodilatation,

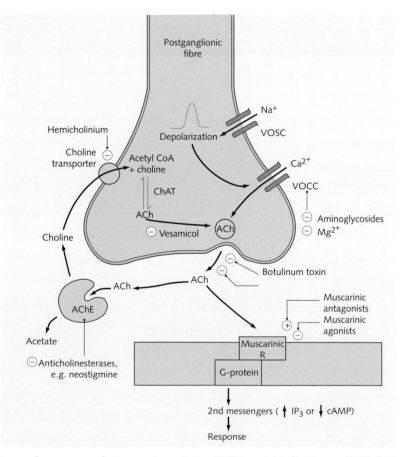

Fig. 4.13 Drugs acting on the parasympathetic nerve transmission. (AChE, acetylcholinesterase; ChAT, choline acetyl transferase; VOCC, voltage-operated calcium channel; VOSC, voltage-operated sodium channel.)

through the release of endothelium-derived relaxing factor (EDRF).

'Eye' M$_4$ receptors

M$_4$ 'eye' receptors are believed to be exclusive to the eye. Their activation causes constriction of the pupil and accommodation for near vision. Transduction is via G-proteins and a decrease in the second messenger cAMP through inhibition of adenylyl cyclase.

Drugs acting on the parasympathetic system

Figure 4.13 summarizes the drugs that act on the parasympathetic system.

Presynaptic agents

For information regarding presynaptic agents, see pp. 55–56.

Anticholinesterases

For information regarding anticholinesterases, see p. 57

Postsynaptic agents

Muscarinic-receptor agonists—These are termed 'parasympathomimetic', they activate postsynaptic receptors (Fig. 4.14).

Muscarinic-receptor antagonists—These are termed 'parasympatholytic' and block postsynaptic receptors (Fig. 4.15).

Non-selective antagonists can be used in anaesthesia to prevent bronchial secretions and vagal slowing of heart rate.

Different tissues respond differently to muscarinic antagonists (Fig. 4.16). Salivary, sweat and bronchial glands are the most sensitive and can be blocked by very low doses of atropine. In contrast, the parietal cells are the most resistant, and the block of gastric acid secretion requires high doses of atropine.

The side-effects of muscarinic antagonists include:

- Dry mouth and skin, and increased body temperature (inhibition of salivary and sweat glands).
- Blurred vision and pupil no longer responsive to light (dilation of pupil).

Fig. 4.14 Muscarinic agonists and their clinical uses

Drug	Muscarinic receptors	Nicotinic receptors	Uses
Carbachol	++	+	Gut and bladder stimulation postoperatively
Methacholine	+++	+	
Bethanechol	+++	—	Gut and bladder stimulation postoperatively
Muscarine	+++	—	
Pilocarpine	++	—	To decrease intraocular pressure in glaucoma

Fig. 4.15 Muscarinic antagonists and their clinical uses

Drug	Muscarinic receptor	Specific uses
Atropine	Non-selective	Reduces GI motility Cardiac arrest
Hyoscine	Non-selective	Motion sickness
Ipratropium	Non-selective	Bronchodilator
Cyclopentolate	M$_4$	Dilation of pupil
Tropicamide	M$_4$	Dilation of pupil
Pirenzepine	M$_1$	Reduces gastric acid secretion
Trihexyphenidyl (benzhexol)	M$_1$	Parkinson's disease

Fig. 4.16 Summary of the opposing effects of sympathetic and parasympathetic nerve stimulation on body tissues

Target tissue	Sympathetic		Parasympathetic		Overall effect
Nerve terminals	α_2	Decreased release	M_2	Decreased release	Decreased transmission
Smooth muscle					
Blood vessels	$\alpha_{1/2}$ β_2	Contraction Relaxation	M_3	Relaxation (via EDRF)	Vasocontriction Vasodilatation
Bronchi	β_2 α_1	Relaxation Contraction	M_3 M_3	Contraction Secretion	Bronchodilation Bronchoconstriction Bronchosecretion
GI tract: non-sphincter sphincter secretions	$\beta/$ α_1 α_1	Relaxation Contraction	M_3 M_3 M_3	Contraction Relaxation Secretion	Increased/decreased motility and tone GI secretions
Parietal cells			M_1	Contraction	Gastric acid secretion
Pancreas			M_3	Contraction	Increased secretions
Uterus	α_1 β_2	Contraction Relaxation	M_3 M_3		
Bladder: detrusor sphincter	β_2 α_1	Relaxation Contraction	M_3 M_3	Contraction Relaxation	Micturition Urine retention
Seminal tract Vas deferens Penis: venous sphincter	α_1 β_2 α_1 α_1	Contraction Relaxation Contraction	M_3	Vasodilatation	Ejaculation Ejaculation Erection
Radial muscle (iris) Ciliary muscle Lacrimal gland	α_1 β_2	Contraction Relaxation	M_4 M_4 M_4	Relaxation Contraction Contraction	Pupil relaxation/ constriction Accommodation Tear secretion
Heart	β_1	Increased rate and force	M_2	Decreased rate and force	
Liver	$\alpha_1/$ β_2	Glygenolysis			
Fat	β_1	Lipolysis			
Salivary glands	$\alpha_1/$ β_1	Secretion of thick saliva	M_3	Abundant secretion of watery saliva	
Platelets	α_2	Platelet aggregation			
Mast cells	β_2	Inhibition of histamine release			

- Paralysis of accommodation: cycloplegia (relaxation of ciliary muscle).
- Urinary retention.
- Central excitation: irritability and hyperactivity.
- Sedation (hyoscine).

NITRERGIC NERVOUS SYSTEM

Nitric oxide is now well recognized as a neurotransmitter in the CNS, and more recently it has been attributed to have numerous roles to play in the peripheral nervous system too.

Nitric oxide is generated by the action of the enzyme nitric oxide synthase (NOS). L-Arginine is the amino acid precursor of nitric oxide synthesis.

Nitric oxide activates the guanylyl cyclase enzyme, which is responsible for generating cyclic guanosine monophosphate (cGMP). The synthesis of cGMP in turn activates a protein kinase, which phosphorylates ion channels in the plasma membrane, and causes hyperpolarization of the smooth muscle cell. Intracellular calcium ions are consequently sequestered into the endoplasmic reticulum, and further calcium influx into the cell inhibited by the closure of calcium channels. The overall effect of a fall in intracellular calcium is a relaxation of the smooth muscle.

The smooth muscle effects of nitric oxide in the peripheral nervous system are now recognized to be important in the gastrointestinal system, and in sexual arousal in both sexes, particularly in the male.

Therapeutic manipulation of the nitrergic nervous system is confined to the male reproductive system at present, and the agents currently used in the management of erectile dysfunction (e.g. sildenafil (Viagra$^{®}$) are discussed in Chapter 6.

Central nervous system 5

● Objectives

After reading this chapter, you will:
● Understand the functions of the central nervous system and the diseases that can occur
● Know the drug classes used to treat these conditions, their mechanisms of action and adverse effects.

BASIC CONCEPTS

The central nervous system consists of the brain and the spinal cord, which are continuous with one another. The brain is composed of the cerebrum (which consists of the frontal, temporal, parietal and occipital lobes), the diencephalon (which includes the thalamus and hypothalamus), the brainstem (which consists of the midbrain, pons and medulla oblongata) and the cerebellum. The brain functions to interpret sensory information obtained about the internal and external environments and send messages to effector organs in response to a situation. Different parts of the brain are associated with specific functions (Fig. 5.1). However, the brain is a complex organ and is not yet completely understood.

PARKINSON'S DISEASE AND PARKINSONISM

Parkinsonism is characterized by a resting tremor, slow initiation of movements (bradykinesia), and muscle rigidity. A patient with parkinsonism will present with characteristic signs including:

● A shuffling gait
● A blank 'mask-like' facial expression
● Speech impairment
● An inability to perform skilled tasks.

Parkinsonism is most commonly caused by Parkinson's disease, though other causes exist.

Parkinson's disease is a progressive neurological disorder of the basal ganglia that occurs most commonly in elderly people.

Aetiology

The cause of Parkinson's disease is unknown in most cases (idiopathic) although both endogenous and environmental neurotoxins are known to be responsible for causing parkinsonism.

Parkinson's disease is progressive, with continued loss of dopaminergic neurons in the substantia nigra correlating with worsening of clinical symptoms. The possibility of a neurotoxic cause has been strengthened by the finding that 1-methyl-4-phenyl-1,2,3, 6-tetrahydropyridine (MPTP), a chemical contaminant of heroin, causes irreversible damage to the nigrostriatal dopaminergic pathway. Thus, this damage can lead to the development of symptoms similar to those of idiopathic Parkinson's disease. Drugs that block dopamine receptors can also induce parkinsonism. Neuroleptic drugs (p. 83) used in the treatment of schizophrenia can produce parkinsonian symptoms as an adverse effect. Rare causes of parkinsonism are cerebral ischaemia (progressive atherosclerosis or stroke), viral encephalitis or other pathological damage.

HINTS AND TIPS

RATS! Symptoms of parkinsonism include *Rigidity*, *Akinesia*, *Tremor* and *Shuffling gait*.

Pathogenesis

Post-mortem analysis of brains of parkinsonian patients shows a substantially reduced concentration of dopamine (less than 10% of normal) in the basal ganglia. The basal ganglia exert an extrapyramidal neural influence that normally maintains smooth voluntary movement.

The main pathology in Parkinson's disease is a progressive degeneration of the dopaminergic neurons of the substantia nigra, which project via the nigrostriatal pathway to the corpus striatum (Fig. 5.2). The inhibitory dopaminergic activity of the nigrostriatal pathway is, therefore, considerably reduced (by 20–40%) in people with Parkinson's disease.

The reduction in the inhibitory dopaminergic activity of the nigrostriatal pathway results in unopposed cholinergic neuron hyperactivity from the corpus

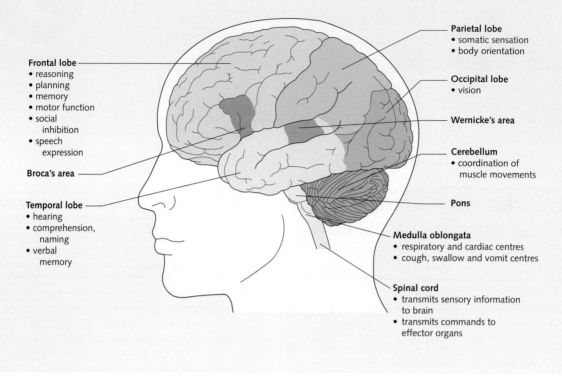

Fig. 5.1 Parts of the brain and their known functions.

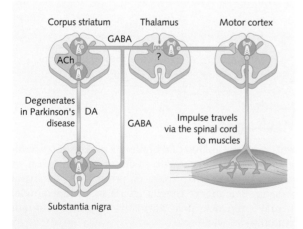

Fig. 5.2 Basal ganglia systems involved in Parkinson's disease. (ACh, acetylcholine; DA, dopamine; GABA, γ-aminobutyric acid.) (Redrawn from Page et al. 2006.)

striatum, which contributes to the pathological features of parkinsonism. Frank symptoms of parkinsonism appear only when more than 80% of the dopaminergic neurons of the substantia nigra have degenerated.

Untreated Parkinson's eventually results in dementia and death.

Treatment of parkinsonism

The treatment of parkinsonism is based on correcting the imbalance between the dopaminergic and cholinergic systems at the basal ganglia (Fig. 5.3). Two major groups of drugs are used: drugs that increase dopaminergic activity between the substantia nigra and the corpus striatum, and anticholinergic drugs that inhibit striatal cholinergic activity.

Drugs that increase dopaminergic activity

Dopamine precursors
An example of a dopamine precursor is levodopa (L-dopa).

Mechanism of action—L-dopa is the immediate precursor of dopamine and is able to penetrate the blood–brain barrier to replenish the dopamine content of the corpus striatum. L-dopa is decarboxylated to dopamine in the brain by dopa decarboxylase, and it has beneficial effects produced through the actions of dopamine on D_2 receptors (see Fig. 5.3). Dopamine itself is not used, owing to its inability to cross the blood–brain barrier.

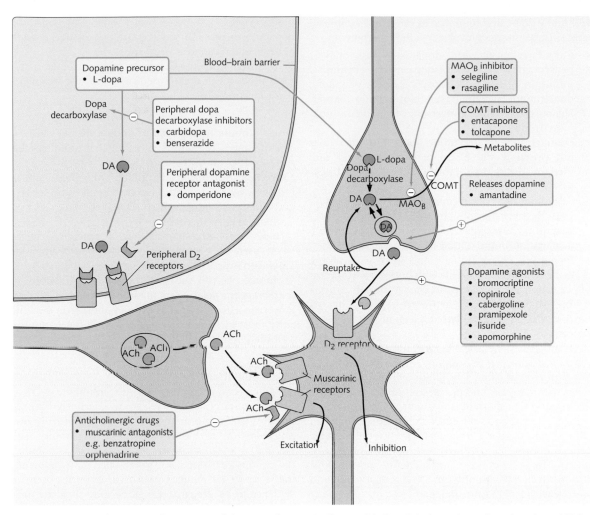

Fig. 5.3 Drugs used to treat parkinsonism and their site of action. (ACh, acetylcholine; DA, dopamine; L-dopa, levodopa; MAOᵦ, monoamine oxidase B; COMT, catechol-O-methyl transferase.)

Route of administration—L-dopa is administered orally. It reaches peak plasma concentrations after 1–2 hours and only 1% reaches the brain, owing to peripheral metabolism.

Indications—L-dopa is used in the treatment of parkinsonism (excluding drug-induced extrapyramidal symptoms).

Contraindications—Closed-angle glaucoma.

Adverse effects—The extensive peripheral metabolism of L-dopa means that large doses have to be given to produce therapeutic effects in the brain. Large doses are more likely to produce adverse effects. These include:

- Nausea and vomiting
- Psychiatric side-effects (schizophrenia-like symptoms)
- Cardiovascular effects (hypotension)
- Dyskinesias.

Nausea and vomiting are caused by stimulation of dopamine receptors in the chemoreceptor trigger zone in the area postrema, which lies outside the blood–brain barrier.

Psychiatric side-effects are common limiting factors in L-dopa treatment; these include vivid dreams, confusion and psychotic symptoms more commonly seen in schizophrenia. These effects are probably a result of increased dopaminergic activity in the mesolimbic area of the brain, possibly similar to that found pathologically in schizophrenia (dopaminergic overactivity is implicated in schizophrenia, p. 82).

Hypotension is common but usually asymptomatic. Cardiac arrhythmias are due to increased catecholamine stimulation following the excessive peripheral metabolism of L-dopa.

Dyskinesias can often develop and tend to involve the face and limbs. They usually reflect over-treatment and respond to simple dose reduction.

Three strategies have been developed to optimize L-dopa treatment, to maximize the central effects of L-dopa within the brain, and minimize its unwanted peripheral effects. These strategies involve co-administration of:

- Carbidopa (given with L-dopa as co-careldopa) or benserazide (given with L-dopa as co-beneldopa), inhibitors of dopa decarboxylase in the periphery, that cannot penetrate the blood–brain barrier. Hence, extracerebral conversion of L-dopa to dopamine is inhibited.
- Domperidone, a dopamine antagonist, that does not penetrate the blood–brain barrier and can, therefore, block the stimulation of dopamine receptors in the periphery.
- Selegiline and entacapone, monoamine oxidase (MAO)$_B$ and catechol-O-methyltransferase (COMT) inhibitors, respectively, which inhibit dopamine degradation in the central nervous system (CNS).

Therapeutic notes—Initially, treatment with L-dopa is effective in 80% of patients with possible restoration of near-normal motor function. Although L-dopa restores dopamine levels in the short term, therapy has no effect on the underlying degenerative disease process.

As progressive neuronal degeneration continues, the capacity of the corpus striatum to convert L-dopa to dopamine diminishes. This affects the majority of patients within 5 years and manifests itself as 'end of dose deterioration' (a shortening of duration of each dose of L-dopa), and the 'on-off effect' (rapid fluctuations in clinical state, varying from increased mobility and a general improvement to increased rigidity and hypokinesia). The latter effect occurs suddenly and for short periods from a few minutes to a few hours, tending to worsen with length of treatment.

Dopamine agonists

Examples of dopamine agonists include bromocriptine, ropinirole, cabergoline, pergolide, pramipexole, lisuride and apomorphine.

Mechanism of action—Bromocriptine, ropinirole, cabergoline (longer acting), pergolide, pramipexole, lisuride and apomorphine are dopamine agonists selective for the D$_2$ receptor (see Fig. 5.3). Apomorphine also has agonist action at D$_1$ receptors. Pramipexole has a high affinity for D$_3$ receptors.

Route of administration—Oral. Apomorphine is given by the subcutaneous route.

Indications—Dopamine agonists are used in combination with L-dopa in an attempt to reduce the late adverse effects of L-dopa therapy ('end of dose deterioration' and 'on-off effect') or when L-dopa alone does not adequately control the symptoms.

Adverse effects—The adverse effects of dopamine agonists are similar to those of L-dopa (i.e. nausea, postural hypotension, psychiatric symptoms), but they tend to be more common and more severe. Apomorphine

produces profound nausea and vomiting. Ergot-derived dopamine agonists (bromocriptine, cabergoline, lisuride and pergolide) can cause fibrosis.

Therapeutic notes—Currently bromocriptine is the most used of the dopamine agonists in the treatment of Parkinson's disease.

Drugs stimulating release of dopamine

Amantadine is an example of a drug that stimulates the release of dopamine (see Fig. 5.3).

Mechanism of action—Facilitation of neuronal dopamine release and inhibition of its reuptake into nerves, and additional muscarinic blocking actions.

Route of administration—Oral.

Indications—Amantadine has a synergistic effect when used in conjunction with L-dopa therapy in Parkinson's disease.

Adverse effects—Anorexia, nausea, hallucinations.

Therapeutic notes—Amantadine has modest antiparkinsonian effects, but it is only of short-term benefit, since most of its effectiveness is lost within 6 months of initiating treatment.

MAO$_B$ inhibitors

Selegiline is an example of a MAO$_B$ inhibitor.

Mechanism of action—Selegiline selectively inhibits the MAO$_B$ enzyme in the brain that is normally responsible for the degradation of dopamine (see Fig. 5.3). By reducing the catabolism of dopamine, the actions of L-dopa are potentiated, thus allowing the dose to be reduced by up to a third. There is evidence to suggest that selegiline may slow the progression of the underlying neuronal degeneration in Parkinson's disease.

Route of administration—Oral.

Indications—MAO$_B$ inhibitors can be used on their own in mild cases of parkinsonism or in conjunction with L-dopa to reduce 'end-of-dose' deterioration in severe parkinsonism.

Adverse effects—The adverse effects of MAO$_B$ inhibitors are those that might be expected by potentiation of L-dopa.

> ### HINTS AND TIPS
>
> Note that with the possible exception of selegiline, none of the drugs used in Parkinson's disease affect the inevitable progressive degeneration of nigrostriatal dopaminergic neurons. The disease process is unaffected, just compensated for by drug therapy.

COMT inhibitors

Entacapone and tolcapone are examples of COMT inhibitors.

Mechanism of action—Dopamine is broken down by a second pathway, in addition to that of MAO_B. The enzyme COMT is responsible for the degradation of dopamine to inactive methylated metabolites. COMT inhibitors specifically inhibit this enzyme.

Route of administration—Oral.

Indications—As an adjunct to L-dopa preparations when 'end-of-dose' is problematic.

Contraindications—Phaeochromocytoma.

Adverse effects—Nausea, vomiting, abdominal pain, diarrhoea.

Therapeutic notes—Due to hepatotoxicity, tolcapone should only be prescribed under specialist supervision.

Drugs that inhibit striatal cholinergic activity

Anticholinergic agents

Benzatropine, procyclidine and orphenadrine are examples of anticholinergic (antimuscarinic) agents.

Mechanism of action—Benzatropine, procyclidine and orphenadrine are antagonists at the muscarinic receptors that mediate striatal cholinergic excitation (see Fig. 5.3). Their major action in the treatment of Parkinson's disease is to reduce the excessive striatal cholinergic activity that characterizes the disease.

Route of administration—Oral.

Adverse effects—Typical peripheral anticholinergic effects, such as a dry mouth and blurred vision, are less common. More often, patients experience a variety of CNS effects, ranging from mild memory loss to acute confusional states.

Therapeutic notes—Termination of anticholinergic treatment should be gradual, as parkinsonism can worsen when these drugs are withdrawn. Anticholinergic drugs are most effective in controlling tremor rather than other symptoms of Parkinson's disease.

Transplantation

The transplantation of cells from the substantia nigra of human fetuses into the putamen of patients with Parkinson's disease has shown some success in controlling parkinsonian symptoms.

Transplantation in the treatment of Parkinson's disease is still experimental, and its role is highly controversial.

DEMENTIA

Alzheimer's disease is a specific process that results in dementia and is unrelated to the dementias associated with stroke, brain trauma and alcohol. Its prevalence increases markedly with age.

Alzheimer's disease is progressive and it is associated with atrophy of the brain substance, loss of neuronal tissue and deposition of amyloid plaques. The clinical features include deterioration in cognitive function, disorientation and generalized confusion.

Loss of neurons in the forebrain is most marked and a relative selective loss of cholinergic neurons most likely accounts for the features of this dementia. The obvious therapeutic target is, therefore, restoration of cholinergic function.

Cholinesterase inhibitors

Donepezil, galantamine and rivastigmine are cholinesterase inhibitors, licensed for use in dementia in the UK.

Mechanism of action—The cholinesterase inhibitors prevent the breakdown of acetylcholine within the synaptic cleft, and they enhance endogenous cholinogenic activity within the CNS and peripheral tissues.

Route of administration—Oral.

Indications—Mild to moderate dementia in Alzheimer's disease.

Contraindications—Pregnancy, breastfeeding, hepatic and renal impairment.

Adverse effects—Nausea, vomiting, diarrhoea, anorexia, agitation.

ANXIETY AND SLEEP DISORDERS

Anxiety and anxiolytics

Anxiety is a state characterized by psychological symptoms such as a diffuse, unpleasant and vague feeling of apprehension, often accompanied by physical symptoms of autonomic arousal such as palpitations, lightheadedness, perspiration, 'butterflies' and, in some people, restlessness.

While occasional anxiety is perfectly normal, it is a common and disabling symptom in a variety of mental illnesses including phobias, panic disorders and obsessive compulsive disorders. Drugs used to treat such anxiety disorders are called anxiolytics.

SLEEP DISORDERS AND HYPNOTICS

Insomnia is a common and non-specific disorder that may be reported by 40–50% of people at any given time.

Causes of insomnia include medical illness, alcohol or drugs, periodic limb movement disorder, sleep apnoea and psychiatric illness. Without an obvious underlying cause, it is known as primary or psychophysiological.

Hypnotics are drugs used to treat psychophysiological (primary) insomnia. The distinction between the treatment of anxiety and that of sleep disorders is not clear-cut, particularly if anxiety is the main impediment to sleep.

γ-Aminobutyric acid receptor

The γ-aminobutyric acid (GABA) receptors of the $GABA_A$ type are involved in the actions of some classes of hypnotic/anxiolytic drugs, notably:

- The benzodiazepines, which are currently the most commonly used clinically
- Newer non-benzodiazepine hypnotics, e.g. zopiclone
- The now obsolete barbiturates.

The $GABA_A$ receptor belongs to the superfamily of ligand-gated ion channels. It consists of several subunits – α, β, γ and δ – which form the $GABA/Cl^-$ channel complex, as well as containing benzodiazepine and barbiturate modulatory receptor sites. The GABA binding site appears to be located on the α and β subunits whereas the benzodiazepine modulatory site is distinct and located on the γ subunit.

GABA released from nerve terminals binds to postsynaptic $GABA_A$ receptors, the activation of which increases the Cl^- conductance of the neuron. Occupation of the benzodiazepine sites by benzodiazepine receptor agonists enhances the actions of GABA on the Cl^- conductance of the neuronal membrane. The barbiturates similarly enhance the action of GABA, but by occupying a distinct modulatory site (Fig. 5.4).

Anxiolytic and hypnotic drugs

The pharmacotherapy of anxiety and sleep disorders involves several different classes of drug, as shown in Figure 5.5, and non-pharmacological management relying on cognitive and behaviour psychotherapy.

Benzodiazepines

Benzodiazepines are drugs with anxiolytic, hypnotic, muscle relaxation and anticonvulsant actions that are used in the treatment of both anxiety states and insomnia.

Benzodiazepines are marketed as either hypnotics or anxiolytics. It is mainly the duration of action that determines the choice of drug (see below).

Mechanism of action—Benzodiazepines potentiate the action of GABA, the primary inhibitory neurotransmitter in the CNS. They do this by binding to a site on $GABA_A$ receptors, increasing their affinity for GABA. This results in an increased opening frequency of these ligand-gated Cl^- channels, thus potentiating the effect of GABA release in terms of inhibitory effects on the postsynaptic cell (Fig. 5.4).

Indications—Benzodiazepines are used clinically in the short-term relief of severe anxiety and severe insomnia, preoperative sedation, status epilepticus and acute alcohol withdrawal.

Route of administration—Oral is the usual route. Intravenous, intramuscular and rectal preparations are available.

Contraindications—Benzodiazepines should not be given to people with bronchopulmonary disease, and they have additive or synergistic effects with other central depressants such as alcohol, barbiturates and antihistamines.

Adverse effects—Benzodiazepines have several adverse effects:

- Drowsiness, ataxia and reduced psychomotor performance are common; therefore, care is necessary when driving or operating machinery.
- Dependence becomes apparent after 4–6 weeks, and is both physical and psychological. The withdrawal syndrome (in 30% of patients) comprises rebound anxiety and insomnia, tremulousness and twitching.

Although in overdose benzodiazepines alone are relatively safe when compared with other sedatives, such as barbiturates, if benzodiazepines are taken in combination with alcohol the CNS-depressant effects

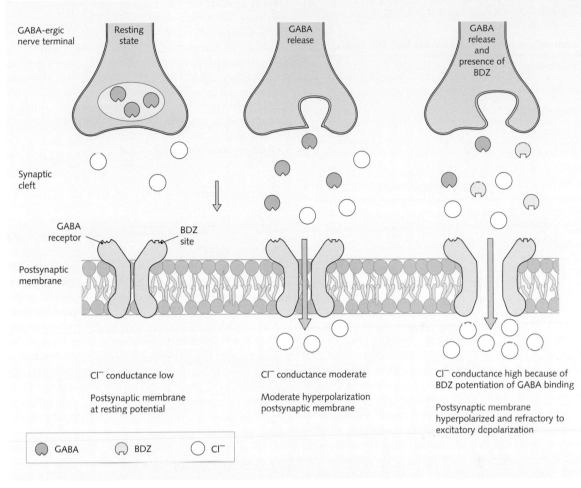

Fig. 5.4 Diagrammatic representation of the GABA$_A$ receptor and how its activity is enhanced by benzodiazepines and similarly by barbiturates. (BDZ, benzodiazepine; Cl$^-$, chloride ion; GABA, γ-aminobutyric acid.) (Redrawn from Page et al. 2006.)

Fig. 5.5 Drugs used to treat anxiety and sleep disorders	
Anxiolytics	**Hypnotics**
Benzodiazepines (act on GABA$_A$ receptors) e.g. diazepam, lorazepam	Benzodiazepines (act on GABA$_A$ receptors) e.g. triazolam, temazepam, lormetazepam, nitrazepam
Acting on serotonergic receptors (act on 5-HT$_{1A}$ or 5-HT$_3$ receptors) e.g. buspirone	Non-benzodiazepine hypnotics (act on GABA$_A$ receptors) e.g. zopiclone, zolpidem and zaleplon
Other drugs e.g. propranolol antidepressants	Other drugs e.g. chloral hydrate clomethiazole barbiturates (obsolete) sedative antidepressants sedative antihistamines
(5-HT, 5-hydroxytryptamine; GABA, γ-aminobutyric acid.)	

Fig. 5.6 Approximate elimination half-lives of the benzodiazepines	
Benzodiazepine	**Approximate half-life (hours)**
Midazolam	2–4
Temazepam	8–12
Lormetazepam	10
Lorazepam	12
Nitrazepam	24
Diazepam	32 (one metabolite is active for up to 200 hours)

are potentiated and fatal respiratory depression can result. Treatment is with the benzodiazepine antagonist flumazenil.

Therapeutic notes—Benzodiazepines are active orally, and they differ mainly in respect of their duration of action (Fig. 5.6). Short-acting agents (e.g. lorazepam and temazepam) are metabolized to inactive compounds, and these are used mainly as sleeping pills because of the relative lack of 'hangover' effects in the morning. Some long-acting agents (e.g. diazepam) are converted to long-lasting active metabolites with a half-life longer than the administered parent drug. With others (e.g. nitrazepam) it is the parent drug itself that is metabolized slowly. Such drugs are more suitable for an anxiolytic effect maintained all day long, or when early morning waking is the problem.

Non-benzodiazepine hypnotics

Zopiclone, zolpidem and zaleplon are the newer-generation hypnotics that have a short duration of action with little or no hangover effect. Although these drugs are not benzodiazepines, they act in a comparable manner to benzodiazepines on the $GABA_A$ receptor, although not at exactly the same sites.

Anxiolytic drugs acting at serotonergic receptors

The serotonergic theory of anxiety suggests that serotonergic transmission is involved in anxiety as, in general, stimulation of this system causes anxiety whereas a reduction in serotonergic neuronal activity reduces anxiety.

The serotonergic theory prompted the development of anxiolytic drugs that act to moderate serotonergic neurotransmission while not causing sedation and incoordination.

5-HT$_{1A}$ agonists
Buspirone is a serotonergic (5-HT$_{1A}$) agonist.

Mechanism of action—In the raphe nucleus the dendrites of serotonergic neurons possess inhibitory presynaptic autoreceptors of the 5-HT$_{1A}$ subtype that, when stimulated, decrease the firing of 5-HT neurons. This class of anxiolytic agents called the azapirones are thought to reduce 5-HT transmission by acting as partial agonists at these 5-HT$_{1A}$ receptors. Buspirone is the first of this new class of anxiolytics.

Route of administration—Oral.

Indications—Buspirone is indicated for the short-term relief of generalized anxiety disorder.

Contraindications—5-HT$_{1A}$ agonists should not be used in people with epilepsy.

Adverse effects—The adverse effects of 5-HT$_{1A}$ agonists include nervousness, dizziness, headache and light-headedness.

In contrast to benzodiazepines, buspirone does not cause significant sedation or cognitive impairment, and it carries only a minimal risk of dependence and withdrawal. It does not potentiate the effects of alcohol.

Therapeutic notes—The anxiolytic effect of buspirone gradually evolves over 1–3 weeks.

5-hydroxytryptamine 3 antagonists
Ondansetron is a 5-HT$_3$ receptor antagonist that is well established for use as an antiemetic drug.

Ondansetron also has anxiolytic properties by virtue of its antagonism at the excitatory postsynaptic 5-HT$_3$ receptor.

β-Adrenoreceptor blockers

β-Adrenoreceptor blockers or β-blockers, e.g. propranolol, can be very effective in alleviating the somatic manifestations of anxiety caused by marked sympathetic arousal, such as palpitations, tremor, sweating and diarrhoea.

Mechanism of action—β-Blockers act by antagonism at β-adrenoreceptors so that excessive catecholamine release does not produce the sympathetic responses of tachycardia, sweating, etc. β-blockers are also used in cardiovascular disease.

Route of administration—Oral.

Indications—β-Blockers are indicated in patients with predominantly somatic symptoms; this, in turn, may prevent the onset of worry and fear. Patients with predominantly psychological symptoms may obtain no benefit. β-blockers can be useful in social phobias and to reduce performance anxiety in musicians, for whom fine motor control may be critical.

Contraindications—β-Blockers should not be used in people with asthma.

Adverse effects—β-Blockers can cause bradycardia, heart failure, bronchospasm and peripheral vasoconstriction.

Barbiturates

Barbiturates are non-selective CNS depressants that produce effects ranging from sedation and reduction of anxiety to unconsciousness and death from respiratory and cardiovascular failure. Barbiturates increase GABA-mediated inhibition by acting on the same receptor as benzodiazepines (the GABA$_A$ receptor), though at a different site.

At low doses, barbiturates prolong the duration of individual Cl$^-$ channel openings triggered by a given GABA stimulus (benzodiazepines increase the frequency of Cl$^-$ channel openings). At high doses, they are far more depressant than benzodiazepines because they start to increase Cl$^-$ conductance directly, thus decreasing the sensitivity of the postsynaptic membrane to excitatory transmitters.

Although very popular until the 1960s as sedative/hypnotic agents, they are now obsolete since they readily lead to psychological and physical dependence, and a relatively small overdose can be fatal. Conversely, benzodiazepines, which have largely replaced barbiturates as sedative/hypnotics, have been taken in huge overdoses without serious long-term effects.

Barbiturates, however, still have a place in anaesthesia and to a lesser extent in the treatment of epilepsy (p. 94).

HINTS AND TIPS

An understanding of the GABA$_A$/Cl$^-$ channel complex is central to the mechanism of action of several classes of hypnotic/anxiolytic drugs. You should be aware what these are.

Miscellaneous agents

A number of miscellaneous hypnotic agents have been used historically and are still prescribed under certain circumstances.

Chloral hydrate and derivatives

Chloral hydrate is metabolized to trichloroethanol, which is an effective hypnotic. It is cheap, but causes gastric irritation and there is no convincing evidence that it has any advantage over the newer benzodiazepines.

Chloral hydrate and its derivatives were previously popular hypnotics for children. Current thinking does not justify the use of hypnotics in children, and these drugs now have very limited uses.

Clomethiazole (chlormethiazole)

Clomethiazole may be a useful hypnotic in elderly people because of the relative freedom from hangover effects. It has no advantage over benzodiazepines in younger adults.

Clomethiazole was once indicated to attenuate the symptoms of acute alcohol withdrawal, though it has been largely replaced by the benzodiazepine, chlordiazepoxide.

Antidepressants

If the underlying cause of insomnia is associated with depression, or particularly in depressed patients exhibiting anxiety and agitation, then tricyclic antidepressants (TCAs) with sedative actions (p. 79), e.g. amitriptyline, may be useful, as they act as hypnotics when given at bedtime. Alternatively, selective serotonin reuptake inhibitors (SSRIs, p. 80) may correct the mood disorder and lessen the symptoms of anxiety or insomnia.

Sedative antihistamines

The older antihistamine drugs, e.g. diphenhydramine, have antimuscarinic actions and pass the blood–brain barrier, commonly causing drowsiness and psychomotor impairment.

Proprietary brands of diphenhydramine are on sale to the public to relieve temporary sleep disturbances, as these drugs are relatively safe.

AFFECTIVE DISORDERS

Affective disorders involve a disturbance of mood (cognitive/emotional symptoms) associated with changes in behaviour, energy, appetite and sleep (biological symptoms). Affective disorders can be thought of as pathological extremes of the normal continuum of human moods, from extreme excitement and elation (mania) to severe depressive states.

There are two types of affective disorder: unipolar affective disorders and bipolar affective disorders.

Monoamine theory of depression

The aetiology of major depressive disorders is not clear. Genetic, environmental and neurochemical influences have all been examined as possible aetiological factors.

The most widely accepted neurochemical explanation of endogenous depression involves the monoamines (noradrenaline; serotonin (5-HT); dopamine). The original hypothesis of depression, 'the monoamine theory', stated that depression resulted from a functional deficit of these transmitter amines, whereas conversely mania was caused by an excess.

The monoamine theory explains why:

- Drugs that deplete monoamines are depressant, e.g. reserpine and methyldopa.
- A wide range of drugs that increase the functional availability of monoamine neurotransmitters improve mood in depressed patients, e.g. tricyclic antidepressants (TCAs) and MAO inhibitors.

- The concentration of monoamines and their metabolites is reduced in the cerebrospinal fluid (CSF) of depressed patients.
- In some post-mortem studies the most consistent finding is an elevation in cortical $5\text{-}HT_2$ binding.

The monoamine theory cannot explain why:

- A number of compounds that increase the functional availability of monoamines, e.g. amphetamines, cocaine and L-dopa, have no effect on the mood of depressed patients.
- Some older, atypical antidepressants e.g. iprindole, worked without manipulating monoaminergic systems.
- There is a 'therapeutic delay' of 2 weeks between the full neurochemical effects of antidepressants and the start of their therapeutic effect.

It is unlikely, therefore, that monoamine mechanisms alone are responsible for the symptoms of depression. Other systems that may be involved in depression include:

- The GABA system
- The neuropeptide systems, particularly vasopressin and the endogenous opiates
- Secondary-messenger systems also appear to have a crucial role in some treatments.

Unipolar affective disorders

A common unipolar affective disorder is depression, which is characterized by misery, malaise, despair, guilt, apathy, indecisiveness, low energy and fatigue, changes in sleeping pattern, loss of appetite and suicidal thoughts. Attempts have been made to classify types of depression as either 'reactive' or 'endogenous' in origin.

Reactive depression is where there is a clear psychological cause, e.g. bereavement. It involves less-severe symptoms and less likelihood of biological disturbance. It affects 3–10% of the population, with the incidence increasing with age, and it is more common in females.

Endogenous depression is where there is no clear cause and more severe symptoms, e.g. suicidal thoughts, and a greater likelihood of biological disturbance, e.g. insomnia, anorexia. It affects 1% of the population, usually starting in early adulthood, and affecting both sexes equally.

The distinction between reactive and endogenous depression is of importance since there is some evidence that depressions with endogenous features tend to respond better to drug therapy.

Treatment of unipolar depressive disorders

The major classes of drug that are used to treat depression, and their mechanisms of action, are summarized in Figure 5.7.

HINTS AND TIPS

Although almost certainly flawed and incomplete, the monoamine theory is probably the best way to rationalize your thinking about affective disorders, and to understand the mechanism of action of the drugs used in their treatment.

Fig. 5.7 Major classes of antidepressant drugs and their mechanisms of action

Class of antidepressant drug	Examples	Mode of action
Tricyclic antidepressants (TCAs)	Amitriptyline Imipramine Lofepramine	Non-specific blockers of monoamine uptake
Selective serotonin reuptake inhibitors (SSRIs)	Fluoxetine Paroxetine Sertraline	Selective blockers of 5-HT reuptake
Serotonin-noradrenaline reuptake inhibitors (SNRIs)	Venlafaxine	Selective blockers of 5-HT and noradrenalline uptake
Monoamine oxidase inhibitors (MAOIs)	Phenelzine Tranylcrpromine	Non-competitive, non-selective irreversible blockers of MAO_A and MAO_B
Reversible inhibitors of MAO_A (RIMAs)	Moclobemide	Reversibly inhibit MAO_A selectively
Atypical	Reboxetine Mirtazapine	Act by various mechanisms that are poorly understood

(5-HT, 5-hydroxytryptamine; MAO, monoamine oxidase.)

TCAs and related drugs

Examples of TCAs and related drugs include amitriptyline, imipramine, dosulepin (dothiepin) and lofepramine.

Mechanism of action—TCAs act by blocking 5-HT and noradrenaline uptake into the presynaptic terminal from the synaptic cleft (Fig. 5.8). They also have a certain affinity for H_1 and muscarinic receptors, and for α_1- and α_2-receptors.

Contraindications—TCAs and related drugs should not be used in:

- Recent myocardial infarction or arrhythmias (especially heart block) since TCAs increase the risk of conduction abnormalities
- Manic phase
- Severe liver disease
- Epilepsy, where TCAs lower the seizure threshold
- Patients taking other anticholinergic drugs, alcohol and adrenaline as TCAs potentiate the effects of these.

Lidocaine is contraindicated in combination with TCAs, owing to a potentially fatal drug interaction.

Adverse effects—Although TCAs are an effective therapy for depression, their adverse effects can reduce patient compliance and acceptability. Side-effects include:

- Muscarinic blocking effects such as a dry mouth, blurred vision, constipation
- α-Adrenergic blocking effects causing postural hypotension
- Noradrenaline uptake block in the heart, increasing the risk of arrhythmias
- Histamine-blocking effects leading to sedation
- Weight gain.

TCAs are relatively dangerous in overdose. Patients present with confusion, mania, and potentially fatal arrhythmias due to the cardiotoxic nature of the drug.

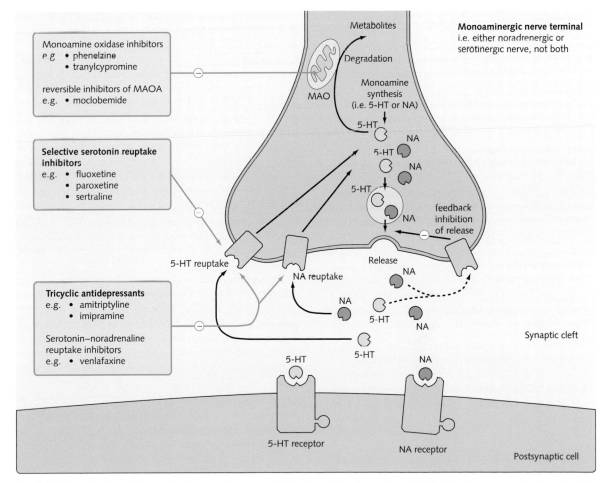

Fig. 5.8 Site of action of the major classes of drug used to treat unipolar depression. (5-HT, 5-hydroxytryptamine (serotonin); MAO, monoamine oxidase; NA, noradrenaline.)

Therapeutic notes—No individual TCA has superior antidepressant activity, and the choice of drug is usually determined by the most acceptable or desired side-effects. For example, drugs with sedative actions, such as amitriptyline or trimipramine, are the TCAs of choice for patients in agitated or anxious states. The most recent TCA is lofepramine, which causes fewer antimuscarinic side-effects, and is less dangerous if taken in overdose.

Therapeutic effects take 2–3 weeks to develop. TCA-related antidepressants should be withdrawn slowly.

Dangerous drug interaction

Tricyclic antidepressants + lidocaine = toxicity

Selective serotonin reuptake inhibitors (SSRIs)

SSRIs are the most recently introduced class of antidepressant agent. Fluoxetine (Prozac®) is an SSRI. Other examples include citalopram, fluvoxamine, paroxetine and sertraline.

Mechanism of action—SSRIs act with a high specificity for potent inhibition of serotonin reuptake into nerve terminals from the synaptic cleft, while having only minimal effects on noradrenaline uptake (see Fig. 5.8). They block serotonin transporters, which belong to a class of Na^+/Cl^--coupled transporters.

Contraindications—SSRIs should not be used with MAO inhibitors as the combination can cause a potentially fatal serotonergic syndrome of hyperthermia and cardiovascular collapse.

Adverse effects—The side-effect profile of SSRIs is much better than that of TCAs and MAO inhibitors as there are no amine interactions, anticholinergic actions, adrenergic blockade or toxic effects in overdose. Adverse effects, however, caused by their effect on serotonergic nerves throughout the body, include nausea, diarrhoea, insomnia, anxiety and agitation. Sexual dysfunction is sometimes a problem.

Therapeutic notes—SSRIs have a similar efficacy to that of TCAs. It is their clinical advantages and lack of side-effects that have led to their popularity. SSRIs are now the most widely prescribed antidepressants.

Serotonin-noradrenaline reuptake inhibitors

Venlafaxine is the most commonly used serotonin-noradrenaline reuptake inhibitor (SNRI)-type antidepressant.

Mechanism of action—SNRIs cause potentiation of neurotransmitter activity in the CNS, by blocking the norepinephrine and serotonin reuptake transporter (see Fig. 5.8).

Contraindications—The drug interactions of SNRIs are much like those of SSRIs; however, extra care must be taken with hypertensive patients as venlafaxine raises blood pressure.

Adverse effects—The adverse effects of SNRIs are similar to those of SSRIs, but they occur with lower frequency.

Therapeutic notes—The pharmacological effects of venlafaxine are similar to those of the TCAs, but adverse effects are reduced because it has little affinity for cholinergic and histaminergic receptors or α-adrenoreceptors.

MAO inhibitors

Examples of irreversible MAO inhibitors include phenelzine, tranylcypromine and isocarboxazid, and an example of reversible inhibitors of MAO_A (RIMAs) is moclobemide.

Mechanism of action—MAO inhibitors block the action of MAO_A and MAO_B, which are neuron enzymes that metabolize the monoamines (noradrenaline, 5-HT and dopamine) (see Fig. 5.8). MAO has two main isoforms, MAO_A and MAO_B. Inhibition of the MAO_A form correlates best with antidepressant efficacy. Both non-selective irreversible blockers of MAO_A and MAO_B, and drugs that reversibly inhibit MAO_A are available.

Adverse effects—Dietary interactions may occur, such as the 'cheese reaction'. MAO in the gut wall and liver normally breaks down ingested tyramine. When the enzyme is inhibited, tyramine reaches the circulation and this causes the release of noradrenaline from sympathetic nerve terminals; this can lead to a severe and potentially fatal rise in blood pressure. Patients on MAO inhibitors must, therefore, avoid foods rich in tyramine, which include cheese, game and alcoholic drinks. Preparations containing sympathomimetic amines (e.g. cough mixtures and nasal decongestants) should also be avoided. MAO inhibitors are not specific, and they reduce the metabolism of barbiturates, opioids and alcohol. Side-effects include CNS stimulation causing excitement and tremor, sympathetic blockade causing postural hypotension, and muscarinic blockade causing a dry mouth and blurred vision. Phenelzine can be hepatotoxic.

Therapeutic notes—Response to treatment may be delayed for 3 weeks or more. Phobic and depressed patients with atypical, hypochondriacal or hysterical features are said to respond best to MAO inhibitors. Because of the dietary and drug restrictions outlined above, MAO inhibitors are largely reserved for depression refractory to other antidepressants and treatment.

Atypical antidepressants

Examples of atypical antidepressants include reboxetine, mirtazapine and tryptophan.

Mechanism of action—Reboxetine is a selective inhibitor of noradrenaline reuptake, increasing the concentration of this mediator in the synaptic cleft. Mirtazapine has α_2-adrenoreceptor-blocking activity, which, by acting on inhibitory α_2-autoreceptors on central noradrenergic nerve endings, may increase the amount of noradrenaline in the synaptic cleft. Tryptophan is an amino acid precursor for serotonin.

Contraindications—The contraindications for atypical antidepressants are similar to those for TCAs.

Adverse effects—Atypical antidepressants generally cause less autonomic side-effects and are less dangerous in overdose, owing to their lower cardiotoxicity compared with TCAs. Mirtazapine may cause agranulocytosis. Tryptophan is associated with eosinophilas Myalgia syndrome.

Therapeutic notes—Mirtazapine is sedative, and it is, therefore, used in depression when a degree of sedation is desirable. Neither reboxetine nor mirtazapine are currently first-line drugs for the treatment of depression. Tryptophan requires specialist supervision due to the stated adverse affect.

Bipolar affective disorder

Bipolar affective disorder presents with mood and behaviour oscillating between depression and mania, and it is, therefore, also known as manic-depressive disorder.

Bipolar affective disorder develops earlier in life than unipolar depressive disorders, and it tends to be inherited. It affects 1% of the population, and it can have associated elements of psychotic phenomena.

> **HINTS AND TIPS**
>
> Mania hardly ever exists in isolation from depression, which is why it is referred to as bipolar affective disorder.

Treatment of bipolar affective disorders

Bipolar affective disorder is treated with a combination of mood stabilizers and antidepressants, and sometimes antipsychotics. Mood stabilizers include lithium and carbamazepine.

Lithium

Lithium is administered as lithium carbonate, and it is the most widely used mood stabilizer, with antimanic and antidepressant activity.

Mechanism of action—The mechanism of action of lithium is unclear, but it probably involves modulation of secondary-messenger pathways of cAMP and inositol triphosphate (IP$_3$). It is known that lithium inhibits the pathway for recapturing inositol for the resynthesis of polyphosphoinositides. It may exert its effect by reducing the concentrations of lipids important in secondary signal transduction in the brain.

Indications—Lithium salts are mainly used in the prophylaxis and treatment of bipolar affective disorder, but also in the prophylaxis and treatment of acute mania and in the prophylaxis of resistant recurrent depression.

Contraindications—Some drugs may interact, causing a rise in plasma lithium concentration and so should be avoided. Such drugs include antipsychotics, non-steroidal anti-inflammatory drugs (NSAIDs), diuretics and cardioactive drugs. Lithium is excreted via the kidney, and caution should be employed in patients with renal impairment.

Adverse effects—Lithium has a long plasma half-life and a narrow therapeutic window; therefore, side-effects are common and plasma concentration monitoring is essential. Early side-effects include thirst, nausea, diarrhoea, tremor and polyuria; late side-effects include weight gain, oedema, acne, nephrogenic diabetes insipidus and hypothyroidism. Toxicity/overdose (serum level >2–3 mmol/L) effects include vomiting, diarrhoea, tremor, ataxia, confusion and coma.

Therapeutic notes—Careful monitoring after initiation of treatment is essential.

Carbamazepine

Carbamazepine is as effective as lithium in the prophylaxis of bipolar affective disorder and acute mania, particularly in rapidly alternating bipolar affective disorder.

Mechanism of action—Carbamazepine is a GABA agonist, and this may be the basis of its antimanic properties. The relevance of its effect in stabilizing neuronal sodium, and on calcium channels, is unclear.

Adverse effects—Drowsiness, diplopia, nausea, ataxia, rashes and headache; blood disorders such as agranulocytosis and leucopenia; and drug interactions with lithium, antipsychotics, TCAs and MAO inhibitors. Many other drugs can be affected by the effect of carbamazepine on inducing hepatic enzymes. Diplopia, ataxia, clonus, tremor and sedation are associated with acute carbamazepine toxicity.

Therapeutic notes—At the start of treatment with carbamazepine, plasma concentrations should be monitored to establish a maintenance dose.

PSYCHOTIC DISORDERS

Psychotic disorders are characterized by a mental state that is out of touch with reality, involving a variety of abnormalities of perception, thought and ideas.

Psychotic illnesses include:

- Schizophrenia
- Schizoaffective disorder
- Delusional disorders
- Some depressive and manic illnesses.

Neuroleptics, or antipsychotics, are drugs used in the treatment of psychotic disorders.

Schizophrenia

Epidemiology

Schizophrenia characteristically develops in people aged 15–45 years; it has a relatively stable cross-cultural incidence affecting 1% of the population; with a greater proportion being male.

Symptoms and signs

Schizophrenia is a psychotic illness characterized by multiple symptoms affecting thought, perceptions, emotion and volition.

Symptoms fall into two groups (positive and negative) that may have different underlying causes.

Positive symptoms include:

- Delusions – false personal beliefs held with absolute conviction.
- Hallucinations – false perceptions in the absence of a real external stimulus; most commonly, these are auditory (hearing voices) and occur in 60–70% of schizophrenics, but they can be visual, tactile or olfactory.
- Thought alienation and disordered thought – belief that one's thoughts are under the control of an outside agency (e.g. aliens, MI5). This type of belief is common, and thought processes are often incomprehensible.

Negative symptoms include:

- Poverty of speech – restriction in the amount of spontaneous speech.
- Flattening of affect – loss of normal experience and expression of emotion.
- Social withdrawal.
- Anhedonia – inability to experience pleasure.
- Apathy – reduced drive, energy, and interest.
- Attention deficit – inattentiveness at work or on interview.

The distinction between the positive and negative symptoms found in schizophrenia is of importance as neuroleptic drugs tend to have most effect on positive symptoms, whereas negative symptoms are fairly refractory to treatment and carry a worse prognosis.

Theories of schizophrenia

The cause of schizophrenia remains mysterious. Any theory of the cause of schizophrenia must take into account the strong, though not invariable, hereditary tendency (50% concurrence in monozygotic twins), as well as the environmental factors known to predispose towards its development.

Many hypotheses have been suggested to explain the manifestations of schizophrenia at the level of neurotransmitters in the brain. The potential role of excessive dopaminergic activity, in particular, has attracted considerable attention. Evidence for this theory includes the following:

- Most antipsychotic drugs block dopamine receptors, the clinical dose being proportional to the ability to block D_2 receptors.
- Single photon emission computed tomography (SPECT) ligand scans show that there are increased D_2 receptors in the nucleus accumbens of schizophrenic patients.
- Psychotic symptoms can be induced by drugs that increase dopaminergic activity, such as some of the antiparkinsonian agents.

However, there is much evidence that the dopaminergic theory fails to explain. Current research indicates a likely role for other neurotransmitters in schizophrenia, including 5-HT, GABA and glutamate. Although the dopamine theory cannot explain many of the features and findings in schizophrenia, most current pharmacological treatment (typical neuroleptics) is aimed at dopaminergic transmission (Fig. 5.9).

COMMUNICATION

Mr Sarhan is a 28-year-old postman who was found at 5 am standing on the edge of Tower Bridge and shouting 'Freedom is through flying'. He was previously seen erratically throwing his mailbag into the River Thames. The police managed to grab him just before he jumped and took him to accident and emergency. The on-call psychiatrist sees him. Mr Sarhan is very agitated and shouting 'They gave me powers to fly! Let me prove it! I can prove it! Don't try to steal my powers, go away!'. A mental state examination supports a diagnosis of schizophrenia. A collateral history is obtained from his parents, who say that he has been acting more and more bizarrely over the past year but they just thought it was due to stress. Shortly after admission, he began shouting abuse and pushing past staff with the intention of leaving despite their discouragement. He was, thus, rapidly tranquillized using haloperidol and sectioned under section 2 of the Mental Health Act.

Treatment of schizophrenia

The treatment of schizophrenia and all other psychotic illnesses involves the use of antipsychotic medication, the neuroleptic drugs. Neuroleptic drugs produce a general improvement in all the acute positive symptoms of

Fig. 5.9 Classes of dopamine receptor

Type	2nd messenger + cellular effects	Location in CNS and postulated function
D_1	cAMP increase	Mainly postsynaptic inhibition Functions unclear
D_2	cAMP decrease K^+ conductance up Ca^{2+} conductance down	Mainly presynaptic inhibition of dopamine synthesis/release in nigrostriatal, mesolimbic and tuberoinfundibular systems Affinity of neuroleptics for D_2 receptors correlates with antipsychotic potency
D_3	Unknown	Localized mainly in limbic and cortical structures concerned with cognitive functions and emotional behaviour Not clear whether antipsychotic effects of neuroleptics are mediated by the D_3 type
D_4	Unknown	Similar to D_3 type; clozapine has particular affinity for D_4 receptors

(cAMP, cyclic adenosine monophosphate; CNS, central nervous system.)

schizophrenia, but it is less clear how effective they are in the treatment of chronic schizophrenia and negative symptoms.

Mechanism of action—Antipsychotic drugs have a variety of structures and fall into various classes (Fig. 5.9 and 5.10). There is a strong correlation between clinical potency and affinity for D_2 receptors among the typical neuroleptics.

Neuroleptics take days or weeks to work, suggesting that secondary effects (e.g. increase in number of D_2 receptors in limbic structure) may be more important than a direct effect of D_2 receptor block.

Most neuroleptics also block other monoamine receptors, and this is often the cause of some of the side-effects of these drugs.

The distinction between typical and atypical groups is not clearly defined, but it rests partly on the incidence of extrapyramidal motor side-effects and partly on receptor specificity. Atypical neuroleptics are less prone to producing motor disorders than other drugs, and they tend to have different pharmacological profiles with respect to dopamine and other receptor specificity.

Route of administration—All the neuroleptic drugs can be given orally, though some of the typical drugs can be given by the intramuscular route, which prolongs their release and aids drug compliance.

Typical neuroleptics

Phenothiazines

This class of compounds is subdivided into three groups by the type of side chain attached to the mother structure (phenothiazine ring) (Fig. 5.10). Side-effect patterns vary with the different side chains:

Fig. 5.10 Classes of neuroleptic drugs

Class	Chemical classification	Examples

Typical anti-psychotics	Phenothiazines:
	    propylamine side chains
	    piperidine side chains
	    piperazine side chains
	Butyrophenones
	Thioxanthines
		Chlorpromazine
		Thioridazine
		Fluphenazine
		Haloperidol
		Flupentixol

Atypical anti-psychotics	Dibenzodiazepines
	Dopamine/5-HT blockers:
	    diphenylbutylpiperidines
	    substituted benzamides
	    benzixasoles
		Clozapine, olanzapine
		Pimozide
		Sulpiride
		Risperidone

(5-HT, 5-hydroxytryptamine.)

- Propylamine side chains – e.g. in chlorpromazine, produce strong sedation, a moderate muscarinic block, and moderate motor disturbance. Indicated for violent patients, owing to their sedative effect.
- Piperidine side chains – e.g. in thioridazine, produce moderate sedation, strong muscarinic block and low motor disturbance. Favoured for use in elderly patients.
- Piperazine side chains – e.g. in fluphenazine, produce low sedation, low muscarinic block and strong motor disturbance. Contraindicated for use in elderly patients, owing to the motor effects.

Butyrophenones and thioxanthenes

The butyrophenone and thioxanthene groups of compounds have the same profile of low sedation, low muscarinic block and high incidence of motor disturbance.

An example of a butyrophenone compound is haloperidol; flupentixol is an example of the thioxanthenes.

Atypical neuroleptics

Dibenzodiazepines

Dibenzodiazepines such as clozapine and olanzapine have a low affinity for the D_2 receptor and a higher affinity for D_1 and D_4 receptors.

Indications—In the UK and US, atypical neuroleptics are indicated only in chronic cases refractory to other drugs, or with severe motor disturbance. This is because of a 1% risk of potentially fatal neutropenia in those patients on these agents.

Adverse effects—Clozapine has a low incidence of adverse motor effects because of its low affinity for the D_2 receptor. Side-effects of dibenzodiazepines include hypersalivation, sedation, weight gain, tachycardia and hypotension.

Therapeutic notes—Olanzapine is similar to clozapine, though carries less risk of agranulocytosis.

Dopamine/5-HT blockers

Examples of dopamine/5-HT blockers include the diphenylbutylpiperidines (e.g. pimozide and sulpiride) and the benzoxasoles (e.g. risperidone).

Sulpiride, and the newer agent pimozide, show high selectivity for D_2 receptors compared with D_1 or other neurotransmitter receptors. Both drugs are effective in treating schizophrenia but, sulpiride is claimed to have less tendency to cause adverse motor effects. Pimozide appears to be similar to conventional neuroleptic agents, but it has a longer duration of action, allowing once-daily medication.

Benzoxasoles such as risperidone show a high affinity for 5-HT receptors and a lower affinity for D_2 receptors. With this class of drugs, extrapyramidal motor side-effects occur with less frequency than with 'classic' neuroleptics.

Quetiapine fumarate is a dibenzothiazepine derivative and acts an as antagonist at the D_1, D_2, 5-HT$_{1A}$ and 5-HT$_2$ receptors.

Aripiprazole appears to mediate its antipsychotic effects primarily by *partial agonism* at the D_2 receptor. It is also a partial agonist at the 5-HT$_{1A}$ receptor, and like the other atypical antipsychotics, aripiprazole displays an antagonist profile at the 5-HT$_{2A}$ receptor, as well as moderate affinity for histamine and α-adrenergic receptors.

Zotepine has good efficacy against negative symptoms of schizophrenia. This is thought to be due to its noradrenaline reuptake inhibition. It also has a high affinity for the *dopamine D_1* and D_2 receptors. It also affects the 5-HT$_{2A}$, 5-HT$_{2C}$, 5-HT$_6$ and 5-HT$_7$ receptors.

Adverse effects of neuroleptics

Neuroleptic drugs cause a variety of adverse effects (Fig. 5.11). The majority of the unwanted effects of neuroleptics can be inferred from their pharmacological actions, such as the disruption of dopaminergic pathways (the major action of most neuroleptics) and the blockade of monoamine and other receptors, including muscarinic receptors, α-adrenoreceptors and histamine receptors.

In addition, individual drugs may cause immunological reactions or have their own characteristic side-effect profile.

Adverse effects on the dopaminergic pathways

There are three main dopaminergic pathways in the brain (Fig. 5.12):

- Mesolimbic and/or mesocortical dopamine pathways running from groups of cells in the midbrain to the nucleus accumbens and amygdala. This pathway affects thoughts and motivation.

Fig. 5.11 Adverse effects of the neuroleptics

- **Acute neurological effects**: acute dystonia, akathisia, parkinsonism
- **Chronic neurological effects**: tardive dyskinesia, tardive dystonia
- **Neuroendocrine effects**: amenorrhoea, galactorrhoea, infertility
- **Idiosyncratic**: neuroleptic malignant syndrome
- **Anticholinergic**: dry mouth, blurred vision, constipation, urinary retention, ejaculatory failure
- **Antihistaminergic**: sedation
- **Antiadrenergic**: hypotension, arrhythmia
- **Miscellaneous**: photosensitivity, heat sensitivity, cholestatic jaundice, retinal pigmentation

Redrawn from Page et al. 2006.

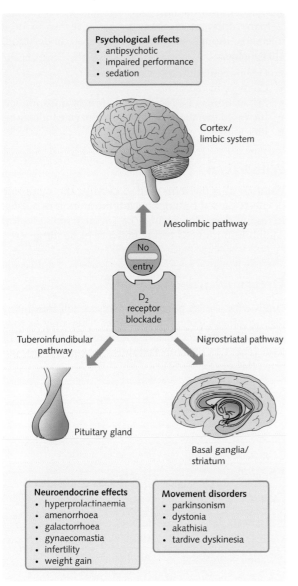

• Psychological effects – due to D_2 receptor blockade of the mesolimbic/mesocortical pathway.
• Movement disorders – due to D_2 receptor blockade of the nigrostriatal pathways.
• Neuroendocrine disorders – due to D_2 receptor blockade of the tuberoinfundibular pathway.

It is by dopaminergic antagonism of the mesolimbic mesocortical pathway that it is thought that typical neuroleptics exert their antipsychotic effects. However, as a side-effect of mesolimbic and mesocortical dopaminergic inhibition, sedation and impaired performance are common.

Blocking of dopamine receptors in the basal ganglia (corpus striatum) frequently results in distressing and disabling movement disorders. Two main types of movement disorder occur. Acute reversible parkinsonian-like symptoms (tremor, rigidity and akinesia) are treated by dose reduction, anticholinergic drugs or switching to an atypical neuroleptic. Slowly developing tardive dyskinesia, often irreversible, and manifesting as involuntary movements of the face, trunk and limbs, appears months or years after the start of neuroleptic treatment. It may be a result of proliferation or sensitization of dopamine receptors. Incidence is unpredictable, and it affects approximately 20% of long-term users of neuroleptics. Treatment is generally unsuccessful. The newer atypical neuroleptics may be less likely to induce tardive dyskinesia.

By reducing the negative feedback on the anterior pituitary, over-secretion of prolactin can result (hyperprolactinaemia). This can lead to gynaecomastia, galactorrhoea, menstrual irregularities, impotence and weight gain in some patients (Fig. 5.12).

Adverse effects from non-selective receptor blockade

The adverse effects of neuroleptics from non-selective receptor blockade include:

• Anticholinergic effects due to muscarinic-receptor blockade, such as dry mouth, urinary retention, constipation, blurred vision, etc.
• Adverse effects due to α-adrenoreceptor blockade. Many neuroleptics have the capacity to block α-adrenoreceptors and cause postural hypotension.
• Adverse effects due to histamine-receptor blockade. Antagonism of central histamine H_1 receptors may contribute to sedation.

Adverse effects due to individual drugs or immune reactions

The neuroleptic drug clozapine can cause neutropenia due to toxic bone marrow suppression, while pimozide can cause sudden death secondary to cardiac arrhythmia.

Immune reactions to neuroleptic drugs can include dermatitis, rashes, photosensitivity and urticaria. Such

Fig. 5.12 Effect of D_2 dopamine receptor blockade on the dopaminergic pathways in the brain.

• Nigrostriatal dopamine pathways running from the midbrain to the caudate nuclei. This pathway is important in smooth motor control.
• Tuberoinfundibular neurons running from the hypothalamus to the pituitary gland, the secretions of which they regulate.

Antagonism of dopamine receptors leads to interference with the normal functioning of these pathways, bringing about unwanted side-effects as well as the desired antipsychotic effect. This antagonism is the cause of the most serious side-effects associated with neuroleptic use, which include:

reactions are more common with the phenothiazines, which can also cause deposits in the cornea and lens.

Neuroleptic malignant syndrome—This is the most lethal adverse effect of neuroleptic use. It is an idiosyncratic reaction of unknown pathophysiology. Symptoms include fever, extrapyramidal motor disturbance, muscle rigidity and coma. Urgent treatment is indicated.

HINTS AND TIPS

Neuroleptics have many side-effects, some related to their principal mechanism of action (dopamine receptor antagonism) and some unrelated to this. Learn these well as they are a popular examination topic.

DRUG MISUSE

Definitions

Drug misuse

Drug misuse is defined as the use of drugs that causes actual physical or mental harm to an individual or to society, or that is illegal. Therefore, drug misuse includes alcohol, nicotine, and the damaging overprescription of tranquillizers, as well as the more obvious illicit drugs such as ecstasy or amphetamines.

Drug dependence

Drug dependence is defined as the compulsion to take a drug repeatedly, with distress being caused if this is prevented. Drugs of dependence all have rewarding effects (this is why they are taken), but they also have unpleasant effects, often as the drug is metabolized and excreted.

Dependence involves psychological factors as well as physical aspects. These are not exclusive and there is a mixture of both in most people who are dependent on drugs. Psychological dependence is when the rewarding effects (positive reinforcement) predominate to cause a compulsion to continue taking the drug. Physical dependence is when the distress on stopping the drug (negative reinforcement) is the main reason for continuing to take it, i.e. avoidance of the 'withdrawal syndrome'.

Drug tolerance

Drug tolerance is the necessity to increase the dose of an administered drug progressively to maintain the effect that was produced by the (smaller) original doses. Drug tolerance is a phenomenon that develops with chronic administration of a drug.

Many different mechanisms can give rise to drug tolerance, though they are rather poorly understood. They include:
- Down-regulation of receptors
- Changes in receptors
- Exhaustion of biological mediators or transmitters
- Increased metabolic degradation (enzyme induction)
- Physiological adaptation.

Withdrawal

Withdrawal is the term used to describe the syndrome of effects caused by stopping administration of a drug. It results from the change of (neuro) physiological equilibrium induced by the presence of the drug.

Drugs of misuse

Drugs with a high potential for misuse fall into many distinct pharmacological categories. They may or may not be used therapeutically and they may be illegal or legal (Fig. 5.13). Controlled drugs are categorized into three classes (Fig. 5.14).

Fig. 5.13 Drugs with high potential for misuse

Drug class	Examples
Central stimulants	Cocaine Amphetamines MDMA (ecstasy) Nicotine
Central depressants	Alcohol Benzodiazepines Barbiturates
Opioid analgesics	Morphine Heroin (diamorphine) Methadone
Cannabinoids	Cannabis Tetrahydrocannabinoids (THCs)
Hallucinogens	LSD Mescaline Psilocybin
Dissociative anaesthetics	Ketamine Phencyclidine

(LSD, lysergic acid diethylamide; MDMA, methylenedioxymethamphetamine.)

Fig. 5.14 Classes of controlled drugs		
Class A drugs	**Class B drugs**	**Class C drugs**
Cocaine	Amphetamines	Benzodiazepines
MDMA	Barbiturates	Cannabis
(ecstasy)	Some weak	Androgenic and
Diamorphine	opioids	anabolic steroids
(heroin) and	Others	Human chorionic
other strong		gonadotrophin
opioids		Others
Lysergic acid		
diethylamide		
(LSD) class B		
substance		
when prepared		
for injection		
Others		

MDMA, methylenedioxymethamphetamine.

HINTS AND TIPS

Always use the correct chemical name when describing drugs of misuse, e.g. amphetamines rather than whizz or speed.

Central stimulants

Amphetamines

Other names—Speed, whizz, billy, base.

Mechanism of action—Amphetamines cause the release of monoamines and the inhibition of monoamine reuptake, especially of dopamine and noradrenaline in neurons.

Route of administration—Amphetamines are administered orally, or 'snorted' as a powder nasally; sometimes used intravenously.

Effects—Increased motor activity; euphoria and excitement; anorexia and insomnia; peripheral sympathomimetic effects, such as hypertension and inhibition of gut motility; and stereotyped behaviour and psychosis, which develop with prolonged usage.

Clinical uses—The clinical uses of amphetamines are for narcolepsy and for hyperkinesis in children. They are no longer recommended as appetite suppressants, owing to their adverse effects.

Tolerance, dependence and withdrawal—Tolerance to the peripheral sympathomimetic stimulant effects of amphetamines develops rapidly, but it develops much more slowly to other effects such as locomotor stimulation. Amphetamines cause strong psychological dependence but no real physical dependence. After stopping chronic use, the individual will usually enter a deep, long sleep ('REM rebound') and awake feeling tired, depressed and hungry. This state may reflect the depletion of the normal monoamine stores.

Adverse effects—Acute amphetamine toxicity causes cardiac arrhythmias, hypertension and stroke. Chronic toxicity causes paranoid psychosis, vasoconstriction, tissue anoxia at sites of injection or snorting, and damage to the fetal brain *in utero*.

Cocaine

Other names—Coke, charlie, snow, crack.

Mechanism of action—Cocaine strongly inhibits the reuptake of catecholamines at noradrenergic neurons, and thus strongly enhances sympathetic activity.

Route of administration—Cocaine hydrochloride is usually snorted nasally. 'Crack' is the free base, which is more volatile and which does not decompose on heating. It can, therefore, be smoked, producing a brief intense 'rush'.

Effects—The behavioural effects produced by cocaine are similar to those produced by amphetamines, such as euphoria. The euphoric effects may be greater, and there is less of a tendency for stereotypical behaviour and paranoid delusions.

The effects of cocaine hydrochloride (lasting about an hour) are not as long lasting as those of amphetamine, while those obtained from crack are brief (minutes).

Clinical uses—Cocaine is occasionally used as a topical anaesthetic by ear, nose and throat specialists.

Tolerance, dependence and withdrawal—Cocaine causes strong psychological dependence but no real physical dependence. Withdrawal causes a marked deterioration in motor performance, which is restorable on provision of the drug.

Adverse effects—Acute cocaine toxicity causes toxic psychosis, cardiac arrhythmias, hypertension and stroke. Chronic toxicity causes paranoid psychosis, vasoconstriction, tissue anoxia at sites of injection or snorting and damage to the fetal brain.

Methylenedioxymethamphetamine (MDMA)

Other names—Ecstasy, E, disco biscuits, pills.

Mechanism of action—MDMA is an amphetamine derivative that has a mechanism of action similar to that of amphetamines (release of monoamines, inhibition of monoamine reuptake). MDMA acts on serotonergic neurons, potentiating 5-HT.

Route of administration—MDMA is usually taken as a pill containing other psychoactive drugs, such as amphetamine or ketamine.

Effects—MDMA has mixed stimulant and hallucinogenic properties, especially in its pure form. Euphoria, arousal and perceptual disturbances are common. Uniquely, MDMA has the effect of creating a feeling of euphoric empathy, so that social barriers are reduced.

Clinical uses—MDMA has no clinical use. Trials have been licensed in the USA for its evaluation as a treatment for people with social avoidant personality disorders.

Tolerance, dependence and withdrawal—It is not currently known to what extent tolerance and dependence occur with MDMA. The withdrawal syndrome is similar to that with amphetamines.

Adverse effects—The most serious acute consequences of acute MDMA toxicity appear to be hyperthermia, exhaustion and dehydration caused indirectly by the hyperexcitability that is induced.

Nicotine

Nicotine is found in cigarettes, cigars, pipes and chewing tobacco.

Mechanism of action—Nicotine exerts its effects by causing nicotinic acetylcholine receptor (nicAChR) excitation leading to neurotransmitter release and nicAChR desensitization.

Route of administration—Nicotine is usually inhaled, although it can be chewed.

Effects—Nicotine has both stimulant and relaxant properties. Physiologically, nicotine increases alertness, decreases irritability and relaxes skeletal muscle tone. Peripheral effects due to ganglionic stimulation include tachycardia, increased blood pressure and decreased gastrointestinal motility

Clinical uses—Nicotine has no clinical use.

Tolerance, dependence and withdrawal—Tolerance to nicotine occurs rapidly, first to peripheral effects but later to central effects.

Nicotine is highly addictive, causing both physical and psychological dependence. Withdrawal from tobacco often leads to a syndrome of craving, irritability, anxiety and increased appetite for approximately 2–3 weeks.

Adverse effects—Acute nicotine toxicity causes nausea and vomiting. Chronic toxicity caused by smoking leads to more morbidity in the UK than all other drugs combined, predisposing to all of the following diseases, often greatly so:

- Cardiovascular diseases, including atherosclerosis, hypertension and coronary heart disease.
- Cancer of the lung, bladder and mouth.
- Respiratory diseases such as bronchitis, emphysema and asthma.
- Fetal growth retardation.

The most successful smoking cures combine psychological and pharmacological treatments.

Pharmacological options largely rely on nicotine replacement, once the patient has stopped smoking, with a gradual reduction in nicotine. The latest drug to be used to help cigarette smokers is bupropion (Zyban®), which is derived from an antidepressant.

Nicotine products

Mechanism of action—Measured doses of nicotine are used to replace nicotine derived from cigarettes once the patient has stopped smoking, meeting the physical nicotine needs. The dose of nicotine is gradually reduced over 10–12 weeks.

Route of administration—Oral (chewing gum, sublingual tablets), transdermal (patches), nasal (spray), inhalation.

Indications—Adjunct to smoking cessation.

Contraindications—Severe cardiovascular disease, recent cerebrovascular accident, pregnancy, breastfeeding.

Adverse effects—Nausea, dizziness, headache and cold, influenza-like symptoms, palpitations.

Therapeutic notes—Nicotine products are available over the counter or GPs can prescribe them for patients intending to stop smoking.

Bupropion (Zyban®)

Mechanism of action—Bupropion is a selective inhibitor of the neuronal uptake of noradrenaline and dopamine. This is believed to reduce nicotine craving and withdrawal symptoms.

Route of administration—Oral.

Indications—Adjunct to smoking cessation.

Contraindications—History of epilepsy and eating disorders, pregnancy, breastfeeding.

Adverse effects—Dry mouth, gastrointestinal disturbances, insomnia, tremor, impaired concentration.

Therapeutic notes—Bupropion is available on the NHS.

Central depressants

Ethanol

Mechanism of action—Ethanol, or alcohol, acts in a similar way to volatile anaesthetic agents, as a general CNS depressant. The cellular mechanisms involved may include inhibition of calcium entry, hence reduction in transmitter release, as well as potentiation of inhibitory GABA transmission.

Route of administration—Ethanol is administered orally.

Effects—The familiar effects of ethanol intoxication range from increased self-confidence and motor incoordination through to unconsciousness and coma. Peripheral effects include a self-limiting diuresis and vasodilatation.

Clinical uses—Ethanol is used as an antidote to methanol poisoning.

Tolerance, dependence and withdrawal—Tolerance, and physical and psychological dependence all occur with ethanol, such that 15 000 people a year are admitted to psychiatric hospital for alcohol dependence and psychosis, and up to 20% of males on a medical ward have alcohol-related disabilities.

The alcohol withdrawal syndrome is a rebound of the nervous system after adaptation to the depression caused by alcohol. This syndrome occurs in two stages:

- Early stage ('hangover') – which is common and starts 6–8 hours after cessation of drinking. It involves tremulousness, nausea, retching and sweating.
- Late stage (delirium tremens) – which is much less common and starts 48–72 hours after cessation of drinking. It involves delirium, tremor, hallucinations and confusion.

Management of these late withdrawal symptoms involves sedation with clomethiazole or benzodiazepines (such as chlordiazepoxide); clonidine may be useful.

Adverse effects—Acute ethanol toxicity causes ataxia, nystagmus, coma, respiratory depression and death. Chronic ethanol toxicity causes neurodegeneration (potentiated by vitamin deficiency), dementia, liver damage, pancreatitis, etc., and accompanying psychiatric illness-depression/psychosis is common.

Benzodiazepines

Mechanism of action—Benzodiazepines exert their effects by potentiation of inhibitory GABA transmission (p. 74).

Route of administration—Benzodiazepines are administered orally.

Effects—The effects of benzodiazepines include sedation, agitation and ataxia.

Clinical uses—Benzodiazepines are heavily prescribed as anxiolytics and hypnotics.

Tolerance, dependence and withdrawal—Benzodiazepines have a potential for misuse – tolerance and dependence are common.

A physical withdrawal syndrome can occur in patients given benzodiazepines, even for short periods. Symptoms include rebound anxiety and insomnia with depression, nausea and perceptual changes that may last from weeks to months.

Adverse effects—The adverse effects of acute benzodiazepine toxicity include hypotension and confusion. Cognitive impairment occurs in chronic benzodiazepine toxicity.

Opioid analgesics

Diamorphine (heroin) and other opioids

Other names—Smack, H, gear, junk, jack, brown.

Mechanism of action—Opioids show agonist action at opioid receptors (p. 139).

Note that the sense of euphoria and well-being produced by strong opioids undoubtedly contributes to their analgesic activity by helping to reduce the anxiety and stress associated with pain. This effect also accounts for the illicit use of these drugs by addicts.

Route of administration—Opioids are generally taken intravenously by misusers as this produces the most intense sense of euphoria ('rush').

Effects—Opioids produce feelings of euphoria and well-being. Other effects are mentioned on p. 139.

Clinical uses—Opioids are used in analgesia for moderate to severe pain.

Tolerance, dependence and withdrawal—Tolerance to opioid analgesics develops quickly in addicts and results in larger and larger doses of the drug being needed to achieve the same effect.

Dependence involves both psychological factors and physical factors. Psychological dependence is based on the positive reinforcement provided by euphoria.

There is a definite physical withdrawal syndrome in addicts following cessation of drug treatment with opioids. This syndrome comprises a complex mixture of irritable and sometimes aggressive behaviour, combined with autonomic symptoms such as fever, sweating, yawning, pupillary dilatation, and piloerection that gives the state its colloquial name of 'cold turkey. Patients are extremely distressed and restless and strongly crave the drug. Symptoms are maximal at 2 days and largely disappear in 7–10 days.

Treatment of withdrawal—Methadone is a long-acting opiate, active orally, that is used to wean addicts from their addiction. The withdrawal symptoms from this longer-acting compound are more prolonged, but less intense than, for example, those of heroin. Treatment usually involves substitution of methadone followed by a slow reduction in dose over time.

Clonidine, an α_2-adrenoreceptor agonist, inhibits firing of locus ceruleus neurons, and it is effective in suppressing some components of the opioid withdrawal syndrome, especially the nausea, vomiting and diarrhoea.

Adverse effects—Acute opioid toxicity causes the following:

- Confusion, drowsiness and sedation. Initial excitement is followed by sedation and finally coma on overdose.
- Shallow and slow respiration – due to reduction of sensitivity of the respiratory centre to CO_2.
- Vomiting – due to stimulation of the chemoreceptor trigger zone.
- Autonomic effects such as tremor and pupillary constriction.
- Bronchospasm, flushing and arteriolar dilatation due to histamine release.

Acute toxicity may be countered by use of an opioid antagonist such as naloxone. The adverse effects of direct chronic toxicity are minor (p. 140).

Cannabinoids

Cannabis

There are two forms of cannabis: marijuana is the dried leaves and flowers of the cannabis plant, and hashish is the extracted resin of the cannabis plant.

Other names—Hashish, weed, skunk, pot, dope, gear, grass, ganja, blow.

Mechanism of action—How cannabis exerts its effects is not clearly defined, but it includes both depressant, stimulant and psychomimetic effects. The active constituent of cannabis is D^9-tetrahydrocannabinol (THC), though metabolites that also have activity may be important.

Route of administration—Cannabis is usually smoked, although it may be eaten.

Effects—Cannabis has several effects:

- Subjectively, users feel relaxed and mildly euphoric.
- Perception is altered, with apparent sharpening of sensory experience.
- Appetite is enhanced.
- Peripheral actions include vasodilatation and bronchodilatation, and a reduction in intraocular pressure.

Clinical uses—Cannabis is not currently licensed for use in the UK. It is being evaluated for palliative or symptomatic relief use in certain conditions in the USA, e.g. for the antiemetic effect of THC, and a possible role in treatment of multiple sclerosis and glaucoma.

Tolerance, dependence and withdrawal—Tolerance to cannabis occurs to a minor degree. It is not dangerously addictive, with only moderate physical and psychological withdrawal effects noted, such as mild anxiety/dysphoria and sleep disturbances.

Adverse effects—Acute cannabis toxicity causes confusion and hallucinations. Chronic toxicity may cause flashbacks, memory loss and 'de-motivational syndrome'. There is a clear correlation between cannabis use and schizophrenia.

Psychotomimetic drugs or hallucinogens

Examples of psychotomimetic drugs include LSD, mescaline and psilocybin.

Street names—Acid, trips, magic mushrooms.

Mechanism of action—How LSD, mescaline and psilocybin produce changes in perception is not well understood, but it seems to involve serotonin. LSD appears to affect serotonergic systems by acting on 5-HT_2 inhibitory autoreceptors on serotonergic neurons to reduce their firing. Whether LSD is an agonist, an antagonist or both is not clear.

Route of administration—Psychotomimetic drugs are administered orally as a liquid, pills or paper stamps.

Effects—Psychotomimetic drugs cause a dramatically altered state of perception-vivid and unusual sensory experiences combined with euphoric sensations. Hallucinations, delusions and panic can occur; this is known as a 'bad trip' and it can be terrifying.

Clinical uses—Psychotomimetic drugs have no clinical uses.

Tolerance, dependence and withdrawal—Tolerance to, dependence on, and withdrawal from psychotomimetic drugs are not significant.

Adverse effects—Acute toxicity from psychotomimetic drugs causes frightening delusions or hallucinations that can lead to accidents or violence. In chronic toxicity, 'flashbacks' (a recurrence of hallucination) may occur long after the 'trip'. Other psychotic symptoms may also occur.

EPILEPSY

Epilepsy is a chronic disease, in which seizures result from the abnormal high-frequency discharge of a group of neurons, starting focally and spreading to a varying extent to affect other parts of the brain. According to the focus and spread of discharges, seizures may be classified as:

- Partial (focal) – which originate at a specific focus and do not spread to involve other cortical areas.
- Generalized – which usually have a focus (often in the temporal lobe) and then spread to other areas.

Different epileptic syndromes can be classified on the basis of seizure type and pattern, with other clinical features (such as age of onset), anatomical location of focus, and aetiology taken into account.

Common types of epileptic syndrome

Epileptic syndromes result from either generalized seizures or focal seizures (Fig. 5.15).

Generalized seizure involves loss of consciousness, and it may be convulsive or non-convulsive:

- Tonic-clonic (grand-mal seizures) – convulsive generalized seizure characterized by periods of tonic muscle rigidity followed later by jerking of the body (clonus).
- Absence (petit-mal seizures) – generalized seizures characterized by changes in consciousness lasting less than 10 seconds. They occur most commonly in children, where they can be confused with day-dreaming.

The effect on the body of focal seizures depends on the location of the abnormal signal focus: e.g. involvement of the motor cortex will produce convulsions whereas involvement of the brainstem can produce unconsciousness. Psychomotor or temporal lobe epilepsy results from a partial seizure with cortical activity localized to the temporal lobe. Such seizures are characterized by features including impaired consciousness or confusion, amnesia, emotional instability, atypical behaviour and outbursts.

Partial motor seizures have their focus in cortical motor regions and they present with convulsive or tonic activity corresponding to the neurons involved, e.g. the left arm.

Another type of epileptic syndrome is status epilepticus. This is a state in which fits follow each other without consciousness being regained. Status epilepticus constitutes a medical emergency because of possible exhaustion of vital centres.

Causes of epilepsy

The aetiology of epilepsy is unknown in 60–70% of cases, but heredity is an important factor. Damage to the brain – for example, by tumours, head injury, infections or cerebrovascular accident – may subsequently cause epilepsy.

The neurochemical basis of the abnormal discharges in epilepsy are not known, but it may involve altered GABA metabolism.

Treatment of epilepsy

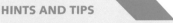

HINTS AND TIPS

Remember that epilepsy is simply aberrant electrical activity spreading throughout an area of, or the whole of, the brain. Antiepileptic medications limit the propagation of this spread and inhibit development of symptoms.

Drugs used to treat epilepsy are termed antiepileptics; the term anticonvulsant is also used.

The aim of pharmacological treatment of epilepsy is to minimize seizure activity/frequency, without producing adverse drug effects.

Mechanisms of action of antiepileptics

Antiepileptic drugs act generically to inhibit the rapid, repetitive neuronal firing that characterizes seizures. There are three established mechanisms of action by which the antiepileptic drugs achieve this (Fig. 5.16).

Inhibition of ionic channels involved in neuronal excitability

Drugs such as phenytoin, carbamazepine and valproate inhibit the 'fast' sodium current. These drugs bind preferentially to inactivated (closed) sodium channels, preventing them from opening. The high-frequency repetitive depolarization of neurons during a seizure increases the proportion of sodium channels in the inactivated state susceptible to blockade. Eventually, sufficient sodium channels become blocked so that the 'fast' neuronal sodium current is insufficient to cause a depolarization. Note that neuronal transmission at normal frequencies is relatively unaffected because a much smaller proportion of the sodium channels are in the inactivated state.

Fig. 5.15 Classification of common epileptic syndromes

Partial (local, focal) seizures	Generalized seizures
Psychomotor (temporal lobe) epilepsy Partial motor epilepsy	Tonic-clonic seizure or grand-mal epilepsy Absence seizure or petit-mal epilepsy

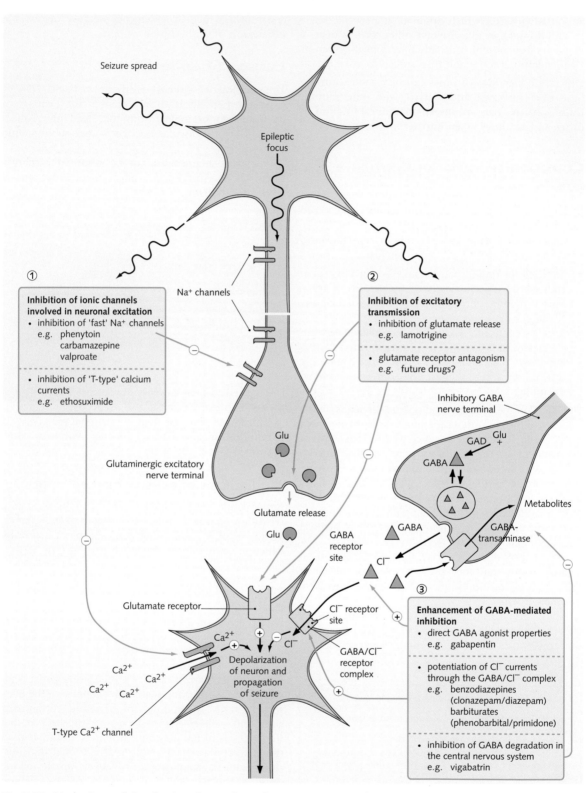

Seizure spread

Epileptic focus

① **Inhibition of ionic channels involved in neuronal excitation**
- inhibition of 'fast' Na+ channels
  e.g. phenytoin
       carbamazepine
       valproate
- inhibition of 'T-type' calcium currents
  e.g. ethosuximide

Na+ channels

② **Inhibition of excitatory transmission**
- inhibition of glutamate release
  e.g. lamotrigine
- glutamate receptor antagonism
  e.g. future drugs?

Inhibitory GABA nerve terminal

Glutaminergic excitatory nerve terminal

Glu

Glutamate release

Glu

GAD Glu +

GABA

Metabolites

GABA

GABA-transaminase

GABA receptor site

Cl−

Glutamate receptor

Cl− receptor site

③ **Enhancement of GABA-mediated inhibition**
- direct GABA agonist properties
  e.g. gabapentin
- potentiation of Cl− currents through the GABA/Cl− complex
  e.g. benzodiazepines
       (clonazepam/diazepam)
       barbiturates
       (phenobarbital/primidone)
- inhibition of GABA degradation in the central nervous system
  e.g. vigabatrin

GABA/Cl− receptor complex

Ca2+

Cl−

Depolarization of neuron and propagation of seizure

Ca2+
Ca2+   Ca2+
Ca2+

T-type Ca2+ channel

Fig. 5.16 Mechanism and site of action of antiepileptic drugs. (GABA, γ-aminobutyric acid; GAD, glutamic acid decarboxylase; Glu, glutamate.)

Ethosuximide inhibits 'T-type' low-threshold, fast-inactivating calcium. Absence seizures involve oscillatory neuronal activity between the thalamus and the cerebral cortex. The oscillation involves 'T-type' calcium channels, which produce low-threshold spikes, thus allowing groups of cells to fire in bursts. It appears that the anti-absence drug ethosuximide reduces this fast-inactivating calcium current, dampening the thalamo-cortical oscillations that are critical in the generation of such absence seizures.

Inhibition of excitatory transmission

Drugs that block excitatory amino acid receptors (N-methyl-D-aspartate (NMDA) antagonists) have been shown to be antiepileptic in animal models. Such drugs may prove useful in the clinical treatment of epilepsy in the future. Lamotrigine, one of the newer antiepileptic agents, inhibits the release of glutamate as one of its actions, and this may contribute to its antiepileptic activity.

Enhancement of GABA-mediated inhibition

This can take any of the following forms:

- Enhancement by direct GABA agonist properties, e.g. by gabapentin, another of the newer antiepileptics, agent which has been designed to mimic GABA in the CNS.
- Potentiation of chloride currents through the $GABA_A/Cl^-$ channel complex, e.g. by benzodiazepines and barbiturates. The increased postsynaptic inhibitory chloride current at $GABA_A$ receptors, hyperpolarizes neurons and makes them refractory to excitation (see Fig. 5.5).
- Inhibition of GABA degradation in the CNS, e.g. by vigabatrin, which is an irreversible inhibitor of GABA transaminase ($GABA_T$), the enzyme normally responsible for metabolism of GABA in the neuron. Inhibition of $GABA_T$, therefore, leads to an increase in synaptic levels of GABA and so enhances GABA-mediated inhibition.

Antiepileptic drugs (anticonvulsants)

Antiepileptic drugs can be classified according to their mechanism of action (Fig. 5.16), but in clinical practice it is useful to think of the drugs according to their use (Fig. 5.17).

Phenytoin

Mechanism of action—This involves use-dependent block of voltage-gated sodium channels. Phenytoin reduces the spread of a seizure. It does not prevent the ignition of an epileptic discharge, but it does stop it spreading and causing overt clinical symptoms.

Route of administration—Oral, intravenous.

Indications—Phenytoin is indicated in all forms of epilepsy except absence seizures; neuralgic pain (p. 142).

Fig. 5.17 Drugs used for epilepsy classified by clinical use

Seizure type	Primary drugs	Secondary drugs
Partial and/or generalized tonic-clonic seizures	Sodium valproate Carbamazepine	Phenytoin Vigabatrin Gabapentin Lamotrigine Phenobarbital
Absence seizures	Ethosuximide Sodium valproate Lamotrigine	Phenobarbital
Status epilepticus	Lorazepam	Diazepam Clonazepam

Contraindications—Phenytoin has many contraindications, mainly because it induces the hepatic cytochrome P_{450} oxidase system, increasing the metabolism of oral contraceptives, anticoagulants, dexamethasone and pethidine.

Adverse effects—The adverse effects of phenytoin may be dosage- or non-dosage-related. The dosage-related effects of phenytoin affect the cerebellovestibular system, leading to ataxia, blurred vision and hyperactivity. Acute toxicity causes sedation and confusion. The non-dosage related effects include collagen effects such as gum hypertrophy and coarsening of facial features; allergic reactions, e.g. rash, hepatitis and lymphadenopathy; haematological effects, e.g. megaloblastic anaemia; endocrine effects, e.g. hirsutism (hair growth); and teratogenic effects (it may cause congenital malformations).

Therapeutic notes—The use of phenytoin is complicated by its zero-order pharmacokinetics, characteristic toxicities, and necessity for long-term administration. Phenytoin has a narrow therapeutic index, and the relationship between dose and plasma concentration is non-linear. This is because phenytoin is metabolized by a hepatic enzyme system that is saturated at therapeutic levels. Small dosage increases may, therefore, produce large rises in plasma concentrations with acute side-effects. Monitoring of plasma concentration greatly assists dosage adjustment. Because of its adverse effects and narrow therapeutic window, phenytoin is no longer a first-line treatment for any of the seizure syndromes.

Sodium valproate

Mechanism of action—Sodium valproate has two mechanisms of action: like phenytoin, it causes use-dependent block of voltage-gated sodium channels; it also increases the GABA content of the brain when given over a prolonged period.

Route of administration—Oral, intravenous.

Indications—Sodium valproate is useful in all forms of epilepsy.

Contraindications—Sodium valproate should not be given to people with acute liver disease or a history of hepatic dysfunction.

Adverse effects—Sodium valproate has fewer side-effects than other antiepileptics; the main problems are gastrointestinal upset and, more importantly, liver failure. Hepatic toxicity appears to be more common when sodium valproate is used in combination with other antiepileptics.

Therapeutic notes—Sodium valproate is well absorbed orally and has a half-life of 10–15 hours. Sodium valproate is now the first-line drug for most types of seizure syndromes.

Carbamazepine

Mechanism of action—Like phenytoin, carbamazepine causes use-dependent block of voltage-gated sodium channels. Oxcarbazepine, another antiepileptic, is structurally a derivative of carbamazepine. It has an extra oxygen atom on the dibenzazepine ring, which helps reduce the impact on the liver of metabolizing the drug, and also prevents the serious forms of anaemia occasionally associated with carbamazepine. It is thought to have the same mechanism of action as carbamazepine.

Route of administration—Oral, rectal.

Indications—Carbamazepine can be used in all forms of epilepsy except absence seizures; neuralgic pain (p. 142).

Contraindications—Like phenytoin, carbamazepine is a strong enzyme inducer and so causes similar drug interactions.

Adverse effects—Ataxia, nystagmus, dysarthria, vertigo, sedation.

Therapeutic notes—Carbamazepine is well absorbed orally with a long half-life (25–60 hours) when first given. Enzyme induction subsequently reduces this half-life.

Ethosuximide

Mechanism of action—Ethosuximide exerts its effects by inhibition of low-threshold calcium currents (T-currents).

Route of administration—Oral.

Indications—Ethosuximide is the drug of choice in simple absence seizures and is particularly well tolerated in children.

Contraindications—Ethosuximide may make tonic-clonic attacks worse.

Adverse effects—The adverse effects of ethosuximide include gastrointestinal upset, drowsiness, mood swings and skin rashes. Rarely, it causes serious bone marrow depression.

Vigabatrin

Mechanism of action—Vigabatrin exerts its effects by irreversible inhibition of GABA transaminase.

Route of administration—Oral.

Indications—Vigabatrin is indicated in epilepsy not satisfactorily controlled by other drugs.

Contraindications—Vigabatrin should not be used in people with a history of psychosis because of the side-effect of hallucinations.

Adverse effects—Drowsiness, dizziness, depression, visual hallucinations.

Therapeutic notes—Vigabatrin is a new drug, used as an adjunct to other therapies.

Lamotrigine

Mechanism of action—Lamotrigine appears to act via an effect on sodium channels, and inhibiting the release of excitatory amino acids.

Route of administration—Oral.

Indications—Monotherapy and adjunctive treatment of partial seizures and generalized tonic-clonic seizures; neuralgic pain (p. 142).

Contraindications—Hepatic impairment.

Adverse effects—Rashes, fever, malaise, drowsiness and, rarely, hepatic dysfunction.

Gabapentin

Mechanism of action—Gabapentin is a lipophilic drug that was designed to act like GABA in the CNS (agonist), though it does not appear to have GABA-mimetic actions. Its mechanism of action remains elusive, but its antiepileptic action almost certainly involves voltage-gated calcium-channel blockade.

Route of administration—Oral.

Indications—As an adjunct to therapy in partial epilepsy with or without secondary generalization.

Contraindications—Avoid sudden withdrawal, in elderly patients and in those with renal impairment.

Adverse effects—Somnolence, dizziness, ataxia, fatigue and, rarely, cerebellar signs.

Barbiturates

Examples of barbiturates include phenobarbital and primidone (which itself, is largely converted to phenobarbital).

Mechanism of action—Barbiturates cause potentiation of chloride currents through the $GABA_A/Cl^-$ channel complex.

Route of administration—Oral, intravenous.

Indications—Barbiturates are used in all forms of epilepsy, including status epilepticus.

Contraindications—Barbiturates should not be used in children, elderly people, and people with respiratory depression.

Adverse effects—The main side-effect of barbiturates is sedation, which limits their use clinically, along with the danger of potentially fatal CNS depression in overdose. Phenobarbital is a good inducer of cytochrome P_{450}, and so it can be involved in drug interactions.

Therapeutic notes—Only the long-acting barbiturates are antiepileptic. Phenobarbital has a plasma half-life of 10 hours. The strong sedating nature of these drugs now limits their use in the management of epilepsy.

Benzodiazepines

Examples of benzodiazepines include clonazepam and clobazam.

Mechanism of action—Benzodiazepines cause potentiation of chloride currents through the $GABA_A/Cl^-$ channel complex (see Fig. 5.5).

Route of administration—Oral, intravenously.

Indications—Clonazepam is occasionally used for tonic-clonic and partial seizures. Lorazepam and diazepam are effective in the management of status epilepticus.

Contraindications—Benzodiazepines should not be used in people with respiratory depression.

Adverse effects—The most common adverse effect of the benzodiazepines is sedation. Intravenous lorazepam and diazepam can depress respiration.

Therapeutic notes—The repeated seizures of status epilepticus can damage the brain and be potentially life-threatening, so they should be controlled by administration of intravenous diazepam. Lorazepam has a longer half-life than diazepam.

Other anticonvulsants

Other agents used as antiepileptics include levetiracetam, tiagabine, topiramate, acetazolamide and piracetam. Their indications and side-effect profiles can be obtained from the *British National Formulary (BNF)*.

COMMUNICATION

Emmett Hezz, a 19-year-old student car mechanic is brought to accident and emergency following a collapse while waiting for a taxi. His fiancée was with him at the time and tells staff that he fell to the ground all of a sudden and that his breathing appeared to stop for about 30 seconds. He then developed jerking movements of his arms and legs and by this time his face had turned blue. He was incontinent of urine and on regaining consciousness was drowsy, confused and complaining of aching muscles. In hospital he was able to explain that 8 months ago, he experienced a similar episode when in a park, but was too embarrassed to tell anybody.

On examination, his pulse is 76 beats per minute and regular. No abnormalities are found, other than a bleeding tongue. The history is very indicative of a tonic-clonic (grand mal) seizure. He is admitted for 24 hours and sent for blood investigations, ECG, head CT and EEG. EEG reveals generalized spike-and-wave activity, but no other abnormality. He is warned not to drive or operate heavy machinery until he has been seizure-free for a year. Emmett agrees to start taking the anticonvulsant sodium valproate and return for a follow-up appointment.

Status epilepticus

Intravenous benzodiazepines (lorazepam or diazepam) are first-line drugs in status epilepticus. If these fail to bring an end to seizure activity, intravenous sodium valproate or phenytoin, or carbamazepine via a nasogastric tube should be attempted, ideally in an intensive care setting. Alternatively intravenous fosphenytoin, a prodrug of phenytoin, can be given more rapidly but requires ECG monitoring. Thiopental can be used as a final option.

THE EYE

The eyeball is a 25 mm sphere made up of two fluid-filled compartments (the aqueous humour and the vitreous humour) separated by a translucent lens, all encased within four layers of supporting tissue (Fig. 5.18). These four layers consist of:

- The cornea and sclera
- The uveal tract, comprising the iris, ciliary body and choroid
- The pigment epithelium
- The retina (neural tissue containing photoreceptors).

Light entering the eye is focused by the lens onto the retina, and the signal reaches the brain via the optic nerve.

Glaucoma

Glaucoma describes a group of disorders characterised by a loss in visual field associated with cupping of the optic disc and optic nerve damage. The glaucomas are the second commonest cause of blindness in the world and the commonest cause of irreversible blindness. Glaucoma is generally associated with raised intraocular pressure (IOP), but can occur when the IOP is within normal limits.

There are two types of glaucoma: open-angle and closed-angle.

Open-angle glaucoma is the most common type of glaucoma and it may be congenital. It is caused by pathology of the trabecular meshwork that reduces the drainage of the aqueous humour into the canal of Schlemm. Treatment involves either reducing the amount of aqueous humour produced (Fig. 5.19) or increasing its drainage.

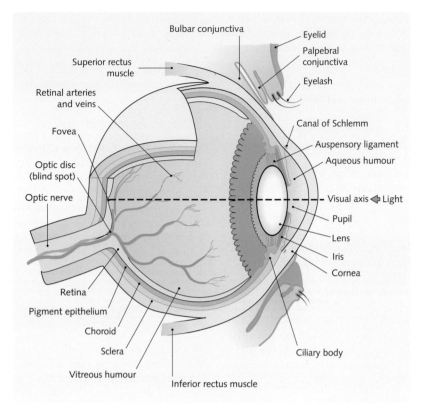

Fig. 5.18 Anatomy of the eye. (Redrawn from Page et al. 2006.)

In closed-angle glaucoma, the angle between the iris and the cornea is very small, and this results in forward ballooning of the iris against the back of the cornea.

Chronic open-angle glaucoma is of insidious onset and often picked up at routine check up, whereas acute closed-angle glaucoma symptoms include painful, red eyes and blurred vision. Acute closed-angle glaucoma is a medical emergency and requires admission to save sight. It is difficult for the patient to notice gradual loss of visual fields associated with chronic open-angle glaucoma and so regular check ups are vital for at-risk groups, such as elderly people.

Treatment of open-angle glaucoma

The most effective way of preventing this damage to the eye is by lowering the IOP. Most drugs used to treat eye disease can be given topically in the form of drops and ointments. To enable these drugs to penetrate the cornea, they must be lipophilic or uncharged.

Drugs used to inhibit aqueous production

β-Adrenoceptor antagonists and prostaglandin analogues are the current choice for first-line treatment.

β-Adrenoceptor antagonists

Timolol and betaxolol are examples of β-adrenoceptor antagonists used in glaucoma.

Mechanism of action—β-Adrenoceptor antagonists block $β_2$-receptors on the ciliary body and on ciliary blood vessels, resulting in vasoconstriction and reduced aqueous production (Fig. 5.19).

Route of administration—Topical.

Indications—Open-angle glaucoma. β-adrenoceptor antagonists are also used in cardiovascular disease (Ch. 2).

Contraindications—β-Adrenoceptor antagonists should not be given to patients with asthma, bradycardia, heart block or heart failure.

Adverse effects—Systemic side-effects include bronchospasm in asthmatic patients, and potentially bradycardia owing to their non-selective action on β-receptors. Other side-effects include transitory dry eyes and allergic blepharoconjunctivitis.

Prostaglandin analogues

Examples include latanoprost and travoprost.

Mechanism of action—Promote outflow of aqueous from the anterior chamber via an alternative drainage route, called the uveoscleral pathway.

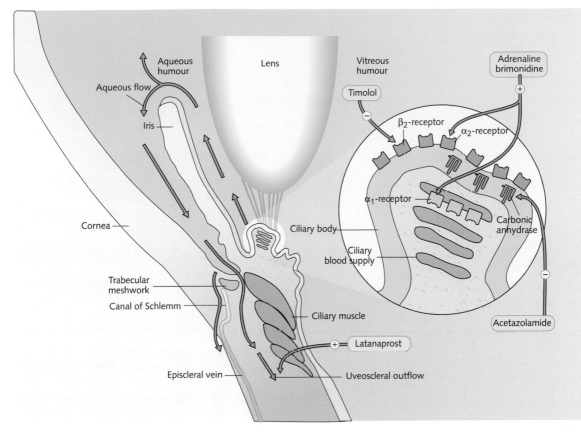

Fig. 5.19 Production and drainage of the aqueous humour. (Redrawn from Page et al. 2006.)

Indications—Open angle glaucoma, ocular hypertension.

Contraindication—Pregnancy.

Adverse effects—Brown pigmentation of the iris may occur.

Sympathomimetics (adrenoceptor agonists)
Adrenaline, dipivefrine and brimonidine are commonly used sympathomimetics.

Mechanism of action—Agonism at α-adrenoceptors is thought to be the principal means by which these agents reduce aqueous production from the ciliary body. Adrenaline may also increase drainage of aqueous humour (see Fig. 5.19).

Route of administration—Topical.

Indications—Open-angle glaucoma. Sympathomimetics are also used in the management of cardiac (Ch. 2) and anaphylactic emergencies and in reversible airways disease (Ch. 3).

Contraindications—Closed-angle glaucoma, hypertension, heart disease.

Adverse effects—Pain and redness of the eye.

Therapeutic notes—Adrenaline is not very lipophilic and, therefore, it does not penetrate the cornea effectively. This can be overcome by administering dipivefrine hydrochloride, a prodrug that crosses the cornea and that is metabolized to adrenaline once inside the eye.

Carbonic anhydrase inhibitors (CAIs)
Acetazolamide and dorzolamide are CAIs.

Mechanism of action—CAIs inhibit the enzyme carbonic anhydrase, which catalyses the conversion of carbon dioxide and water to carbonic acid, which dissociates into bicarbonate and H^+. Bicarbonate is required by the cells of the ciliary body, and underproduction of bicarbonate limits aqueous secretion (Fig. 5.19). CAIs given systemically have a weak diuretic effect (Ch. 7).

Route of administration—Oral, topical, intravenous.

Indications—Open-angle glaucoma.

Contraindications—Hypokalaemia, hyponatraemia, renal impairment. These effects can be reduced if the drug is given in a slow-release form.

Adverse effects—Irritation of the eye, nausea, vomiting, diarrhoea, diuresis.

Drugs used to increase the drainage of aqueous humour

Miotics–muscarinic agonists

Pilocarpine is a muscarinic agonist.

Mechanism of action—Pilocarpine causes contraction of the constrictor pupillae muscles of the iris, constricting the pupil, and allowing aqueous to drain from the anterior chamber into the trabecular meshwork (Fig. 5.19).

Route of administration—Topical.

Indications—Open-angle glaucoma.

Contraindications—Acute iritis, anterior uveitis.

Adverse effects—Eye irritation, headache and browache, blurred vision, hypersalivation. May exacerbate asthma.

Treatment of closed-angle glaucoma

Drugs to treat closed-angle glaucoma are used in emergencies as a temporary measure to lower IOP.

Pilocarpine and a carbonic anhydrase inhibitor are often first-line treatments, with mannitol and glycerol being administered systemically and reduce IOP for resistant or more serious cases.

YAG (yttrium-aluminium-garnet) laser surgery provides a permanent cure for closed-angle glaucoma. A hole is made in the iris (iridectomy) to allow increased flow of aqueous humour.

> ### HINTS AND TIPS
>
> Stimuli that cause the pupils to dilate, such as sitting awake in a dark room, increase the tightness of the angle between the iris and the cornea and can thus precipitate an attack of acute closed-angle glaucoma.

Examining the eye

Mydriatic drugs dilate the pupil, i.e. cause mydriasis, while cycloplegic drugs cause paralysis of the ciliary muscle, i.e. cycloplegia. Mydriatic and cycloplegic drugs are used in ophthalmoscopy to allow a better view of the interior of the eye.

Mydriasis and cycloplegia reduce the drainage of the aqueous humour, and they should, therefore, be avoided in patients with closed-angle glaucoma.

Muscarinic antagonists

The most effective mydriatics are the muscarinic antagonists. These block the parasympathetic control of the iris sphincter muscle.

The type of muscarinic antagonist chosen will depend on the length of the procedure and on whether or not cycloplegia is required.

The most commonly used muscarinic antagonists, their duration of action, and their mydriatic and cycloplegic effects are summarized in Fig. 5.20.

α-Adrenoceptor agonists

α-Adrenoceptor agonists can cause mydriasis by stimulating the sympathetic control of the iris dilator muscle. The sympathetic system does not control the ciliary muscle, however, and, therefore, these drugs do not produce cycloplegia. The α-agonist most commonly used to produce mydriasis is phenylephrine.

Muscarinic agonists and α-antagonists

A muscarinic agonist such as pilocarpine, or an α-antagonist such as moxisylyte may be used to reverse mydriasis at the end of an ophthalmic examination. This is not usually necessary.

Fig. 5.20 Mydriatic and cycloplegic effects of the commonly used muscarinic antagonists

Drug	Duration (h)	Mydriatic effect	Cycloplegic effect
Tropicamide	1–3	++	+
Cyclopentolate	12–24	+++	+++
Atropine	168–240	+++	+++

Endocrine and reproductive systems

6

Objectives

After reading this chapter, you will:
- Understand the main functions of the endocrine and reproductive systems
- Know which drugs affect the functioning of these systems and how
- Be aware of indications, contraindications and adverse drug reactions.

THE THYROID GLAND

Basic concepts

Production of thyroid hormones

The thyroid gland secretes three hormones, triiodothyronine (T_3), thyroxine (T_4) and calcitonin.

The principal effects of the thyroid hormones are: determination of basal metabolic rate and influence of growth through stimulation of growth hormone synthesis and action. Other effects are summarized in Figure 6.1.

The follicular cells of the thyroid gland synthesize and glycosylate thyroglobulin before secreting it into their lumen. Iodination of the tyrosine residues on this molecule is catalysed by thyroid peroxidase and results in the formation of monoiodotyrosine (MIT) or diiodotyrosine (DIT), according to the position on the ring at which this occurs. The coupling of MIT with DIT produces T_3, and the coupling of two DIT molecules produces T_4. Coupling is also catalysed by thyroid peroxidase.

Thyroglobulin, now known as colloid, is endocytosed into the follicular cells, where it is broken down to release T_3, T_4, MIT and DIT T_3 and T_4 are secreted into the plasma; MIT and DIT are metabolized within the cells and their iodide is recycled (Fig. 6.2).

The iodine required for the synthesis of T_3 and T_4 comes mainly from the diet in the form of iodide. Through the action of a thyrotrophin-dependent pump, iodide is concentrated in the follicular cells, where it is converted into iodine by thyroid peroxidase.

Control of thyroid hormone secretion

The hypothalamus contains thyroid-hormone receptors that are able to detect and respond to decreased levels of T_3 and T_4 by causing the release of thyrotrophin-releasing hormone (TRH). TRH reaches the anterior pituitary via the portal circulation and stimulates TRH receptors on thyrotroph cells which in turn secrete thyroid-stimulating hormone (TSH).

TSH reaches the thyroid gland through the systemic circulation where it stimulates thyroid hormone secretion (Fig. 6.3). Both T_3 and T_4 bind to proteins in the plasma (mostly thyroxine-binding globulin), and less than 1% of total thyroid hormones are free. It is the free thyroid hormones which exert the physiological effects. T_3 is about five times more biologically active than T_4, and T_4 is converted to T_3 in some peripheral tissues.

T_3 and T_4 exert negative feedback on the hypothalamus and pituitary.

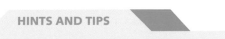

HINTS AND TIPS

Most modern laboratory thyroid function tests measure just TSH, although levels of free and total T_3 and T_4 can be measured as well as thyroxine-binding globulin.

Thyroid dysfunction

Hypothyroidism

Hypothyroidism, thyroid insufficiency, is relatively common in adults and associated with tiredness and lethargy, weight gain, intolerance to cold, dry skin, bradycardia and mental impairment. Children with hypothyroidism manifest delayed bone growth, whereas a deficiency in utero also results in mental retardation – this condition is known as cretinism.

Hashimoto's thyroiditis is an autoimmune disease resulting in fibrosis of the thyroid gland. It is the most common cause of hypothyroidism and, like most autoimmune diseases, is more prevalent in women. Myxoedema is also immunological in origin, and represents the most severe form of hypothyroidism, sometimes causing coma.

Thyroid-hormone resistance and reduced TSH secretion will also produce the symptoms of hypothyroidism.

The causes of hypothyroidism are summarized in Figure 6.4.

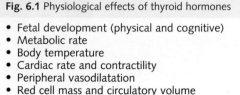

Fig. 6.1 Physiological effects of thyroid hormones

- Fetal development (physical and cognitive)
- Metabolic rate
- Body temperature
- Cardiac rate and contractility
- Peripheral vasodilatation
- Red cell mass and circulatory volume
- Respiratory drive
- Peripheral nerves (reflexes)
- Hepatic metabolic enzymes
- Bone turnover
- Skin and soft tissue effects

From Page et al. 2006.

Management of hypothyroidism

Levothyroxine

Thyroxine is given as levothyroxine sodium in maintenance therapy. It has a half-life of 6 days and a peak onset of 9 days.

Mechanism of action—Levothyroxine is converted to T_3 in vivo.

Route of administration—Oral.

Indications—Hypothyroidism.

Contraindications—Levothyroxine should not be given to people with thyrotoxicosis, and should be used with caution in those who have cardiovascular disease.

Adverse effects—Arrhythmias, tachycardia, anginal pain, cramps, headache, restlessness, sweating, weight loss.

Therapeutic regimen—The starting dose of levothyroxine sodium should be no greater than 100 µg daily (reduce in the elderly or those with cardiovascular disease) and increase by 25–50 µg every 4 weeks until a dose of 100–200 µg is reached.

Liothyronine sodium (L-triiodothyronine sodium)

As liothyronine is bound only slightly by thyroid binding globulin, it has a more rapid onset of effects and a shorter duration of action than levothyroxine.

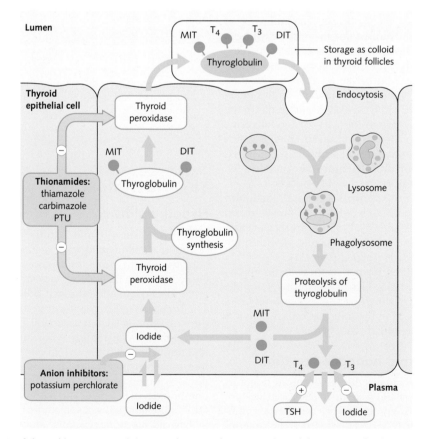

Fig. 6.2 Synthesis of thyroid hormones and the site of action of some antithyroid drugs. (DIT, diiodotyrosine; MIT, monoiodotyrosine; PTU, propylthiouracil; T_3, triiodothyronine; T_4, thyroxine; TSH, thyroid-stimulating hormone.) (From Page et al. 2006.)

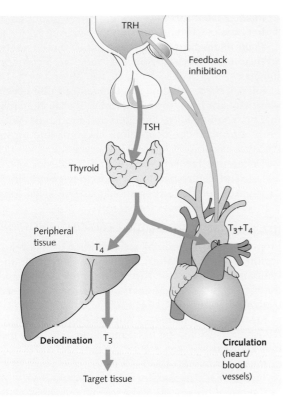

Fig. 6.3 Hypothalamic–pituitary–thyroid axis: control of thyroid hormone synthesis. (T_3, triiodothyronine; T_4, thyroxine; TSH, thyroid-stimulating hormone; TRH, thyrotrophin-releasing hormone.) (Redrawn from Page et al. 2006.)

Contraindications—Liothyronine should not be given to people with cardiovascular disorders.

Adverse effects—Arrhythmias, tachycardia, anginal pain, cramps, headache, restlessness, sweating, weight loss.

Therapeutic regimen—The dosage of liothyronine sodium should be gradually increased as with levothyroxine sodium (20 μg liothyronine sodium is equivalent to 100 μg levothyroxine sodium). Intravenous liothyronine is the drug of choice in the emergency treatment of myxoedema (hypothyroid) coma.

Hyperthyroidism

Hyperthyroidism, thyroid excess, results either from the overproduction of endogenous hormone or exposure to excess exogenous hormone. Symptoms include increased basal metabolic rate (BMR) with consequent weight loss, increased appetite, increased body temperature, and sweating, as well as nervousness, tremor, tachycardia and classic ophthalmic signs.

Graves' disease (diffuse toxic goitre) is the most common cause of hyperthyroidism. It is an autoimmune disease caused by the activation of TSH receptors by antibodies. This results in an enlargement of the gland and therefore excess hormone production.

Toxic nodular goitre is the second most common cause of hyperthyroidism. It is due to either a single adenoma (hyperfunctioning adenoma) or multiple adenomas (multinodular goitre).

The causes of hyperthyroidism are summarized in Figure 6.5.

Fig. 6.4 Causes of hypothyroidism	
Primary	Chronic lymphocytic thyroiditis (Hashimoto's disease)
	Subacute thyroiditis
	Painless thyroiditis (postpartum thyroiditis)
	Radioactive iodine ingestion
	Post thyroidectomy
	Iodine deficiency or excess
	Inborn errors of thyroid hormone synthesis
Secondary	Pituitary disease
Target tissues	Thyroid hormone resistance

From Page et al. 2006.

Mechanism of action—Liothyronine is rapidly metabolized in vivo to T_3. It has a half-life of 2–5 days and a peak onset of 1–2 days.

Route of administration—Oral, intravenous.

Indications—Liothyronine is given for severe hypothyroidism where a rapid effect is needed.

Fig. 6.5 Causes of hyperthyroidism
• Excess exogenous thyroid hormone
• Diffuse toxic goitre (Graves' disease)
• Hyperfunctioning adenoma (toxic nodule)
• Toxic multinodular goitre
• Painless thyroiditis
• Subacute thyroiditis
• Thyroid-stimulating hormone (TSH)-secreting adenoma
• Human chorionic gonadotropin (hCG)-secreting tumours

From Page et al. 2006.

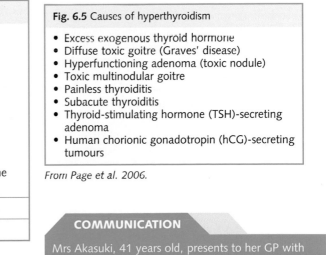

COMMUNICATION

Mrs Akasuki, 41 years old, presents to her GP with tremor and weight loss of 6.5 kg (1 stone) over 4 weeks, despite increased appetite. She admits to feeling hot and sweaty both day and night, which has affected her sleep. On examination a diffuse goitre is seen. Her pulse is rapid and she has noticeable exophthalmos. A pregnancy test is negative. A blood sample is taken and reveals an elevated serum T_3 and T_4 with suppressed TSH levels. Mrs Akasuki is diagnosed as having hyperthyroidism. She is given propanolol for her symptoms and is started on carbimazole to suppress her thyroid. After 4 weeks she is reviewed and checked for neutropenia, a possible dangerous side-effect of carbimazole treatment.

Management of hyperthyroidism

Thioureylenes

The thioureylenes are the first-line drugs for treatment of hyperthyroidism. Carbimazole, thiamazole, and propylthiouracil (PTU) are examples of thioureylenes.

In the body, carbimazole is rapidly converted to active compound thiamazole.

Mechanism of action—The thioureylenes cause inhibition of thyroid peroxidase with a consequent reduction in thyroid hormone synthesis and storage (see Fig. 6.2). The effects of PTU may take several weeks to manifest as the body has stores of T_3 and T_4. PTU also inhibits the peripheral deiodination of T_4 to T_3.

Route of administration—Oral.

Indications—Thioureylenes are used for hyperthyroidism. Patients sensitive to carbimazole are given PTU.

Contraindications—Thioureylenes should not be given to people with a large goitre. PTU should be given at a reduced dose in patients with renal impairment.

Adverse effects—Nausea and headache; allergic reactions, including rashes; hypothyroidism; and, rarely hepatotoxicity, bone marrow suppression, alopecia.

Therapeutic regimen—Carbimazole is given at 20–60 mg daily until the patient is euthyroid (4–11 weeks later), then the dose is progressively reduced to a maintenance level of 5–15 mg daily. Treatment is usually given for 18 months. PTU is given at 300–600 mg daily until the patient is euthyroid, then the dose is progressively reduced to a maintenance level of 50–150 mg daily.

Anion inhibitors

Iodine, iodide and potassium perchlorate are examples of anion inhibitors.

Potassium perchlorate inhibits the uptake of iodine by the thyroid (see Fig. 6.2), but is no longer used owing to the risk of aplastic anaemia.

Iodide is the most rapidly acting treatment against thyrotoxicosis and is given in thyrotoxic crisis (thyroid storm).

Mechanism of action—Iodine and iodide cause inhibition of conversion of T_4 to T_3, of organification, and of hormone secretion. They also reduce the size and vascularity of the gland, which is evident after 10–14 days.

Route of administration—Oral.

Indications—Thyrotoxicosis; preoperatively.

Contraindications—Iodine and iodide should not be given to breastfeeding women as they cause goitre in infants.

Adverse effects—Iodine and iodide can cause hypersensitivity reactions including rashes, headache, lacrimation, conjunctivitis, laryngitis and bronchitis. With long-term treatment, depression, insomnia and impotence can occur.

Therapeutic regimen—Iodine and iodide are given 10–14 days before partial thyroidectomy, with either carbimazole or PTU. They should not be given long term as iodine becomes less effective.

β-Adrenoceptor antagonists

Propranolol and atenolol are examples of β-adrenoceptor antagonists. They are used to attenuate the symptoms of increased thyroid hormone levels, and the effect of increased numbers of adrenoceptors caused by thyroid hormone.

Mechanism of action—β-Adrenoceptor antagonists reduce tachycardia, the basal metabolic rate, nervousness and tremor.

Route of administration—Oral.

Indications—Thyrotoxic crisis; preoperatively.

Contraindications—β-Adrenoceptor antagonists should not be given to people with asthma.

Adverse effects—The side-effects of β-Adrenoceptor antagonists are given in Chapter 2.

Radioiodine

The use of radioactive iodine to treat hyperthyroidism is not classically considered pharmacology, although it is used in the management of thyroid disorders.

THE ENDOCRINE PANCREAS AND DIABETES MELLITUS

Control of plasma glucose

Blood glucose levels are maintained at a concentration of about 5 mmol/L, and usually do not exceed 8 mmol/L. A plasma glucose concentration of 2.2 mmol/L or less may result in hypoglycaemic coma and death due to a lack of energy reaching the brain. A plasma glucose concentration of more than 10 mmol/L exceeds the renal threshold for glucose and means that glucose will be present in the urine. Osmotic diuresis then occurs.

The islets of Langerhans, located in the pancreas, contain glucose receptors and secrete the hormones glucagon and insulin. These hormones are short-term regulators of plasma glucose levels with opposite effects. In addition, their release can be influenced by gastrointestinal hormones and autonomic nerves.

Glucose receptors are also found in the ventro-medial nucleus and lateral areas of the hypothalamus. These are able to regulate appetite and feeding, and also indirectly stimulate the release of a variety of hormones, including adrenaline, growth hormone and cortisol, all of which affect glucose metabolism.

The hormones involved in blood glucose regulation target the liver, skeletal muscle and adipose tissue.

Insulin

Insulin is a 51 amino acid peptide made up of an α- and a β-chain linked by disulphide bonds. It has a half-life of 3–5 minutes and is metabolized to a large extent by the liver (40–50%), but also by the kidneys and muscles.

In response to high blood glucose levels (as occurs after a meal), as well as to glucosamine, amino acids, fatty acids, ketone bodies and sulphonylureas, the β-cells of the endocrine pancreas secrete insulin along with a C-peptide.

Insulin release is mediated by ATP-dependent potassium channels, located in the membrane of the β-cells. These close in response to elevated cytoplasmic ATP and decreased cytoplasmic ADP levels, resulting in depolarization of the membrane. This triggers calcium entry into the cell through voltage-dependent calcium channels, and subsequent insulin release (Fig. 6.6).

Insulin release is inhibited by low blood glucose levels, growth hormone, glucagon, cortisol and sympathetic nervous system activation.

The insulin receptor consists of two α and two β subunits linked by disulphide bonds. Insulin binds to the extracellular α subunits, resulting in the internalization of the receptor and its subsequent breakdown. The β subunits display tyrosine kinase activity on the binding of insulin to the receptor. Autophosphorylation of the β subunits ensues, resulting in the phosphorylation of phospholipase C with subsequent liberation of diacylglycerol (DAG) and inositol triphosphate (IP_3).

The effects of insulin are summarized in Figure 6.7.

Fig. 6.7 Metabolic effects of insulin on fuel homeostasis	
Carbohydrates	Increase glucose transport Increase glycogen synthesis Increase glycolysis Inhibit gluconeogenesis
Fats	Increase lipoprotein lipase activity Increase fat storage in adipocytes Inhibit lipolysis (hormone-sensitive lipase) Increase hepatic lipoprotein synthesis Inhibit fatty acid oxidation
Proteins	Increase protein synthesis Increase amino acid transport

From Page et al. 2006.

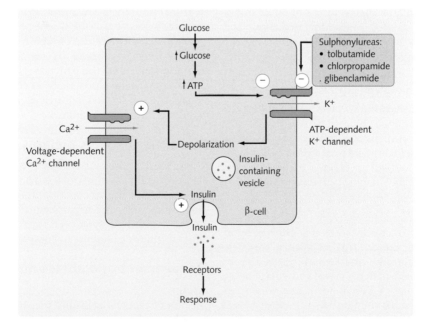

Fig. 6.6 Mechanism of insulin secretion from pancreatic β-cells.

Mrs Raye, 26 years, is 25 weeks into her first pregnancy. Her body mass index (BMI) is 30 and there is a family history of both diabetes and stroke. She is found to have glucose in her urine on routine testing. She has an oral glucose tolerance test. Her fasting plasma glucose is 4.7 mmol/L and her 2 hours post glucose load level is 12.1 mmol/L, indicative of diabetes. The test should be repeated to confirm the result, however, prompt action is also required to prevent harm to the fetus. There is a higher chance of congenital abnormalities with elevated plasma glucose concentrations. Fetal ultrasound is used to exclude this. Mrs Raye is told to try a diabetic diet with small and frequent meals. Since she is overweight, her diet should also be calorie-restricted. After 4 days it is noted this has not worked and insulin injections are started. Her insulin regimen is insulin aspart (rapid and short action), before meals and isophane insulin (delayed onset and intermediate length of action), at breakfast and bedtime. She is warned about symptoms of hypoglycaemia and told to eat if she recognizes them.

Fig. 6.8 Features of type 1 and type 2 diabetes mellitus

Type 1 diabetes (IDDM)	Type 2 diabetes (NIDDM)
0.5% prevalence in adults	5% prevalence in adults
Juvenile onset (<30 years)	Maturity onset (>30 years)
Absolute lack of insulin	Relative lack of, or excess, insulin
Not associated with obesity	Often associated with obesity
Insulin therapy	Oral agents (sulphonylureas) usually suffice
Ketoacidosis frequent	Ketoacidosis uncommon
Linked to the presence of islet cell antibody and genetic markers (HLA antigens)	No known autoimmune origin

Diabetes mellitus

Diabetes mellitus is characterized by an inability to regulate plasma glucose within the normal range. There is an absolute or relative insulin deficiency leading to hyperglycaemia, glycosuria (glucose in the urine), polyuria (production of large volumes of dilute urine) associated with cellular potassium depletion and polydipsia (intense thirst).

There are two types of diabetes mellitus:

- Insulin-dependent (Type 1; IDDM)
- Non-insulin-dependent (Type 2; NIDDM).

The differences between the two types are summarized in Figure 6.8.

The long-term consequences of both types of diabetes are similar, and include increased risk of cardiovascular and cerebrovascular events, peripheral and autonomic neuropathy, nephropathy and retinopathy.

Type 1 diabetes

In type 1 diabetes, pancreatic β-cells are destroyed by an autoimmune T-cell attack. This leads to a complete inability to secrete insulin and ketoacidosis is a problem. Some untreated patients have a plasma glucose concentration of up to 100 mmol/L due to insulin deficiency. In this situation, lipolysis is increased, as is the production of ketone bodies from fatty acids. This leads to ketonuria and metabolic acidosis; body fluids become hypertonic, resulting in cellular dehydration, and eventually in hyperosmolar coma.

Type 1 diabetes is apparent at a young age.

Type 2 diabetes

In type 2 diabetes, insulin is often secreted as on average 50% of the β-cells remain active, although there is also peripheral resistance to insulin. Unlike type 1 diabetes, this is relatively common in all populations enjoying an affluent life-style. The prevalence of type 2 diabetes increases with age and the degree of obesity.

Ketosis is not a feature of type 2 diabetes as ketone production is suppressed by the small amounts of insulin produced by the pancreas. Hyperosmolar non-ketotic coma is the type 2 diabetes equivalent to ketoacidosis, and can be fatal if untreated, although responds rapidly to fluids and insulin.

Secondary diabetes mellitus

Not to be confused with type 2 diabetes, secondary diabetes mellitus accounts for less than 2% of all new cases of diabetes, and is most commonly due to pancreatic disease (pancreatitis, carcinoma, cystic fibrosis), endocrine disease (Cushing's syndrome, acromegaly) or drug-induced (thiazide diuretics or corticosteroid therapy).

Management of diabetes mellitus

Insulin

The aim of exogenous insulin preparations is to mimic basal levels of endogenous insulin and meal-induced increases in insulin.

Nowadays the insulin preparation used is mostly the human (recombinant) insulin (however, insulin preparations of bovine origin are also available). Insulin is available as short-, intermediate-, and long-acting preparations (Figure 6.9).

Short-acting insulins are soluble. These preparations most resemble endogenous insulin, and can be given intravenously in hospital. The rapid-acting insulins aspart and lispro have a faster onset and shorter duration of action than the traditional short-acting insulin. Exubera® is a short-acting insulin in the form of an inhaled powder, which could potentially eliminate the need for multiple injections. However, as yet it has not replaced the standard route of administration. Furthermore, patients must have stopped smoking for 6 months prior to commencement of Exubera® and must not also have severe lung disease.

Intermediate- and long-acting insulins are not as soluble as the short-acting preparations. Their solubility is decreased by precipitating the insulin with zinc or protamine (a basic protein), which prolongs their release into the blood stream.

Mechanism of action—Insulin preparations mimic endogenous insulin.

Route of administration—Insulin must always be given parenterally (intravenously, intramuscularly or subcutaneously), as it is a peptide and thus destroyed in the gastrointestinal tract. Short-acting insulin is given intravenously in emergencies, but administration of the insulin preparations in maintenance treatment is usually subcutaneous.

Indications—Type 1 diabetes; type 2 diabetes uncontrolled by other means.

Adverse effects—Local reactions and, in overdose, hypoglycaemia. Protamine can cause allergic reactions. Rarely, there may be immune resistance.

Therapeutic regimen—Different regimens are used according to the patient's needs and age:

- Short-acting insulin three times daily (before breakfast, lunch and dinner) and intermediate-acting insulin at bedtime.
- Short-acting insulin and intermediate-acting insulin mixture twice daily before meals.
- Short-acting insulin and intermediate-acting insulin mixture before breakfast, short-acting insulin before dinner, and intermediate-acting insulin before bedtime.
- Short-acting insulin and intermediate-acting insulin mixture before breakfast is adequate for some type 2 diabetes patients needing insulin.

Therapeutic notes—Preparations are now available which contain mixtures of short and intermediate- and long-acting insulins, allowing patients to inject themselves only once each time they administer their insulin.

Oral hypoglycaemics

Oral hypoglycaemics act to lower plasma glucose. The sulphonylureas and the biguanides are the main drugs used from this class, but newer drugs are also now available.

Sulphonylureas

Gliclazide, tolbutamide, chlorpropamide and glibenclamide are examples of sulphonylureas.

Mechanism of action—Sulphonylureas block ATP-dependent potassium channels in the membrane of the pancreatic β-cells, causing depolarization, calcium influx and insulin release.

Route of administration—Oral.

Indications—Sulphonylureas are given for diabetes mellitus, in patients with residual β-cell activity.

Contraindications—Breastfeeding women, or people with ketoacidosis. Long-acting sulphonylureas (chlorpropamide, glibenclamide) should be avoided in elderly people and in those with renal and hepatic insufficiency, as these drugs can induce hypoglycaemia.

Adverse effects—Weight gain; sensitivity reactions, including rashes; gastrointestinal disturbances; headache; hypoglycaemia.

Therapeutic regimen—Tolbutamide is given at 500 mg two or three times daily and lasts for 6 hours; chlorpropamide is given at 100–250 mg daily and lasts for 12 hours; and glibenclamide is given at 2.5–15 mg daily and lasts for 12 hours.

Fig. 6.9 Insulin preparations			
Insulin preparation	Action	Peak activity (h)	Duration (h)
Rapid-acting insulin	Very rapid	0–2	3–4
Short-acting insulin	Rapid	1–3	3–7
Isophane insulin	Intermediate	2–12	12–22
Insulin zinc suspension	Prolonged	4–24	24–28

Biguanides

Metformin is the only drug in this class.

Mechanism of action—Metformin increases the peripheral utilization of glucose, by increasing uptake, and decreasing gluconeogenesis. To work, metformin requires the presence of endogenous insulin; thus, patients must have some functioning β-cells.

Route of administration—Oral.

Indications—Type 2 diabetes where dieting and sulphonylureas have proved ineffective.

Contraindications—Metformin should not be given to patients with hepatic or renal impairment (owing to the risk of lactic acidosis) or heart failure.

Adverse effects—Anorexia, headache, nausea and vomiting, lactic acidosis and decreased vitamin B_{12} absorption.

Therapeutic regimen—Metformin is given at 1 g two or three times daily. It can be used alone or with sulphonylureas. Metformin should be taken with or after food.

Other antidiabetics

α-Glucosidase inhibitors

Acarbose is the only available drug in this class.

Mechanism of action—Acarbose inhibits intestinal α-glucosidases, and delays the absorption of starch and sucrose.

Route of administration—Oral.

Indications—Diabetes mellitus inadequately controlled by diet alone or in combination with other oral hypoglycaemics.

Contraindications—Pregnancy, breastfeeding, bowel disease.

Adverse effects—Flatulence, diarrhoea.

Therapeutic notes—Like metformin, acarbose is particularly useful in the obese diabetic patient.

Thiazolidinediones

Rosiglitazone and pioglitazone belong to the thiazolidinediones.

Mechanism of action—These agents are believed to reduce peripheral insulin resistance, leading to a reduction in plasma glucose.

Route of administration—Oral.

Indications—Type 2 diabetes inadequately controlled by diet alone or in combination with other oral hypoglycaemics.

Contraindications—Hepatic impairment, history of heart failure.

Adverse effects—Gastrointestinal disturbance, weight gain. Potentially liver failure.

Therapeutic notes—The thiazolidinediones should only be prescribed by a physician experienced in treating type 2 diabetes, and are currently only licensed for use in combination with either a sulphonylurea or metformin.

Diet and fluid replacement

Dietary control

Dietary control is important for both type 1 and type 2 diabetes.

The diet should aim to derive its energy from the following constituents, in the following amounts:

- 50% carbohydrate (slowly absorbed forms)
- 35% fat
- 15% protein.

This regimen aims to reduce total fat intake, increase protein intake, and increase the intake of high fibre foods, which slow the rate of absorption from the gut.

Simple sugars, as found in sweet drinks and cakes, should be avoided. Meals should be small and regular, thus avoiding large swings in blood glucose levels.

Rehydration therapy

In the acute diabetic patient the fluid deficit can be as high as 7–8 L. Rehydration therapy is essential to regain fluid and electrolyte balance and takes precedence over the administration of insulin.

> **HINTS AND TIPS**
>
> It is essential to know about the management of the acute diabetic patient. Not only is this a very common exam question, you will also encounter such patients on the wards.

Untreated diabetic patients have hyperkalaemia as potassium requires insulin to enter cells. As soon as insulin is administered, however, potassium follows glucose into cells, and hypokalaemia becomes the danger. The rehydration fluid should therefore contain potassium, but plasma K^+ should be measured hourly.

Diabetic patients are also at risk of metabolic acidosis due to excessive ketone production. If the acidosis is severe (pH < 7.0), bicarbonate can be administered intravenously, although evidence to support this is weak.

Hypoglycaemia

Hypoglycaemia is an uncommon presentation in the untreated diabetic patient, although very common in those taking insulin, and sulphonylureas.

The symptoms of hypoglycaemia are driven by the sympathetic nervous system and include:

- Sweating
- Tremor
- Anxiety
- Altered consciousness.

The history may reveal the patient has not eaten as scheduled, exercised or taken too much insulin.

Management depends on the consciousness of the patient. If the patient is alert, glucose can be given orally as a syrup, or as simple sugar. If consciousness is altered, oral administration of glucose is dangerous, and there is a risk of the patient aspirating. In this situation, glucose should be administered intravenously or glucagon can be given by intramuscular or intravenous injection.

Glucose (dextrose monohydrate)

Glucose is administered parenterally as dextrose monohydrate.

Mechanism of action—Dextrose mimics endogenous glucose and is utilized by cells.

Route of administration—Intravenous.

Indications—Hypoglycaemia, as part of rehydration therapy.

Contraindications—Hyperglycaemia.

Adverse effects—Venous irritation, thrombophlebitis. Hypokalaemia may occur.

Therapeutic notes—Glucose is also available in numerous oral preparations, although the patient must be alert and conscious before these are administered as aspiration can occur.

Glucagon

Glucagon is a polypeptide hormone, normally secreted by the pancreatic α-cells.

Mechanism of action—Glucagon acts on the liver to convert glycogen to glucose, and to synthesize glucose from non-carbohydrate precursors (gluconeogenesis). The overall effect is to raise plasma glucose levels.

Route of administration—Parenteral.

Indications—Insulin-induced hypoglycaemia.

Contraindications—Phaeochromocytoma.

Adverse effects—Nausea, vomiting, diarrhoea, hypokalaemia.

Therapeutic notes—Unlike intravenous glucose, glucagon can be administered easily by non-medical personnel, and can be carried by the patient as a prefilled syringe-pen.

HINTS AND TIPS

In an acute hyperglycaemic attack, it is essential that fluids and soluble insulin are given intravenously to rehydrate the patient rapidly and decrease blood sugar levels.

ADRENAL CORTICOSTEROIDS

Basic concepts

The adrenal cortex secretes several steroid hormones into the bloodstream. These are categorized by their actions into two main classes – mineralocorticoids and glucocorticoids.

Aldosterone is the main mineralcorticoid and is synthesized in the zona glomerulosa. It affects water and electrolyte balance, and possesses salt-retaining activity.

Hydrocortisone (cortisol) and cortisone are the main glucocorticoids and are synthesized in the zona fasciculata and zona reticularis. These affect carbohydrate, fat and protein metabolism, and suppress inflammatory and immune responses. Cortisol and cortisone also possess some mineralocorticoid activity.

Small quantities of some sex steroids, mainly androgens, are also produced by the adrenal cortex.

Synthesis and release

Adrenal corticosteroids are not pre-formed, but are synthesized when required from cholesterol (Fig. 6.10).

Glucocorticoids

The release of cortisol is controlled by negative feedback to the hypothalamic–pituitary–adrenal axis (Fig. 6.10). There is a diurnal pattern of activity with an early morning peak in cortisol release.

A variety of sensorineural inputs regulate the release of corticotrophin-releasing factor (CRF) in the hypothalamus; examples include physiological and psychological 'stress', injury and infection. CRF, a 41-amino acid polypeptide, reaches the anterior pituitary in the hypothalamo-hypophysial portal system where it stimulates the release of adrenocorticotrophic hormone (ACTH). ACTH is formed from a larger molecule, pro-opiomelanocortin, and is released into the circulation where it stimulates the synthesis and release of cortisol from the adrenal cortex.

Natural and artificial glucocorticoids circulating in the blood exert a negative feedback effect on the production of both CRH and ACTH.

Mineralocorticoids

Aldosterone release is also partially controlled by ACTH, but other factors, especially the renin–angiotensin system (RAS), and plasma potassium levels, are more important.

Mechanism of action of corticosteroids

Endogenous and synthetic corticosteroids act in a similar way. The hormone or drug circulates to peripheral tissues where it enters cells (steroids are lipid soluble) and binds to cytosolic corticosteroid receptors. After hormone binding, these receptors are translocated to the nucleus where they interact with DNA and lead to the transcription of corticosteroid-responsive genes (CRG).

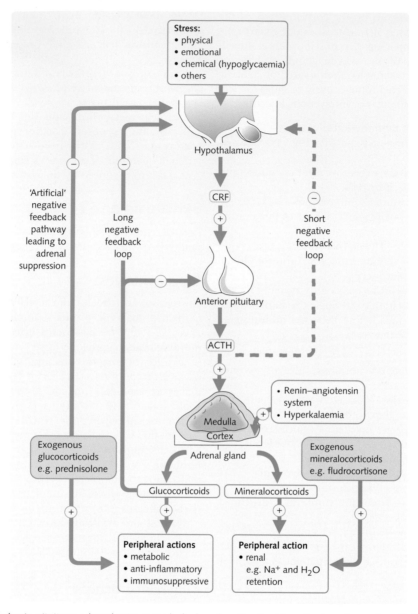

Fig. 6.10 Hypothalamic–pituitary–adrenal axis: control of adrenal corticosteroid synthesis and secretion. (ACTH, adrenocorticotrophic hormone; CRF, corticotrophin-releasing factor.)

The products of these CRGs have diverse effects on the target tissues (Fig. 6.11). The actions of corticosteroids are divided into effects on inorganic metabolism (mineralocorticoid effects) and effects on organic metabolism (glucocorticoid effects).

Therapeutic use of corticosteroids

Corticosteroids have wide-ranging and powerful effects on human physiology. There are two main areas where these properties are taken advantage of in the therapeutic use of corticosteroids – physiological replacement therapy of corticosteroid deficiency, and anti-inflammatory therapy and immunosuppression (Chs 10 and 11).

Exogenous corticosteroids

Both naturally occurring, and a number of synthetic corticosteroids are available for clinical use. These vary in their potency, half-life and the balance between glucocorticoid versus mineralocorticoid activity (Fig. 6.12).

Mechanism of action—Exogenous corticosteroids imitate endogenous corticosteroids.

Fig. 6.11 Major effects of corticosteroids	
Glucocorticoids	
Immunological	• Decreased production of T and B lymphocytes and macrophages, involution of lymphoid tissue • Decreased function of T and B lymphocytes, and reduced responsiveness to cytokines • Inhibition of complement system
Anti-inflammatory	• Profound generalized inhibitory effects on inflammatory response • Reduced production of acute inflammatory mediators, especially the eicosanoids (prostaglandins, leukotrienes, etc.), owing to production of lipocortin, an enzyme that inhibits phospholipase A_2, thus blocking the formation of arachidonic acid and its metabolites (see Ch. 10) • Reduced numbers and activity of circulating immunocompetent cells, neutrophils, and macrophages • Decreased activity of macrophages and fibroblasts involved in the chronic stages of inflammation, leading to decreased inflammation and decreased healing
Carbohydrate metabolism	• Increased gluconeogenesis, decreased cellular uptake and utilization of glucose, increased storage of glycogen in the liver (hyperglycaemic actions)
Fat metabolism	• Redistribution of lipid from steroid-sensitive stores (limbs) to steroid-resistant stores (face, neck, trunk)
Protein metabolism	• Increased catabolism, decreased anabolism, leading to protein degradation
Cardiovascular	• Increased sensitivity of vascular system to catecholamines, reduced capillary permeability leading to raised blood pressure
Central nervous system	• High levels can cause mood changes (euphoria/depression) or psychotic states, perhaps due to electrolyte changes
Anterior hypothalamus and pituitary	• Negative feedback effect of CRF and ACTH with the result that endogenous secretion of glucocorticoids is reduced, and may remain so after prolonged glucocorticoid therapy ('adrenal suppression')
Mineralocorticoids	
Kidney	• Increased permeability of the apical membrane of cells in the distal renal tubule to sodium • Stimulation of the Na^+/K^+ ATPase pump leading to reabsorption of Na^+ and loss of K^+ in the urine • Water is passively reabsorbed owing to sodium retention; thus extracellular fluid and blood volume are increased (raising blood pressure)

Fig. 6.12 Examples of therapeutically used corticosteroids		
Glucocorticoids		**Mineralocorticoids**
'Natural hormones'	**Synthetic**	**Synthetic**
Hydrocortisone (cortisol)	Prednisolone Betamethasone Dexamethasone Beclomethasone Triamcinolone	Fludrocortisone Deoxycortone

Corticosteroid replacement therapy is necessary when endogenous hormones are deficient, as happens in:

• Primary adrenocortical destruction (Addison's disease)
• Secondary adrenocortical failure due to deficient ACTH from the pituitary or post adrenalectomy
• Suppression of the hypothalamic–pituitary–adrenal axis due to prolonged glucocorticoid therapy.

As all the actions of natural corticosteroids are required, a glucocorticoid with mineralocorticoid activity (cortisol) or separate glucocorticoid and mineralocorticoid are given.

The anti-inflammatory and immunosuppressive effects of glucocorticoids are used to treat a wide variety of conditions (Fig. 6.13). In these cases, synthetic glucocorticoids with little mineralocorticoid activity are used (Ch. 10).

Indications—The therapeutic use of corticosteroids falls into the two main categories of physiological replacement therapy, and anti-inflammatory therapy and immunosuppression.

Fig. 6.13 Examples of conditions in which corticosteroids are used for their anti-inflammatory and immunosuppressive effects

Systemic uses	Topical uses	
Acute inflammatory conditions e.g. anaphylaxis, status asthmaticus, fibrosing alveolitis, angioneurotic oedema	Asthma	Aerosol
Chronic inflammatory conditions e.g. rheumatoid arthritis, inflammatory bowel disease, systemic lupus erythematosus, glomerulonephritis	Allergic rhinitis	Nasal spray
Neoplastic disease myelomas, lymphomas, lymphatic leukaemias	Eczema	Ointment or cream
Miscellaneous organ transplantation	Inflammatory bowel disease	Foam enema

Contraindications—Exogenous corticosteroids should not be given to people with systemic infection, unless specific antimicrobial therapy is being given.

Route of administration—Replacement therapy is given orally twice a day at physiological doses to try to mimic as closely as possible the level and rhythm of natural corticosteroid secretion.

When used to suppress inflammatory and immune responses, corticosteroids may be given orally or intravenously, but, depending on the condition, the topical administration of glucocorticoids is preferred, if feasible, as it can deliver high concentrations to the target site while minimizing systemic absorption and adverse effects (Fig. 6.13).

At high doses, even topically administered glucocorticoids can achieve systemic penetration.

Adverse effects—Overdosage or prolonged use of corticosteroids may exaggerate some of their normal physiological actions, leading to mineralocorticoid and glucocorticoid side-effects. Many of these effects are similar to those seen in Cushing's syndrome, a condition caused by excess secretion of endogenous corticosteroids (Fig. 6.14).

The metabolic side-effects of glucocorticoids include:

- Central obesity and a 'moon' face, as fat is redistributed.
- Hyperglycaemia, which may lead to clinical diabetes mellitus, due to disturbed carbohydrate metabolism.
- Osteoporosis, due to catabolism of protein matrix in bone.
- Loss of skin structure, with purple striae, and easy bruising, due to altered protein metabolism.
- Muscle weakness and wasting, due to protein catabolism.
- Suppression of growth in children.

Corticosteroid therapy suppresses endogenous secretion of adrenal hormones via negative feedback on the hypothalamic–pituitary–adrenal axis.

Adrenal atrophy can persist for years after withdrawal from prolonged corticosteroid therapy. Replacement corticosteroid therapy is needed to compensate for the lack of sufficient adrenocortical response in times of stress (e.g. illness, surgery). Steroid therapy must be withdrawn slowly after long-term treatment, as sudden withdrawal can lead to an acute adrenal insufficiency crisis.

With glucocorticoid therapy, the modification of inflammatory and immune reactions leads to an increased susceptibility to infections. This can progress unnoticed because of the suppression of normal indicators of infection, such as inflammation. Increased susceptibility occurs to usually pathogenic and opportunistic bacterial, viral and fungal organisms. Re-activation of latent infections (e.g. tuberculosis, herpes viruses) can occur.

The effects are most serious when corticosteroids are being used systemically, although topical use can exacerbate superficial skin infections, and inhaled corticosteroids can encourage oropharyngeal thrush etc.

The other effects of glucocorticoids include mood changes – euphoria and, rarely, psychosis, peptic ulceration due to inhibition of gastrointestinal prostaglandin synthesis, and eye problems such as cataracts and exacerbation of glaucoma.

Fluid retention, hypokalaemia and hypertension can all be side-effects of any corticosteroids that possess significant mineralocorticoid activity.

HINTS AND TIPS

You must know the adverse effects of corticosteroid therapy as they are numerous, common and a popular exam question. Some of the adverse effects caused by corticosteroids are logical exaggerations of their normal physiological actions, others are more unexpected and must therefore be learned individually.

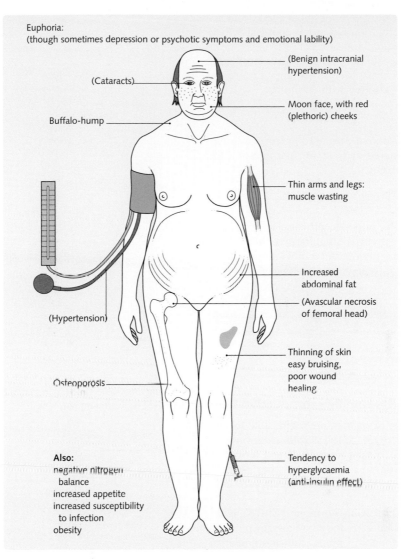

Euphoria:
(though sometimes depression or psychotic symptoms and emotional lability)

(Cataracts)

(Benign intracranial hypertension)

Buffalo-hump

Moon face, with red (plethoric) cheeks

Thin arms and legs: muscle wasting

(Hypertension)

Increased abdominal fat

(Avascular necrosis of femoral head)

Osteoporosis

Thinning of skin easy bruising, poor wound healing

Also:
negative nitrogen balance
increased appetite
increased susceptibility to infection
obesity

Tendency to hyperglycaemia (anti-insulin effect)

Fig. 6.14   Effects of prolonged corticosteroid use – the Cushingoid appearance.

Therapeutic notes on specific steroid agents

Glucocorticoids

Hydrocortisone (cortisol):

- Is administered orally for adrenal replacement therapy and possesses mineralocorticoid activity
- Is administered intravenously in status asthmaticus and anaphylactic shock
- Is applied topically for eczema, inflammatory bowel conditions, etc.

Prednisolone:

- Is predominantly glucocorticoid in activity
- Is the oral drug most widely used in allergic and inflammatory diseases.

Deflazacort:

- Derived from prednisolone, with high glucocorticoid activity
- Administered orally, and indicated in inflammatory and allergic disorders.

Betamethasone and dexamethasone:

- Have very high glucocorticoid activity with insignificant mineralocorticoid activity.
- Are very potent drugs used orally and by injection to suppress inflammatory and allergic disorders, and to reduce cerebral oedema – they do not possess salt- or water-retaining actions.

Beclometasone:

- Is the dipropionate ester of betamethasone

- Is a very potent drug with no mineralocorticoid activity that is useful topically, as it is poorly absorbed through membranes and skin
- Is used as an aerosol in asthma, and as a cream and ointment in eczema to provide high local anti-inflammatory effects with minimal systemic penetration.

Triamcinolone:

- Is a moderately potent drug used in severe asthma
- Is also administered by intra-articular injection for rheumatoid arthritis.

Mineralocorticoids

Fludrocortisone:

- Has such high mineralocorticoid activity that glucocorticoid activity is insignificant
- Is administered orally, in combination with a glucocorticoid, in replacement therapy.

THE REPRODUCTIVE SYSTEM

Hormonal control of the reproductive system

Physiology of the female reproductive tract

The female gonads, or ovaries, are responsible for oogenesis and the secretion of the steroid sex hormones, namely oestrogens (mainly oestradiol) and progesterone. The production of the female sex hormones is controlled by the hypothalamic–pituitary–ovarian axis (Fig. 6.15).

Gonadotrophin-releasing hormone (GnRH) is secreted by the hypothalamus and stimulates the pulsatile secretion of the gonadotrophins, follicle-stimulating hormone (FSH) and luteinizing hormone (LH) by the anterior pituitary. In turn, these act upon the ovaries to stimulate the release of oestradiol, progesterone and other ovarian hormones.

The ovarian hormones are able to exert a negative feedback on the hypothalamus and/or the pituitary. Some of these are selective in their inhibition; for example, inhibin selectively inhibits FSH release from the pituitary, activin selectively stimulates FSH release from the pituitary, and gonadotrophin-surge-attenuating factor selectively inhibits LH secretion from the pituitary.

Menstrual cycle

The menstrual cycle is divided into a follicular phase (days 1–14) and a luteal phase (days 14–28). The cycle proceeds as follows (numbers refer to Fig. 6.16):

1. Day 1 is the first day of menstruation, which involves the shedding of the uterine endometrium.

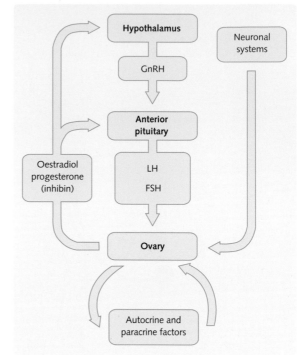

Fig. 6.15 Hypothalamic-pituitary-ovarian axis. (FSH, follicle-stimulating hormona; GnRH, gonadotrophin-releasing hormone; LH, luteinizing hormone.)

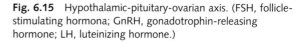
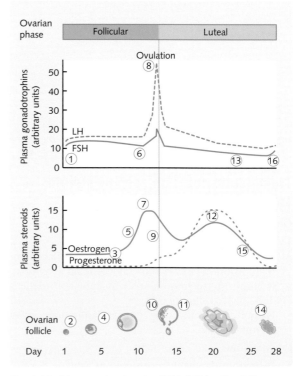

Fig. 6.16 The menstrual cycle. (FSH, follicle-stimulating hormone; LH, luteinizing hormone.)

Plasma oestrogen levels are low and thus little negative feedback occurs. As a result, the secretion of LH and FSH begins to increase.

2. 10–25 pre-antral follicles start to enlarge and secrete oestrogen.

3. FSH stimulates the granulosa cells to secrete oestrogen, the levels of which rise.

4. About 1 week into the cycle, one of the follicles becomes dominant, and the others undergo atresia. The dominant follicle secretes increasingly larger amounts of oestrogen.

5. Plasma oestrogen levels rise significantly as a result of increased sensitivity of the granulosa cells to FSH.

6. Elevated oestrogen levels provide negative feedback, and FSH secretion decreases.

7. Plasma oestrogen levels are now so high (> 200 pg/mL) that they exert a positive feedback on gonadotrophin secretion. This occurs for about 2 days, during which FSH stimulates the appearance of LH receptors on the granulosa cells.

8. An LH surge occurs. This results in a decrease in oestrogen secretion, an increase in progesterone secretion by the granulosa cells, and the resumption of meiosis in the egg.

9. Oestrogen levels decline after ovulation.

10. The first meiotic division is completed.

11. On day 14, ovulation, the release of the ovum, occurs. This is approximately 18 hours after the LH surge.

12. The granulosa cells are transformed into the corpus luteum, which secretes both oestrogen and progesterone in large quantities.

13. There is a rise in the levels of oestrogen and progesterone. As a result, FSH and LH secretion is suppressed, and their levels fall.

14. If fertilization does not take place, the corpus luteum degenerates after about 10 days.

15. Oestrogen and progesterone levels fall; menstruation is imminent.

16. FSH and LH secretion increase once more, and the 28-day cycle begins again.

Physiology of the male reproductive tract

The male gonads, or testes, are responsible for spermatogenesis and the secretion of the steroid sex hormone testosterone. Spermatogenesis takes place in the lumen of the seminiferous tubules of the testis. The production of the male sex hormones is controlled by the hypothalamic–pituitary axis (Fig. 6.17).

The Sertoli cells are connected to one another by tight junctions, and extend from the basement membrane of the seminiferous tubules into the lumen. Under the influence of FSH, these synthesize testosterone receptors and inhibin.

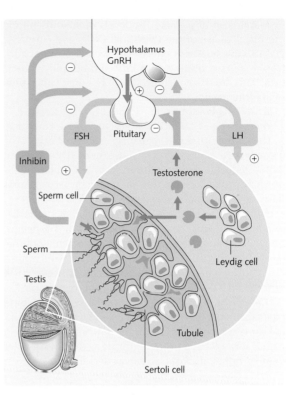

Fig. 6.17 Hormonal control of Sertoli, Leydig and sperm cell function. (FSH, follicle-stimulating hormone; GnRH, gonadotrophin-releasing hormone; LH, luteinizing hormone.) (Redrawn from Page et al. 2006.)

The Leydig cells are found in the connective tissue between the tubules. Under the influence of LH, these synthesize testosterone. Testosterone acts locally to increase sperm production, and also peripherally on the testosterone-sensitive tissues of the body.

Testosterone and inhibin are able to exert negative feedback control over the anterior pituitary, the former decreasing LH secretion and the latter decreasing FSH secretion. In addition, testosterone and inhibin act on the hypothalamus to decrease GnRH secretion.

Drugs that affect the reproductive system

Oral contraceptives

Combined oral contraceptive pill

The combined oral contraceptive pill (COCP) contains both an oestrogen (usually ethinylestradiol, 20–50 μg) and a progestogen (an analogue of progesterone).

COCPs provide a highly effective form of contraception. Their efficacy is reduced by some broad-spectrum antibiotics, which reduce enterohepatic recirculation of oestrogen by killing gut flora.

Mechanism of action—The levels of steroids mimic the luteal phase of the menstrual cycle, and suppress, via negative feedback effects, the secretion of gonadotrophins. As a result, follicular selection and maturation, the oestrogen surge, the LH surge, and thus ovulation, do not take place.

Route of administration—Oral.

Indications—Contraception and menstrual symptoms.

Contraindications—Pregnancy, breastfeeding, or those with a history of heart disease or hypertension, hyperlipidaemia or any prothrombotic coagulation abnormality, diabetes mellitus, migraine, breast or genital tract carcinoma or liver disease.

Adverse effects—Nausea, vomiting and headache, weight gain, breast tenderness, impaired liver function, impaired glucose tolerance in diabetic women, 'spotting' (slight bleeding at the start of the menstrual cycle), thrombosis and hypertension, a slightly increased risk of cervical cancer, and a possibly increased risk of breast cancer.

Therapeutic regimen—COCPs are taken for 21 days (starting on the first day of the menstrual cycle) at about the same time each day, with a 7-day break to induce a withdrawal bleed. If the delay in taking the pill is greater than 12 hours, the contraceptive effect may be lost.

☠ Dangerous drug interaction

Combined oral contraceptive pill+certain antibiotics=reduced efficacy

Progesterone-only pill (minipill)

The minipill consists of low-dose progestogen; ovulation still takes place and menstruation is normal. The minipill is not as effective as the COCP.

Mechanism of action—The minipill causes thickening of cervical mucus preventing sperm penetration. It also causes suppression of gonadotrophin secretion, and occasionally ovulation, but the latter effect does not occur in the majority of women.

Route of administration—Oral.

Indications—Contraception. It is more suitable for heavy smokers and patients with hypertension or heart disease, diabetes mellitus and migraine, or in those who have other contraindications for oestrogen therapy.

Contraindications—Pregnancy, arterial disease, liver disease, breast or genital tract carcinoma.

Adverse effects—Menstrual irregularities, nausea, vomiting and headache, weight gain, breast tenderness.

Therapeutic regimen—The minipill is taken as one tablet daily, at the same time, starting on day 1 of the menstrual cycle and then continuously. If the delay in taking the pill is greater than 3 hours, the contraceptive effect may be lost.

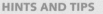

Other contraceptive regimens

Depot-progesterone

Examples of depot-progesterone drugs include medroxyprogesterone acetate and the etonogestrel-releasing implant. These provide long-term contraception.

Mechanism of action—Depot-progesterone causes thickening of cervical mucus. It also causes suppression of gonadotrophin secretion, and occasionally ovulation, but the latter effect does not occur in the majority of women.

Route of administration—Medroxyprogesterone acetate is administered intramuscularly. The etonogestrel-releasing implant system relies on a hormone rod placed subdermally

Indications—Contraception.

Contraindications—Pregnancy arterial disease, liver disease, osteoporosis, breast or genital tract carcinoma.

Adverse effects—Menstrual irregularities, nausea, vomiting and headache, weight gain, breast tenderness.

Therapeutic notes—Medroxyprogesterone acetate provides protection for about 12 weeks. The etonogestrel-implant system provides protection for 3 years.

Emergency contraception ('morning-after' pill)

The 'morning-after' pill, levonorgestrel, provides a form of emergency contraception.

Mechanism of action—High doses of a progestogen alone, or a progestogen with an oestrogen prevent implantation of the fertilized egg. This is 75% effective. Contractions of the smooth muscle are induced, and these accelerate the movement of the fertilized egg into the unprepared uterine endometrium.

Route of administration—Oral.

Indications—The morning-after pill is used for emergency contraception after unprotected intercourse.

Contraindications—Preparations containing oestrogens should not be used in patients who have contraindications to oestrogens (see above).

Adverse effects—Nausea, vomiting and headache, dizziness, menstrual irregularities.

Therapeutic regimen—The morning-after pill regimen depends upon the type of pill being taken, but commonly consists of one or two tablets within 72 hours of intercourse, and one or two tablets 12 hours later. Consult the *British National Formulary (BNF)* for details.

Oestrogens and antioestrogens

Oestrogen agonists

The adverse symptoms of the menopause can be attributed to decreased levels of oestrogen that occur as the ovaries begin to fail. Evidence suggests that oestrogen given in low doses to menopausal women will reduce postmenopausal osteoporosis, vaginal atrophy and the incidence of stroke and myocardial infarction.

A progestogen is co-administered with oestrogen to inhibit oestrogen-stimulated endometrial growth and thus reduce the risk of uterine cancer and fibroids

*Examples of oestrogen agonists include estradiol and estriol.

Mechanism of action—Oestrogen agonists mimic premenopausal endogenous oestrogen levels.

Route of administration—Oral, or by transdermal patches, gels or subcutaneous implants.

Indications—Oestrogen agonists are used alone for hormone replacement therapy (HRT) in menopausal women who have undergone a hysterectomy, and in conjunction with a progestogen if the patient has a uterus.

Contraindications—Pregnancy, oestrogen-dependent cancer, active or previous thromboembolic disease.

Adverse effects—Increased risk of endometrial cancer and possibly an increased risk of breast cancer after many years of treatment.

Therapeutic regimen—Oestrogen agonists are given for several years, starting in the perimenopausal period.

Oestrogen antagonists

Examples of oestrogen antagonists include tamoxifen, clomifene and toremifene.

Mechanism of action—Anti-oestrogens act at oestrogen receptors in oestrogen-sensitive tissues, such as the breast, bone endometrium, and also feedback to the pituitary, antagonizing endogenous oestrogen.

Route of administration—Tamoxifen is administered orally or by intravenous or subcutaneous injection whereas clomifene is administered orally.

Indications—Oestrogen antagonists are used for female infertility and breast cancer.

Contraindications—Hepatic disease, ovarian cysts, endometrial carcinoma.

Adverse effects—Multiple pregnancies and hot flushes. Withdrawal causes visual disturbances and ovarian hyperstimulation.

Progestogens and anti-progestogens

Progestogen agonists

Examples of progestogen agonists include progesterone, medroxyprogesterone, dydrogesterone, hydroxyprogesterone and norethisterone.

Mechanism of action—Progestogen agonists mimic endogenous progesterone.

Route of administration—Oral, or by transdermal patches, gels or subcutaneous implants.

Indications—Progestogen agonists are given for premenstrual symptoms, severe dysmenorrhoea, menorrhagia, endometriosis, contraception and as part of HRT.

Contraindications—Pregnancy or to those with arterial disease, liver disease or breast or genital tract carcinoma.

Adverse effects—Menstrual irregularities, nausea, vomiting and headache, weight gain, breast tenderness.

Progestogen antagonists

Mifepristone is an example of a progestogen antagonist.

Mechanism of action—Progestogen antagonists bind to progesterone receptors but exert no effect. They sensitize the uterus to prostaglandins and can therefore be used in combination with prostaglandins in the termination of early pregnancy.

Route of administration—Oral.

Indications—Progestogen antagonists are used in the termination of pregnancy.

Contraindications—Progestogen antagonists should not be given to pregnant women (64 days gestation or more), to women with adrenal failure or haemorrhagic disorders, or to those on anticoagulant or long-term corticosteroid treatment, or to smokers aged 35 years and over.

Adverse effects—Vaginal bleeding, faintness, nausea and vomiting.

Androgens and antiandrogens

Androgen agonists

Testosterone and mesterolone are examples of androgen agonists.

Mechanism of action—Androgen agonists mimic endogenous androgens.

Route of administration—Oral, intramuscularly or by implant or cutaneous patch.

Indications—Androgen agonists are given as androgen-replacement therapy in castrated men, for pituitary or testicular disease causing hypogonadism, and for breast cancer.

Contraindications—Androgen agonists should not be given to men with breast or prostate cancer, to people with hypercalcaemia, or to women who are pregnant or breast-feeding.

Adverse effects—Sodium retention causing oedema, hypercalcaemia, suppression of spermatogenesis, virilism in women and premature closure of epiphyses in prepubertal boys. The incidence of prostate abnormalities and prostate cancer is also increased.

Androgen antagonists

Cyproterone is an androgen antagonist that is a progesterone derivative. Both oestrogens and progestogens have anti-androgenic properties.

Mechanism of action—Androgen antagonists are partial agonists at androgen receptors, and act on the hypothalamus to reduce the synthesis of gonadotrophins. They inhibit spermatogenesis, causing reversible infertility, but are not contraceptives.

Route of administration—Oral.

Indications—Androgen antagonists are used for male hypersexuality and sexual deviation, prostate cancer, acne, female hirsutism, and precocious puberty.

Contraindications—Androgen antagonists should not be given to people with hepatic disease or severe diabetes, or to those aged 18 and under as their bones are not fully matured.

Adverse effects—Fatigue and lethargy, and hepatotoxicity

Therapeutic notes—Finasteride is technically an anti-androgen, although it inhibits the enzyme 5α-reductase which metabolizes testosterone to the more potent androgen dihydrotestosterone. Finasteride is indicated in benign prostatic hyperplasia and is administered orally.

> **HINTS AND TIPS**
>
> Like breast cancer in women, prostate cancer in men is most often hormone dependent. Exogenous androgens can promote, and anti-androgens can suppress, tumour growth.

Anabolic steroids

Nandrolone and stanozolol are examples of anabolic steroids.

Mechanism of action—Anabolic steroids are androgenic; stimulate protein synthesis and promote wound and fracture healing.

Route of administration—Nandrolone is administered by deep intramuscular injection and stanozolol orally.

Indications—Anabolic steroids can be used for osteoporosis in post-menopausal women, aplastic anaemias and chronic biliary obstruction.

Contraindications—Hepatic impairment, men with prostate or breast cancer, pregnant women.

Adverse effects—Acne, sodium retention causing oedema, virilization in women, amenorrhoea, inhibition of spermatogenesis, liver tumours.

GnRH agonists and antagonists

Agonists

Goserelin, leuprolide and buserelin are examples of GnRH agonists.

Mechanism of action—GnRH agonists are given intermittently, and mimic endogenous GnRH. Continuous use desensitizes the GnRH receptors on the gonadotrophs and inhibits gonadotrophin synthesis.

Route of administration—Buserelin is administered intranasally whereas goserelin and leuprolide are administered by subcutaneous injection.

Indications—GnRH agonists are used for ovulation induction in those with GnRH deficiency, endometriosis, precocious puberty, and sex-hormone-dependent cancers and prostate cancer.

Adverse effects—Menopause-like symptoms, including hot flushes, palpitations, and decreased libido due to hypo-oestrogenism, and breakthrough bleeding.

Therapeutic regimen—Pulsatile administration of GnRH agonists is every 90 minutes for a few minutes. The treatment must not exceed 6 months, and should not be repeated.

Antagonists

Danazol and gestrinone are examples of a GnRH antagonists.

Mechanism of action—GnRH antagonists inhibit the release of GnRH and the gonadotrophins. They bind to the sex steroid receptors, displaying androgenic, anti-oestrogenic, and anti-progestogenic effects.

Route of administration—Oral.

Indications—GnRH antagonists are given for endometriosis, menstrual disorders, including menorrhagia, cystic breast disease, gynaecomastia.

Contraindications—Pregnancy, hepatic, renal or cardiac impairment, vascular disease.

Adverse effects—Nausea and vomiting, weight gain, androgenic effects such as acne and hirsutism.

Therapeutic notes—Cetrorelix and ganirelix are luteinizing hormone releasing hormone antagonists, inhibiting the release of the gonadotrophins. They are administered parenterally and are used for infertility in specialist centres.

Oxytocic drugs

The oxytocic drugs, oxytocin, ergometrine, prostaglandins E and F (e.g. gemeprost (PGE_1 analogue), dinoprostone (PGE_2) and carboprost (15-methyl PGF_{2a})) all cause uterine contractions.

Oxytocin is a posterior pituitary hormone that acts on uterine muscle to induce powerful contractions. It does this directly and also indirectly by stimulating the muscle to synthesize prostaglandins.

In addition, prostaglandins ripen and soften the cervix, further aiding the expulsion of a uterine mass.

Mechanism of action—Oxytocin acts on oxytocin receptors. The mechanism for ergometrine is not well understood, but may be via partial agonist action at α-adrenoceptors or 5-hydroxytryptamine receptors. The prostaglandins act at prostaglandin receptors.

Route of administration—Gemeprost and dinoprostone are administered by vaginal pessary; dinoprostone can also be administered extra-amniotically; oxytocin is administered by slow intravenous infusion, and oxytocin and ergometrine together are injected intramuscularly. Prostaglandins can be administered by intravenous infusion.

Indications—Prostaglandins are used to induce abortion. Oxytocin and dinoprostone are used for the induction of labour while oxytocin, ergometrine and carboprost (in those unresponsive to oxytocin and ergometrine) are used for the management of the third-stage of labour and prevention and treatment of postpartum haemorrhage.

Contraindications—Oxytocic drugs should not be given to women with vascular diseases; ergometrine should not be used to induce labour.

Adverse effects—Nausea and vomiting, vaginal bleeding, uterine pain. Oxytocin can cause hypotension and tachycardia.

BONE AND CALCIUM

Bone and calcium physiology

Bone is a tissue comprised mainly of calcium, phosphates and a protein meshwork, in addition to the components of the bone marrow.

Bone functions to provide support and enables us to carry out various physiological processes such as respiration and movement. Bone is also an active tissue and crucial in the homeostasis of calcium and phosphate.

Serum calcium is ultimately controlled by the peptide, parathyroid hormone (PTH), derived from the parathyroid glands. PTH maintains serum calcium by acting on the kidney to reabsorb calcium from the tubular filtrate, and to stimulate the activation of vitamin D. PTH also acts directly on bone, mobilizing calcium. Activated vitamin D (1,25-dihydroxycholecalciferol) promotes absorption of calcium from the gut. PTH is secreted in response to low serum calcium.

Calcitonin, from the thyroid gland, inhibits calcium mobilization from bone, and decreases reabsorption from the renal tubules.

Disorders of bone and calcium

Osteoporosis is an overall loss of bone mass, and commonly occurs in women after the menopause, when oestrogens fall, and bone mobilisation slowly increases. Other causes of osteoporosis include thyrotoxicosis, and excessive glucocorticoids (exogenous or endogenous).

Osteodystrophy occurs in renal failure and is driven by secondary hyperparathyroidism. Rickets (vitamin D deficiency) is now rare in the West, although the adult variant, osteomalacia, is not uncommon. Hypercalcaemia is a medical emergency, and is most often due to malignancy.

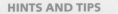

HINTS AND TIPS

Rehydration therapy is as important in hypercalcaemia as it is in ketoacidosis (hyperglycaemia), as fluid will be lost in the urine due to osmotic diuresis.

Drugs used in bone and calcium disorders

COMMUNICATION

Mrs Price, 73 years old, weighing 44 kg, presents with a painful, swollen and 'dinner fork-like' deformity of her wrist. Radiography shows she has fractured both radial and ulnar styloid processes (Colles' fracture). The doctor was concerned that she had poor bone density and sent her for a DEXA (dual energy X-ray absorptiometry) scan. The scan indicated Mrs Price had developed early osteoporosis. Her bones are manually aligned and put in a cast to be reviewed in 6 weeks. She is put on alendronate, a bisphosphonate, to increase her bone density and thus help prevent further fractures. Also, she is put on calcium and vitamin D supplements.

Bisphosphonates

Disodium etidronate, alendronate and disodium pamidronate are examples of bisphosphonates.

Mechanism of action—Bisphosphonates inhibit and potentially destroy osteoclasts, which are responsible for mobilizing calcium from bone.

Route of administration—Oral, parenteral.

Indications—Prevention of postmenopausal osteoporosis and corticosteroid-induced osteoporosis, and for the management of hypercalcaemia of malignancy.

Contraindications—Renal impairment, hypocalcaemia.

Adverse effects—Nausea, oesophageal reactions (with oral preparations), hypocalcaemia.

Calcium salts

Calcium gluconate and calcium lactate are calcium salts.

Mechanism of action—Calcium supplementation replaces calcium deficiencies.

Route of administration—Oral, intravenous.

Indications—Hypocalcaemia, calcium deficiency, osteoporosis.

Contraindications—Hypercalcaemia.

Adverse effects—Mild gastrointestinal disturbance, bradycardia, arrhythmias.

Therapeutic notes—If calcium is given parenterally, serum calcium should be repeatedly monitored.

Vitamin D

Vitamin D can be administered in its inactive form as ergocalciferol, or in its active form as calcitriol.

Mechanism of action—Vitamin D acts on the gut to absorb calcium from the diet.

Route of administration—Oral, parenteral.

Indications—Vitamin D deficiency, hypocalcaemia secondary to hypoparathyroidism, renal failure and postmenopausal osteoporosis.

Contraindications—Hypercalcaemia.

Adverse effects—Symptoms of overdosage include anorexia, lassitude, nausea and vomiting, weight loss, hypercalcaemia.

Therapeutic notes—Serum calcium should be monitored closely once vitamin D therapy has started, and if symptoms of hypercalcaemia appear.

Calcitonin

Mechanism of action—Calcitonin binds specific receptors on osteoclasts inhibiting their mobilisation of bone, and acts on the kidney to limit calcium reabsorption from the proximal tubules.

Route of administration—Subcutaneous or intramuscular.

Indications—Hypercalcaemia, Paget's disease of bone, bone pain in neoplastic disease.

Contraindications—Caution if history of allergy, or renal impairment.

Adverse effects—Nausea, vomiting, flushing, diarrhoea, tingling of hands.

Selective oestrogen receptor modulator

The drug is called raloxifene.

Mechanism of action—Raloxifene has both oestrogen antagonistic (uterine endometrium and breast tissue) and agonistic properties (bone and lipid metabolism).

Route of administration—Oral.

Indications—Treatment and prevention of postmenopausal osteoporosis.

Contraindications—History of venous thromboembolism, undiagnosed uterine bleeding, hepatic or severe renal impairment, pregnancy, breastfeeding.

Adverse effects—Venous thromboembolism, thrombophlebitis, hot flushes, leg cramps, peripheral oedema, flu-like symptoms.

Therapeutic notes—It may reduce the incidence of oestrogen-receptor positive breast cancer and cardiovascular events but there is no clear evidence of this as yet.

Future drugs

Denosumab is licensed for use in osteoporosis in postmenopausal women at risk of fracture. It is currently being considered for use in men receiving hormone ablation therapy for prostate cancer. It has been proved to be as effective as bisphosphonate in the treatment of bone loss and only has to given subcutaneously every 6 months.

Kidney and urinary system 7

● **Objectives**

After reading this chapter, you will:
- Understand the function of the kidney and urinary system
- Know which drugs affect kidney and urinary function and how they do so
- Be aware of drug indications, contraindications and adverse reactions.

BASIC CONCEPTS

Despite making up only 1% of total body weight, the kidneys receive approximately 25% of the cardiac output.

The volume of plasma filtered by the kidneys is termed the glomerular filtration rate (GFR) and is equal to approximately 180 L/day for a person weighing 70 kg. This means that the entire plasma volume is filtered about 60 times a day. The kidneys have a large functional reserve and the loss of one kidney normally produces no ill-effects. The ureters transport the urine from the kidney to the bladder, where urine is stored. Urine leaves the bladder through the urethra. In women, this is a short tube that opens just in front of the vagina. In men, the tube is longer, passing through the prostate and the penis. The kidneys have the most complex functions (see below), the bladder functions as a storage sac, and the ureter and urethra mainly act as conduits for the transportation of urine.

THE KIDNEY

Functions of the kidney

The kidney has several functions. These include:
- Regulation of body water content
- Regulation of body mineral content and composition
- Regulation of body pH
- Excretion of metabolic waste products, e.g. urea, uric acid and creatinine
- Excretion of foreign material, e.g. drugs
- Secretion of renin, erythropoietin and 1,25-dihydroxyvitamin D_3
- Gluconeogenesis.

The nephron

Each kidney is made up of approximately one million functional units, known as 'nephrons' (Fig. 7.1). Each nephron consists of:
- A renal corpuscle which comprises a glomerulus and a Bowman's capsule.
- A tubule which comprises a proximal tubule, loop of Henle, distal convoluted tubule and collecting duct system.

Blood supply

Blood reaches each kidney via the renal artery, which divides into numerous branches before forming the afferent arterioles. These afferent arterioles enter the glomerular capillaries (the glomeruli) and leave as the efferent arterioles.

The efferent arteriole leaving most nephrons immediately branches into a set of capillaries known as the 'peritubular capillaries'. These branch extensively and form a network of capillaries surrounding the tubules in the cortex into which reabsorption from the tubule occurs, and from which various substances are secreted into the tubule.

Glomerular filtration

During glomerular filtration, the fluid fraction of blood in the glomerulus is forced through the capillary endothelium, a basement membrane, and the epithelium of the Bowman's capsule, to enter a fluid-filled space known as the 'Bowman's space'.

Approximately 20% of the plasma entering the glomerulus is filtered. The filtered fluid is known as the glomerular filtrate and consists of protein-free plasma.

Tubular function

The tubules are involved in reabsorption and secretion. Important components of plasma tend to be reabsorbed more or less completely, e.g. sodium and glucose are

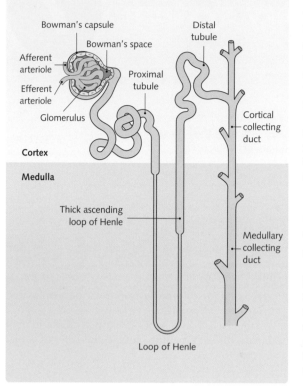

Fig. 7.1 Structure of the juxtaglomerular nephron. (Redrawn from Page et al. 2006.)

99–100% reabsorbed. Waste products are only partially reabsorbed, e.g. approximately 45% of urea is reabsorbed.

The tubules secrete hydrogen and potassium ions, as well as organic species such as creatinine, and drugs such as penicillin.

Sodium and water reabsorption

Approximately 99% of filtered water and sodium is reabsorbed, but none is secreted.

Sodium is pumped out of tubular cells into the interstitium by the Na^+/K^+ ATPase pump in their basolateral membrane. This forms a concentration gradient of sodium; high concentration within the filtrate of the tubule lumen, and a low concentration of sodium within the cytoplasm of the tubular cells. This gradient forms the basis of most reabsorption and secretion processes that subsequently occur. Sodium reabsorption from the lumen varies according to the section of the tubule (see Figs 7.2–7.5).

Water is reabsorbed by passive diffusion, following the movement of sodium ions, and through specific water channels (aquaporins) in the collecting tubules, which greatly increases the reabsorption of water.

Proximal tubule

The Bowman's capsule extends into the proximal tubule, which is made up of an initial convoluted section and a straight section. The proximal tubule is permeable to water and ions and is the site into which many drugs are secreted. Approximately two-thirds of the filtrate volume is reabsorbed back into the blood in the proximal tubule.

Sodium movement into the cell is coupled with that of glucose and amino acids, whereas chloride movement is by passive diffusion (Fig. 7.2). Reabsorption of bicarbonate also takes place in the proximal tubule.

Loop of Henle

The loop of Henle consists of a descending limb, a thin ascending limb and a thick ascending limb.

Twenty-five per cent of filtered sodium is reabsorbed in the thick ascending limb (see Fig. 7.3), but this portion of the tubule is impermeable to water. Increase in the solute load (sodium) in the interstitium between the ascending loop and the collecting tubules sets up an osmotic gradient which subsequently permits water reabsorption from the collecting tubules – the countercurrent multiplier system.

Juxtaglomerular apparatus

Where the afferent and efferent arterioles enter the glomerulus, a group of specialized cells, the macula densa, are situated, in what is named the juxtaglomerular apparatus. These cells secrete renin, which is a fundamental part of renin–angiotensin system. The renin–angiotensin system is involved directly in vascular tone and in the release of aldosterone (Ch. 2).

Distal convoluted tubule and collecting tubule

The distal tubule is continuous with the collecting duct. The collecting duct is the site at which the tubules of many nephrons merge before draining into the renal pelvis. The renal pelvis is continuous with the ureter.

The late distal tubule and collecting duct contain two cell types (see Fig. 7.5):

- Principal cells, which incorporate sodium and potassium channels
- Intercalated cells, which incorporate H^+ATPases that secrete hydrogen ions.

Sodium movement into the principal cells exceeds potassium movement out of the cells, so that a negative potential difference is established. Sodium is transported across the basolateral membrane by Na^+/K^+ ATPase and potassium is moved into the cell before being forced out by the negative potential.

This part of the tubule is the major site for potassium secretion.

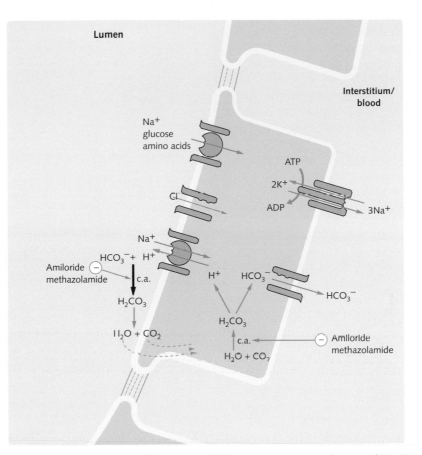

Fig. 7.2 The proximal tubule is one of the sites of bicarbonate (HCO_3-) reabsorption. Carbonic acid (H_2CO_3) is formed in the cytoplasm from the action of carbonic anhydrase (c.a.) on carbon dioxide (CO_2) and water. H_2CO_3 immediately dissociates into HCO_3-, which moves down its concentration gradient across the basolateral membrane, and H^+, which is secreted into the lumen in exchange for Na^+. In the lumen, H^+ combines with filtered HCO_3- to form H_2CO_3 and subsequently CO_2 and water, which are able to diffuse back into the cell. (Redrawn from Page et al. 2006.)

The late distal tubule and collecting duct also contain mineralocorticoid receptors. When aldosterone binds to these, it produces an increase in the synthesis of Na^+ and K^+ channels, Na^+/K^+ ATPase, and ATP, so that Na^+ reabsorption is increased, and K^+ and H^+ secretion are also increased.

The collecting tubule is also the site for water reabsorbing via specific water channels named aquaporins. Fine-tuning of the amount of water to be reabsorbed is controlled by the hypothalamus, which governs how much anti-diuretic hormone (ADH or vasopressin) is released from the pituitary gland. Release of ADH results in more aquaporins being inserted into the luminal membrane, and more water being reabsorbed (Ch. 2).

Atrial natriuretic peptide, derived from the atria of the heart in response to fluid overload, is believed to act on the distal nephron causing a water and solute diuresis. This is a potential target for future therapeutic manipulation.

HINTS AND TIPS

Several different sodium channels exist in the renal tubule, which is why the various diuretic drugs act at different sites along its course, and have different molecular actions and clinical side-effects.

DIURETICS

COMMUNICATION

Mrs Hurst, 77 years old, has developed increasing dyspnoea and fatigue. She has also noticed ankle swelling preventing her from wearing her favourite wellington boots. She has a past medical history of angina, takes aspirin regularly and glyceryl trinitrate when required. Following ECG and B type natriuretic peptide testing, she was diagnosed as having heart failure.

Her symptoms, being caused by pulmonary and peripheral oedema, were treated with the loop diuretic furosemide with the aim of decreasing her fluid overload. Enalapril (an angiotensin-converting enzyme (ACE) inhibitor) and carvedilol (a β-blocker) were started concurrently, because they have been shown to improve symptoms and decrease mortality.

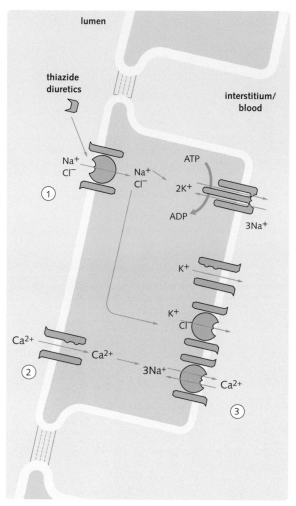

Fig. 7.4 Transport mechanisms in the early distal tubule. Thiazide diuretics increase the excretion of Na^+ and Cl^- by inhibiting the Na^+/Cl^- co-transporter (1). The reabsorption of Ca^{2+} (2) is increased by these drugs by a mechanism that may involve stimulation of Na^+/Ca^{2+} countertransport (3) due to an increase in the concentration gradient for Na^+ across the basolateral membrane. (Redrawn from Page et al. 2006.)

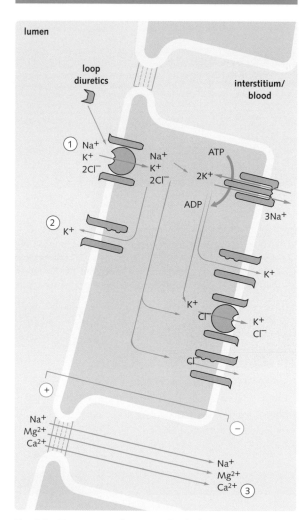

Fig. 7.3 Transport mechanism in the thick ascending loop of Henle. Loop diuretics block the $Na^+/K^+/2Cl^-$ co-transporter (1) thereby increasing the excretion of Na^+ and Cl^-. These drugs also decrease the potential difference across the tubule cell, which arises from the recycling of K^+ (2), and this leads to increased excretion of Ca^{2+} and Mg^{2+} by inhibiting paracellular diffusion (3). (Redrawn from Page et al. 2006.)

Diuretics are drugs that work on the kidneys to increase urine volume by reducing salt and water reabsorption from the tubules. They are prescribed in the treatment of oedema, where there is an increase in interstitial fluid volume leading to tissue swelling.

Oedema occurs when the rate of fluid formation exceeds that of fluid reabsorption from the interstitial fluid into the capillaries. The commonest causes for systemic oedema are:

- Congestive cardiac failure
- Hypoalbuminaemia (including liver failure and the nephrotic syndrome).

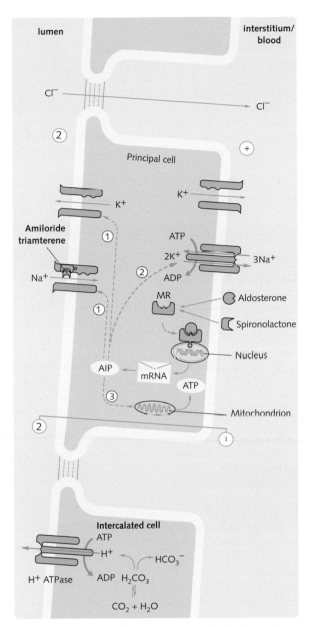

Fig. 7.5 Transport mechanisms in the late distal tubule and collecting duct. Amiloride and triamterene block the luminal Na$^+$ channels, which reduces the lumen-negative potential difference across the principal cell and decreases the driving force for K$^+$ secretion from the principal cell and H$^+$ secretion from the intercalated cell. The net effect is increased Na$^+$ excretion and decreased K$^+$ and H$^+$ excretion. Aldosterone binds to a cytoplasmic mineralocorticoid receptor (MR) stimulating the production of aldosterone-induced proteins (AIP), which (1) activate and increase the synthesis of Na$^+$ and K$^+$ channels; (2) increase the synthesis of Na$^+$/K$^+$ ATPase, and (3) increase mitochondrial production of adenosine triphosphate (ATP). The effect of aldosterone is to decrease Na$^+$ excretion and increase K$^+$ and H$^+$ excretion in urine, whereas spironolactone, an aldosterone antagonist, has the opposite effects. (Redrawn from Page et al. 2006.)

Loss of fluid from the intravascular space into the interstitial compartment results in an apparent hypovolaemic state. Poor perfusion of the kidneys activates the renin–angiotensin system, which causes sodium and water retention. This exacerbates the problem of oedema.

Types of diuretics

Loop diuretics

Furosemide, bumetanide, torsemide are examples of loop diuretics.

Loop diuretics cause the excretion of 15–25% of filtered sodium as opposed to the normal 1% or less. This can result in a profound diuresis.

Site of action—Loop diuretics act at the thick ascending segment of the loop of Henle.

Mechanism of action—Loop diuretics inhibit the Na$^+$/K$^+$/2Cl$^-$ co-transporter in the luminal membrane (Fig. 7.3). This increases the amount of sodium reaching the collecting duct and thereby increases K$^+$ and H$^+$ secretion. Calcium and magnesium reabsorption is also inhibited, owing to the decrease in potential difference across the cell normally generated from the recycling of potassium.

Loop diuretics additionally have a venodilator action, which often brings about relief of clinical symptoms prior to the onset of diuresis.

Route of administration—Oral, intravenous or intramuscular. Intravenous route is used in emergencies as therapeutic effect is much quicker (about 30 minutes compared with 4–6 hours for an oral dose).

Indications—Acute pulmonary oedema, oliguria due to acute renal failure, and resistant congestive heart failure (CHF) and hypertension.

Contraindications—Loop diuretics should not be given to those with severe renal impairment. They should be given only with extreme caution to patients receiving:

- cardiac glycosides (as the hypokalaemia caused by loop diuretics potentiates the action of cardiac glycosides and consequently increases the risk of cardiac glycoside-induced arrhythmias)
- aminoglycoside antibiotics, as these interact with loop diuretics and increase the risk of ototoxicity and potential hearing loss.

Adverse effects—Hypokalaemia, hyponatraemia, hyperuricaemia, hypotension, hypovolaemia. Metabolic alkalosis may occur due to increased hydrogen secretion and thus excretion. Hypocalcaemia and hypomagnesaemia are also possible.

HINTS AND TIPS

Most diuretic drugs block sodium reabsorption from the renal tubule. High solute load in the tubule results in an osmotic diuresis.

Thiazide and related diuretics

Bendroflumethiazide, chlortalidone, metolazone and indapamide are examples of thiazide or related diuretics.

Thiazides produce a moderately potent diuresis, causing the excretion of 5–10% of filtered sodium.

Site of action—Thiazide diuretics act on the early distal tubule.

Mechanism of action—Thiazide diuretics inhibit the Na^+/Cl^- co-transporter in the luminal membrane (Fig. 7.4). Like loop diuretics, they increase the secretion of K^+ and H^+ into the collecting ducts but, in contrast, they decrease Ca^{2+} excretion by a mechanism possibly involving the stimulation of a Na^+/Ca^{2+} exchange across the basolateral membrane; this is due to reduced tubular cell sodium concentration.

Route of administration—Oral, peak effect at 4–6 hours.

Indications—Hypertension, and oedema secondary to CHF, liver disease or nephrotic syndrome. Occasionally used for prophylaxis of calcium-containing renal stones.

Contraindications—Hypokalaemia, hyponatraemia, hypercalcaemia. Caution when prescribing to those taking cardiac glycosides, or to those with diabetes mellitus (thiazides may cause hyperglycaemia).

Adverse effects—Hypokalaemia, hyperuricaemia, hyponatraemia, and hypermagnesaemia, hypercalcaemia, metabolic alkalosis.

Potassium-sparing diuretics

Spironolactone, amiloride and triamterene are all potassium-sparing diuretics.

Potassium-sparing diuretics produce mild diuresis and cause the excretion of 2–3% of filtered sodium.

Site of action—Potassium-sparing diuretics work at the late distal tubule and collecting duct (Fig. 7.5).

Mechanism of action—There are two classes of potassium-sparing diuretics:

- **Sodium-channel blockers:** E.g. amiloride and triamterene. These drugs block sodium reabsorption by the principal cells, thus reducing the potential difference across the cell and reducing K^+ secretion. Secretion of H^+ from the intercalated cells is also decreased.
- **Aldosterone antagonists:** E.g. spironolactone. Spironolactone is a competitive antagonist at aldosterone receptors, and thus reduces Na^+ reabsorption and therefore K^+ and H^+ secretion. The degree of diuresis depends on aldosterone levels.
  Route of administration—Oral.

Indications—In conjunction with other diuretics (thiazides, loop diuretics) in managing heart failure or hypertension, to maintain normal serum potassium levels.

Aldosterone antagonists are used in the treatment of hyperaldosteronism, which can be primary (Conn's syndrome) or secondary (as a result of CHF, liver disease or nephrotic syndrome).

Contraindications—Potassium-sparing diuretics interact with angiotensin-converting enzyme inhibitors, increasing the risk of hyperkalaemia. They should not be given to patients with renal failure.

Adverse effects—Gastrointestinal disturbances, hyperkalaemia, hyponatraemia. Aldosterone antagonists have a wide range of adverse effects, including gynaecomastia, menstrual disorders and male sexual dysfunction.

Therapeutic notes—Low-dose spironolactone has beneficial effects in CHF. Several preparations exist which combine a potassium-sparing diuretic with either a thiazide or a loop diuretic, for example co-amilofruse which contains amiloride and furosemide; such drugs are listed in the *British National Formulary (BNF)*.

Osmotic diuretics

Mannitol is an osmotic diuretic.

Site of action—Osmotic diuretics exert their effects in tubular segments that are water permeable; proximal tubule, descending loop of Henle, and the collecting ducts.

Mechanism of action—Osmotic diuretics are freely filtered at the glomerulus, but only partially, if at all, reabsorbed. Passive water reabsorption is reduced by the presence of this non-reabsorbable solute within the tubule lumen. The net effect is increased water loss, with a relatively smaller loss of sodium.

Route of administration—Mannitol is administered intravenously.

Indications—Osmotic diuretics are used mainly for raised intracranial, and rarely raised intraocular, pressure (glaucoma).

Contraindications—Congestive cardiac failure, pulmonary oedema.

Adverse effects—Chills and fever.

Therapeutic notes—Osmotic diuretics are seldom used in heart failure as expansion of blood volume can be greater than the degree of diuresis produced.

THE URINARY SYSTEM

Urinary retention

Acute urinary retention is treated with urethral catheterization. Chronic urinary retention is usually painless, and management depends upon the underlying cause. In men, the commonest cause for chronic urinary retention is benign prostatic hyperplasia (BPH). Surgery is the definitive treatment, though many patients can be treated medically. Three classes of drugs can be used to treat bladder outflow obstruction secondary to BPH. These are:

- α-Blockers
- Parasympathomimetics
- Anti-androgens.

α-Blockers

Doxazosin and prazosin are examples of α-blockers, and act by relaxing the smooth muscle at the urethra opening of the bladder, increasing the flow of urine. Since the α-blockers are also used as vasodilators in cardiovascular disease (Ch. 2), hypotension can be a side-effect, though are otherwise well tolerated.

Parasympathomimetics

Parasympathomimetics, such as bethanechol, act by increasing detrusor muscle contraction. Their effect is most marked when there is bladder outlet obstruction, and they have no role in the relief of acute urinary retention. Side-effects include sweating, bradycardia and intestinal colic. They are now used infrequently, being superseded by catheterization.

Anti-androgens

Finasteride is a specific inhibitor of the enzyme 5α-reductase, which converts testosterone to the more potent androgen dihydrotestosterone. This inhibition leads to a reduction in prostate size, and improvement of urinary flow. The anti-androgens are described in Chapter 6.

Urinary incontinence

COMMUNICATION

Mr Raheem, 80 years old, presents with a history of increasing nocturia, urgency and reduced urinary flow for the past 2 years. Urinalysis was negative. Renal function and ultrasound were normal. His urine flow rate showed moderate impairment. Digital rectal examination revealed a smooth, enlarged prostate, suggestive of benign prostatic hyperplasia. Prostate serum antigen was normal, supporting a diagnosis of benign prostatic hyperplasia (rather than prostatic cancer). Since the patient was reluctant to undergo an operation and declined transurethral resection of the prostate (TURP), he was managed medically by tamsulosin, an α-adrenergic blocker.

Urinary incontinence by definition is the inability to prevent the discharge of urine. There are three main types of urinary incontinence:

- True incontinence
- Stress incontinence
- Urge incontinence.

Urge incontinence is the only type that is practically amenable to pharmacological intervention, mostly with antimuscarinic drugs.

Antimuscarinics

Oxybutynin is the most widely used antimuscarinic for urge incontinence.

Mechanism of action—Oxybutynin relaxes the detrusor muscle of the bladder.

Route of administration—Oral, transdermal (patches).

Indications—Urinary frequency, urgency, urge incontinence.

Contraindications—Intestinal obstruction, significant bladder outflow obstruction, glaucoma.

Adverse effects—Dry mouth, constipation, blurred vision, nausea and vomiting.

Therapeutic notes—The main side-effects are typically due to the anticholinergic effect, and are commonly dose related.

Erectile dysfunction

Erectile dysfunction (impotence) is a common problem worldwide and has numerous causes.

The penis is innervated by autonomic (involuntary) and somatic (voluntary) nerves. Parasympathetic innervation brings about erection, and sympathetic innervation is responsible for ejaculation. Nonadrenergic, noncholinergic neurotransmission (NANC) also appears to promote erection.

Nitric oxide is believed to be the principal mediator of inducing and sustaining an erection. This highly reactive species activates the guanylyl cyclase enzyme, which subsequently generates cyclic guanosine monophosphate (cGMP).

The synthesis of cGMP in turn activates a protein kinase, which phosphorylates ion channels in the plasma membrane, and causes hyperpolarisation of the smooth muscle cell. Intracellular calcium ions are consequently sequestered into the endoplasmic reticulum, and further calcium influx into the cell inhibited by the closure of calcium channels. The overall effect of a fall in intracellular calcium is a relaxation of the smooth muscle, and increased blood flow to the penis.

While nitric oxide has a very short half-life and is molecularly unstable, cGMP is broken down by a specific group of enzymes, the phosphodiesterases, which subsequently results in the penis returning to its flaccid state. Phosphodiesterase type 5 is thought to be the principal species within the penis, and clearly a target for therapeutic manipulation.

Phosphodiesterase inhibitors

Sildenafil is a selective inhibitor of phosphodiesterase type 5.

Mechanism of action—Inhibition of phosphodiesterase-mediated degradation of cGMP. Higher intracellular levels of cGMP result in continual relaxation of penile smooth muscle and maintenance of an erection.

Route of administration—Oral.

Indications—Erectile dysfunction. There are strict guidelines in the UK as to which groups of patients can be prescribed sildenafil on the National Health Service. These include patients with: diabetes, multiple sclerosis, Parkinson's disease, poliomyelitis, prostate cancer, severe pelvic injury, single gene neurological disease, spina bifida or spinal cord injury. For a comprehensive list of criteria, consult the *BNF*.

Contraindications—Concurrent treatment with nitrates. Conditions in which vasodilation or sexual activity are inadvisable.

Adverse effects—Dyspepsia, headache, flushing, visual disturbances.

Therapeutic notes—Non-specific inhibition of phosphodiesterase type 6 in the retina is responsible for occasional colour disturbances in some patient's vision. Erection will not occur unless there is sexual stimulation.

Prostaglandin E_1

Alprostadil is a synthetic prostaglandin E_1 analogue.

Mechanism of action—It has a similar effect on penile smooth muscle as nitric oxide.

Route of administration—Direct injection into the corpus cavernosum of the penis, or applied into the urethra.

Indications—Erectile dysfunction.

Contraindications—Predisposition to prolonged erection, urethral stricture and use of other agents for erectile dysfunction.

Adverse effects—Penile pain, priapism.

HINTS AND TIPS

Phosphodiesterase enzymes degrade the cyclic nucleotides cAMP and cGMP. Inhibitors of the phosphodiesterases, such as sildenafil, and the less specific xanthines such as theophylline, result in accumulation of these mediators, which brings about the physiological effects of these drugs.

Objectives

After reading this chapter, you will:
• Understand the function of the gastrointestinal system
• Know which drugs affect gastrointestinal function
• Be aware of drug indications, contraindications and adverse reactions.

THE STOMACH

Basic concepts

The stomach not only acts as a sac to store food, but also helps in its breakdown both mechanically and chemically (through hydrochloric acid and digestive enzymes). Peptic ulceration and gastro-oesophageal reflux disease (GORD) are two of the common problems that can occur in the stomach.

Peptic ulceration

The gastric epithelium secretes several substances – hydrochloric acid (HCl) (parietal cells), digestive enzymes (peptic cells) and mucus (mucus-secreting cells). The acid and enzymes convert food into a thick semi-liquid paste called chyme. The mucus protects the stomach from its own corrosive secretions.

Peptic ulceration results from a breach in the mucosa lining the alimentary tract caused by acid and enzyme attack. Unprotected mucosa rapidly undergoes auto-digestion leading to a range of damage – inflammation or gastritis, necrosis, haemorrhage, and even perforation as the erosion deepens.

Gastric and duodenal ulcers differ in their location, epidemiology, incidence and aetiology but present with similar symptoms and treatment is based on similar principles. Peptic ulcer disease is chronic, recurrent and common, affecting at least 10% of the population in developed countries. *Helicobacter pylori* plays a role in the pathogenesis of a significant proportion of peptic ulcer disease.

COMMUNICATION

Mr Springfields is a 40-year-old city worker, who presents to accident and emergency with epigastric pain relieved by eating, smelling heavily of alcohol and smoke. He has vomited dark-coloured blood and this is evident on his shirt. He admits to melaena and recent weight loss. Mr Springfields has a 20-pack year smoking history and a 1-year past medical history of back pain, for which he takes ibuprofen. He is pale and tachycardic, with a blood pressure of 110/65 mmHg. Upper gastrointestinal flexible endoscopy reveals a shallow ulcer overlying a blood clot. Biopsy is taken to test for *H. pylori* and returns positive. His management includes being given oxygen and blood transfusions. He is also given *H. pylori* eradication therapy (a proton pump inhibitor and antibiotics) consisting of omeprazole, amoxicillin and metronidazole.

Protective factors

The mucosal defences against acid/enzyme attack consist of:

• The mucous barrier (approximately 500 mm thick), a mucous matrix into which bicarbonate ions are secreted, producing a buffering gradient.
• The surface epithelium, which requires prostaglandins E_2 and I_2, synthesized by the gastric mucosa. These are thought to exert a cytoprotective action by increasing mucosal blood flow.

Acid secretion

The regulation of acid secretion by parietal cells is especially important in peptic ulceration and constitutes a major target for drug action (Fig. 8.1). Acid is secreted from gastric parietal cells by a unique proton pump that catalyses the exchange of intracellular H^+ for extracellular K^+. The secretion of HCl is controlled by the activation of three main receptors on the basolateral membrane of the parietal cell. These are:

• Gastrin receptors, which respond to gastrin secreted by the G cells of the stomach antrum

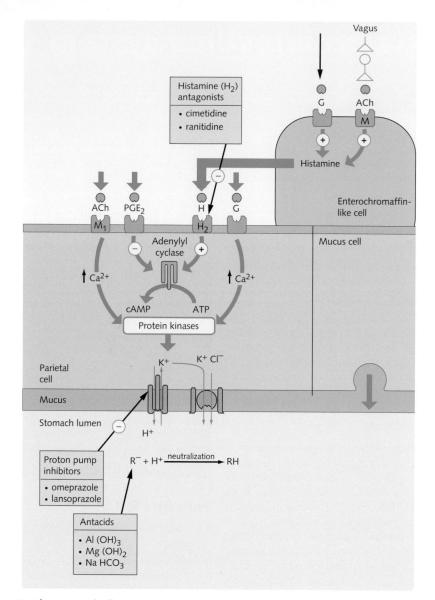

Fig. 8.1 Acid secretion from parietal cells is reduced by muscarinic antagonists, histamine (H_2) antagonists and the proton pump inhibitors. Gastrin (G) and acetylcholine (Ach) stimulate the parietal cell directly to increase acid secretion and also stimulate enterochromaffin-like cells to secrete histamine, which then acts upon the H_2 receptors of the parietal cell. Antacids raise the luminal pH by neutralizing hydrogen ions. Mucosal strengtheners adhere to and protect ulcer craters and may kill *Helicobacter pylori*. (Redrawn from Page et al. 2006.)

- Histamine (H_2) receptors, which respond to histamine secreted from the enterochromaffin-like paracrine cells that are adjacent to the parietal cell
- Muscarinic (M_1, M_3) receptors on the parietal cell, which respond to acetylcholine (ACh) released from neurons innervating the parietal cell.

Although the parietal cells possess muscarinic and gastrin receptors, both ACh and gastrin mainly exert

their acid secretory effect indirectly, by stimulating nearby enterochromaffin-like cells to release histamine. Histamine then acts locally on the parietal cells where activation of the H_2 receptor results in the stimulation of adenylyl cyclase and the subsequent secretion of acid. Excessive production of gastrin from a rare tumour, a gastrinoma, can result in excess acid production, and in peptic ulceration, a condition known as Zollinger–Ellison syndrome.

Gastro-oesophageal reflux

Stomach contents are normally prevented from re-entering the oesophagus by the lower oesophageal sphincter (LOS). Loss of tone of the LOS, or a rise in intra-abdominal pressure are the commonest causes of GORD, of which heartburn is the major symptom. Conservative treatment options include weight loss and raising the head of the patient's bed. Precipitating factors should be avoided, as should excess smoking and alcohol. The drugs used in GORD are the same as for other acid-related disorders (Fig. 8.2).

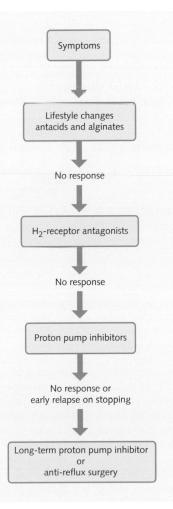

Fig. 8.2 Treatment of gastro-oesophageal reflux disease: a stepwise approach. (Adapted from Haslett et al. *Davidson's Principles and Practice of Medicine*, 18th edition, Churchill Livingstone, Edinburgh, 1999.)

Prevention and treatment of acid-related disease

Drugs that are effective in the treatment of peptic ulcers either reduce/neutralize gastric acid secretion or increase mucosal resistance to acid-pepsin attack. Peptic ulcers thus treated will heal rapidly, but recurrence is common unless *H. pylori* is eliminated.

Reduction of acid secretion

Proton pump inhibitors (PPI)

Omeprazole and lansoprazole are examples of PPIs.

Mechanism of action—PPIs cause irreversible inhibition of H^+/K^+ ATPase that is responsible for H^+ secretion from parietal cells (see Fig. 8.1). They are inactive prodrugs and are converted at acidic pH to sulphonamide, which combines covalently and thus irreversibly with -SH groups on H^+/K^+ ATPase. This inhibition is highly specific and localized.

Route of administration—Oral. Some PPIs can be given intravenously.

Indications—Short-term treatment of peptic ulcers, eradication of *H. pylori*, severe GORD, confirmed oesophagitis, Zollinger–Ellison syndrome.

Contraindications—No important contraindications are reported.

Adverse effects—Gastrointestinal upset, nausea, headaches. There might be a risk of gastric atrophy with long-term treatment.

Histamine H_2-receptor antagonists

Examples of H_2-receptor antagonists include cimetidine and ranitidine.

Mechanism of action—H_2-receptor antagonists competitively block the action of histamine on the parietal cell by their antagonism of H_2 receptors (Fig. 8.1).

Route of administration—Oral. Some antihistamines can be given intravenously.

Indications—H_2-receptor antagonists are the first-line treatment of peptic ulcer disease and GORD.

Contraindications—Cimetidine should be avoided by patients stabilized on warfarin, phenytoin and theophylline.

Adverse effects—Dizziness, fatigue, gynaecomastia, rash.

Therapeutic notes—H_2-receptor antagonists do not reduce acid production to the same extent as proton pump inhibitors, but do relieve the pain of ulcer and promote healing. The drugs are administered at night when acid buffering by food is at its lowest. The usual regimen is twice daily for 4–8 weeks. Cimetidine inhibits the P_{450} enzyme system, reducing the metabolism of drugs such as warfarin, phenytoin, theophylline and MDMA ('ecstasy'), potentiating their pharmacological effect.

Mucosal strengtheners

Misoprostol

Mechanism of action—Misoprostol is a synthetic analogue of prostaglandin E. It imitates the action of endogenous prostaglandins (PGE_2 and PGI_2) in maintaining the integrity of the gastroduodenal mucosal barrier, and promotes healing (Fig. 8.1).

Route of administration—Oral.

Indications—Ulcer healing and ulcer prophylaxis with non-steroidal anti-inflammatory drug (NSAID) use.

Contraindications—Misoprostol should not be given to people with hypotension, or to women who are pregnant or breastfeeding.

Adverse effects—Diarrhoea, abdominal pain.

Therapeutic notes—Misoprostol is most effective at correcting the deficit caused by NSAIDs that inhibit cyclooxygenase-1 and reduce prostaglandin synthesis (Ch. 10). Misoprostol can prevent NSAID-associated ulcers, and therefore is particularly useful in elderly people in whom NSAIDs cannot be withdrawn.

Chelates

Bismuth chelate and sucralfate appear to help protect the gastric mucosa by several means, including inhibiting the action of pepsin, promoting synthesis of protective prostaglandins and stimulating the secretion of bicarbonate. They are administered orally and are generally well tolerated.

Antacids

Examples of antacids include aluminium hydroxide and magnesium carbonate.

Mechanism of action—Antacids consist of alkaline Al^{3+} and Mg^{2+} salts that are used to raise the luminal pH of the stomach. They neutralize acid and, as a result, may reduce the damaging effects of pepsin, which is pH dependent (Fig. 8.1). Additionally, Al^{3+} and Mg^{2+} salts bind and inactivate pepsin.

Route of administration—Oral.

Indications—Symptomatic relief of ulcers, non-ulcer dyspepsia and GORD.

Contraindications—Aluminium hydroxide and magnesium hydroxide should not be given to people with hypophosphataemia.

Adverse effects—Constipation, diarrhoea.

Therapeutic notes—Antacids are still useful for the relief of symptoms of ulceration; frequent high dosing can promote ulcer healing but this is rarely practical.

Alginates

Alginate-containing antacids are administered orally, and form an impenetrable raft which floats on the surface of the gastric contents. This layer prevents gastric acid from refluxing into the oesophagus, and is therefore most useful in GORD. This class of drug is very well tolerated, but does not have any effect on acid secretion, or on preventing or healing of peptic ulcers.

Helicobacter pylori eradication regimens

H. pylori plays a significant role in the pathogenesis of peptic ulcer disease. It does not cause ulcers in everyone it infects (50–80% of the population) but, of those who develop ulcers, 90% can be found to have an *H. pylori* infection in their antrum.

Treatment of peptic ulcer disease should include eradication of *H. pylori*. The rate of recurrence of duodenal ulcer after healing can be as high as 80% within 1 year when *H. pylori* eradication is not part of the treatment, but less than 5% when *H. pylori* is eradicated.

The ideal treatment for *H. pylori* eradication is not yet clear. Current regimens under evaluation include:

- The 'classic' triple therapy – 1 or 2 weeks' treatment with omeprazole, metronidazole and amoxicillin or clarithromycin. This eliminates *H. pylori* in 90% of patients but adverse effects, compliance and resistance can be problematic.
- Quadruple therapy – Omeprazole, two antibiotics and bismuth chelate.

> **HINTS AND TIPS**
>
> Peptic ulcer disease is very common, and potentially life-threatening. Always check with patients if they have an ulcer or ulcer-like symptoms before prescribing NSAIDs.

NAUSEA AND VOMITING

Basic concepts

The commoner causes for nausea and vomiting are shown in Figure 8.3. The act of vomiting is coordinated in the vomiting centre within the brainstem. This centre receives neuronal input from several sources, though fibres from the chemoreceptor trigger zone (CTZ) of the fourth ventricle appear fundamental in bringing about emesis. The CTZ lies outside the blood–brain barrier, and is sensitive to many stimuli, such as drugs and endogenous and potentially exogenous chemical mediators. The CTZ contains numerous dopamine receptors, which partially explains why anti-Parkinsonian drugs (dopaminergic drugs) often induce nausea and vomiting, whereas some antidopaminergic drugs are used as antiemetics.

Fig. 8.3 Commoner causes of nausea and vomiting

- Gastrointestinal irritation
- Motion sickness
- Vestibular disease
- Hormone disturbance
- Drugs and radiation
- Exogenous toxins
- Pain
- Psychogenic factors
- Intracranial pathology

Emetic drugs

It is advantageous, occasionally, to induce emesis (vomiting) to empty the stomach of an ingested toxic substance. Ipecacuanha is given as a liquid, and causes gastric irritation resulting in emesis. There is no evidence to support its use, however, and gastric lavage is the preferred method.

Antiemetic drugs

H₁-receptor antagonists

Cyclizine and cinnarizine are antiemetic antihistamines.

Mechanism of action—These antihistamines have little effect on nausea and vomiting induced by substances acting directly upon the CTZ, though appear effective antiemetics in motion sickness and vestibulocochlear disease.

Route of administration—Cyclizine – oral, intramuscular, intravenous. Cinnarizine – oral.

Indications—Motion sickness, vestibular disorders, vertigo.

Adverse effects—Drowsiness, dry mouth, blurred vision.

Therapeutic notes—Antihistamines have significant antimuscarinic activity, and should be used with caution in prostatic hypertrophy, urinary retention and glaucoma.

Phenothiazines

Prochlorperazine is the most widely used antiemetic drug in this class, though the phenothiazines are also used for their antipsychotic properties (Ch. 5).

Mechanism of action—Numerous effects. Block dopamine, histamine and muscarinic receptors.

Route of administration—Oral, rectal, intramuscular.

Indications—Nausea and vomiting, vertigo, psychosis (Ch. 5).

Contraindications—May exacerbate existing parkinsonian symptoms.

Adverse effects—Sedation, postural hypotension, increased prolactin levels, extrapyramidal effects.

Dopamine antagonists

Domperidone and metoclopramide are examples of the antiemetic dopamine antagonists.

Mechanism of action—Domperidone and metoclopramide block dopamine receptors, and act on the CTZ. Their central antiemetic effect is enhanced as they also promote gastric emptying and small intestine peristalsis.

Route of administration—Metoclopramide – oral, intramuscular, intravenous. Domperidone – oral, rectal.

Indications—Nausea and vomiting, functional dyspepsia.

Contraindications—Metoclopramide is not routinely given to patients under the age of 20 as there is an increased risk of extrapyramidal side-effects in the young.

Adverse effects—Extrapyramidal effects, hyperprolactinaemia.

5-HT₃ receptor antagonists

Ondansetron is an example of 5-HT₃ receptor antagonists.

Mechanism of action—Antagonism of the 5-HT₃ (serotonin) receptor in the CTZ is believed to be responsible for the antiemetic effects of this class of drugs.

Route of administration—Oral, rectal, intramuscular, intravenous.

Indications—Nausea and vomiting, especially associated with administration of cytotoxic drugs.

Adverse effects—Constipation, headache.

Other antiemetics

The synthetic cannabinoid nabilone has antiemetic properties where there is direct stimulation of the CTZ. Hyoscine is a muscarinic-receptor antagonist, and like the antihistamines is most effective in the treatment of motion sickness. Betahistine dihydrochloride is used in Ménière's disease, though its prime effects are assumed to be on the vestibulocochlear nerve.

THE INTESTINES

Basic concepts

Intestinal motility

Normal motility, or peristalsis, of the intestinal tract acts to mix bowel contents thoroughly and to propel them in a caudal direction. Regulation of normal intestinal motility is under neuronal and hormonal control.

Neuronal control

Two principal intramural plexuses form the enteric nervous system. These are:

- The myenteric plexus (Auerbach's plexus) – located between the outer longitudinal and middle circular muscle layers.
- The submucous plexus (Meissner's plexus) – on the luminal side of the circular muscle layer.

Together, these autonomic ganglionated plexuses control the functioning of the gastrointestinal tract through complex local reflex connections between sensory neurons, smooth muscle, mucosa and blood vessels.

Extrinsic parasympathetic fibres from the vagus are excitatory and extrinsic sympathetic fibres are inhibitory. The enteric autonomic nervous system is a major target in the pharmacological therapy of gastrointestinal disorders.

Hormonal control

The activity of the gastrointestinal tract is influenced both by endocrine (e.g. gastrin) and paracrine (e.g. histamine, secretin, cholecystokinin, vasoactive intestinal peptide) secretions.

Drugs that affect intestinal motility

Four classes of drug are used clinically for their effects on gastrointestinal motility (Fig. 8.4). These are:

- Motility stimulants
- Antispasmodics
- Laxatives (purgatives)
- Antidiarrhoeals.

Motility stimulants

Agents that increase the motility of the gastrointestinal tract without a laxative effect are used for motility disorders such as GORD and gastric stasis (slow

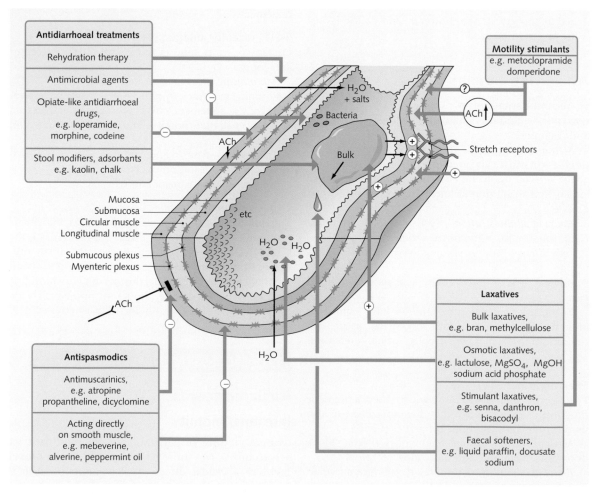

Fig. 8.4 Intestinal motility: control and site of drug action.

stomach emptying), or for diagnostic techniques such as duodenal intubation. Domperidone and metoclopramide in addition to their antiemetic effects, both act to increase gastric and intestinal motility, though their mechanism of action for the latter remains unclear.

Antispasmodics

The smooth muscle relaxant properties of antispasmodic drugs may be useful as adjunctive treatment in non-ulcer dyspepsia, irritable bowel syndrome and diverticular disease.

There are two classes of antispasmodic drug. These are:

- Antimuscarinics
- Drugs acting directly on smooth muscle.

Antimuscarinics

Examples of antimuscarinics include atropine, propantheline and dicyclomine.

Mechanism of action—Antimuscarinics act by inhibiting parasympathetic activity causing relaxation of gastrointestinal smooth muscle.

Route of administration—Oral.

Indications—Non-ulcer dyspepsia, irritable bowel syndrome, diverticular disease.

Contraindications—Antimuscarinics tend to relax the lower oesophageal sphincter and should be avoided in GORD. Other contraindications include angle-closure glaucoma, myasthenia gravis, paralytic ileus and prostatic enlargement.

Adverse effects—Anticholinergic effects – dry mouth, blurred vision, dry skin, tachycardia, urinary retention.

Drugs acting directly on smooth muscle

Mebeverine, alverine and peppermint oil are examples of drugs that act directly on smooth muscle.

Mechanism of action—Mebeverine, alverine and peppermint oil are believed to be direct relaxants of smooth muscle.

Route of administration—Oral.

Indications—Irritable bowel syndrome and diverticular disease.

Contraindications—Paralytic ileus.

Adverse effects—Nausea, headache, heartburn are occasional problems.

> **HINTS AND TIPS**
>
> Irritable bowel syndrome is extremely common in all age groups and in both sexes, and is often self-limiting over time. Sinister pathology should be excluded, and the patient reassured. Dietary modification and antispasmodics form the mainstay of treatment.

Laxatives

Laxatives are drugs used to hasten transit time in the gut and encourage defacation. Laxatives are used to relieve constipation (an infrequent or difficult passage of stool) and to clear the bowel prior to medical and surgical procedures.

It should be remembered that individual bowel habit can vary considerably. The frequency and volume of stool are best regulated by diet, but drugs may be necessary. The passage of food through the intestine can be hastened by:

- Bulk-forming laxatives
- Osmotic laxatives
- Stimulant laxatives
- Faecal softeners.

Bulk-forming laxatives

Bran, methylcellulose and ispaghula husk are examples of bulk-forming laxatives.

Mechanism of action—Bulk-forming laxatives increase the volume of the non-absorbable solid residue in the gut, distending the colon and stimulating peristaltic activity

Route of administration—Oral.

Indications—Constipation, particularly when small hard stools are present.

Contraindications—Dysphagia, intestinal obstruction, colonic atony, faecal impaction.

Adverse effects—Flatulence, abdominal distension and gastro-intestinal obstruction.

Therapeutic notes—Adequate fluid intake should be encouraged, and clinical effects may take several days to develop.

Osmotic laxatives

Examples of osmotic laxatives include lactulose and saline purgatives.

Mechanism of action—Osmotic laxatives are poorly absorbed compounds that increase the water content of the bowel by osmosis. Lactulose is a semi-synthetic disaccharide that is not absorbed from the gastro-intestinal tract. Similarly, magnesium and sodium salts are poorly absorbed and are osmotically active.

Route of administration—Oral.

Indications—Constipation, hepatic encephalopathy

Contraindications—Intestinal obstruction.

Adverse effects—Flatulence, cramps, abdominal discomfort.

Stimulant laxatives

Senna, danthron, bisacodyl and sodium picosulphate are examples of stimulant laxatives.

Mechanism of action—Stimulant laxatives increase gastrointestinal peristalsis and water and electrolyte secretion by the mucosa, possibly by stimulating enteric nerves.

Route of administration—Oral.

Indications—Constipation and bowel evacuation prior to medical/surgical procedures.

Contraindications—Intestinal obstruction.

Adverse effects—In the short term, side-effects of stimulant laxatives include intestinal cramp. Prolonged use can lead to damage to the nerve plexuses resulting in the deterioration of intestinal function and atonic colon. Danthron is potentially carcinogenic, hence its limited use.

Therapeutic notes—Stimulant laxatives should be given for short periods only, and danthron is indicated for use only in the terminally ill.

Faecal softeners

Liquid paraffin and docusate sodium are examples of faecal softeners.

Mechanism of action—Faecal softeners promote defaecation by softening (e.g. docusate sodium) and/ or lubricating (e.g. liquid paraffin) faeces to aid their passage through the gastrointestinal tract.

Route of administration—Oral. Docusate sodium can be administered rectally.

Indications—Constipation, faecal impaction, haemorrhoids, anal fissures.

Contraindications—Should not be given to children younger than 3 years.

Adverse effects—The prolonged use of liquid paraffin may impair the absorption of fat-soluble vitamins A and D and cause 'paraffinomas'.

Therapeutic notes—Prolonged use of faecal softeners is not recommended.

Antidiarrhoeal drugs

Diarrhoea is the passage of frequent, liquid stools. Causes of diarrhoea include infections, toxins, drugs, chronic disease and anxiety.

There are four approaches to the treatment of severe acute diarrhoea. These are:

- Maintenance of fluid and electrolyte balance through oral rehydration therapy (ORT)
- Use of antimicrobial drugs
- Use of opiate-like antimotility drugs
- Use of stool modifiers/adsorbents.

Maintenance of fluid and electrolyte balance through ORT

ORT should be the first priority in the treatment of acute diarrhoea of all causes, and can be life-saving.

ORT solutions are isotonic or slightly hypotonic; they vary in their composition but a standard formula would contain NaCl, KCl, sodium citrate and glucose in appropriate concentrations.

Intravenous rehydration therapy is needed if dehydration is severe.

Use of antimicrobial drugs

Antibiotic treatment of diarrhoea is useful only when a pathogen has been identified or is highly suspected. Acute infectious diarrhoea is usually self-limiting. Antibiotic therapy itself carries certain risks:

- Spreading antibiotic resistance among enteropathogenic bacteria
- Destroying normal commensal gut flora, allowing overgrowth of the bacterium *Clostridium difficile*, which can result in pseudomembranous colitis, a potentially fatal condition.

Antibiotic treatment is indicated in:

- Severe cholera or *Salmonella typhimurium* infection – tetracycline
- *Shigella* species infections – ampicillin
- *Campylobacter jejuni* – erythromycin or ciprofloxacin.

Antibiotics are discussed in detail in Chapter 11.

Use of opiate-like antimotility drugs

Examples of opiate-like antimotility drugs include loperamide and codeine.

Mechanism of action—Opiate-like antimotility drugs act on μ-opiate receptors in the myenteric plexus, which increases the tone and rhythmic contraction of the intestine, but lessens propulsive activity. Loperamide and codeine also have an antisecretory action.

Route of administration—Oral.

Indications—Opiate-like antimotility drugs have a limited role as an adjunct to fluid and electrolyte replacement in acute diarrhoea. They are also used as adjunctive therapy in some chronic diarrhoeal conditions.

Contraindications—Opiate-like antimotility drugs should not be given to people with diarrhoeal conditions such as acute ulcerative colitis or antibiotic-associated colitis. They are not recommended for children.

Adverse effects—Nausea, vomiting, abdominal cramps, constipation, drowsiness.

Therapeutic notes—Loperamide is the most appropriate opioid for local effects on the gut.

COMMUNICATION

Mr Sandhu, a 27-year-old medical student, went to India for 2 weeks and developed cramps in his lower abdomen, loose, watery and explosive stools, a feeling of general malaise, nausea and occasional vomiting. He self-diagnosed himself with traveller's diarrhoea. Mr Sandhu started taking loperamide, which he had brought with him and noticed some improvement almost immediately. However, he stayed unwell and went to seek medical advice. He was given oral rehydration therapy because he had lost a lot of fluid through diarrhoea and vomiting. This helped and he was well again after 4 days.

Use of stool modifiers/adsorbents

Examples of stool modifiers/adsorbents include kaolin, chalk, charcoal and methylcellulose.

Mechanism of action—It has been suggested that stool modifiers/adsorbents act by absorbing toxins or by coating and protecting the intestinal mucosa, though there is no evidence to support this.

Route of administration—Oral.

Indications—There is little evidence to recommend adsorbents at all.

Contraindications—Adsorbents are not recommended for acute diarrhoea.

Adverse effects—Stool modifiers/adsorbents may reduce the absorption of other drugs.

Therapeutic notes—Adsorbents are popular 'remedies' for the treatment of diarrhoea, although there is little evidence of their benefits.

> **HINTS AND TIPS**
>
> Diarrhoea can be life-threatening, especially in children. Management in most cases relies on fluid replacement, prior to treating the underlying cause.

Inflammatory bowel disease

The main two inflammatory bowel diseases are Crohn's disease and ulcerative colitis. Crohn's disease can affect the entire gut and inflammation occurs throughout the full thickness of the bowel wall, while ulcerative colitis affects only the large bowel and inflammation is limited to bowel mucosa. Symptoms often relapse and remit, and their aetiology remains unclear.

Treatment of these conditions is not only pharmacological but also depends on psychological support, correction of nutritional deficiencies and often surgical resection.

Drug treatment is aimed at controlling inflammation and bringing about remission, and the mainstay of drug treatment for these diseases are:

- Glucocorticoids
- Aminosalicylates
- Immunosuppressives, cytotoxics and antibiotics.

Glucocorticoids

Examples of glucocorticoids include prednisolone, budesonide and hydrocortisone.

Mechanism of action—Glucocorticoids have an anti-inflammatory effect (Ch. 10).

Route of administration—In localized disease glucocorticoids may be administered rectally as enemas, suppositories or foams. In extensive or severe disease, oral or intravenous therapy may be required.

Indications—Glucocorticoids are given for acute relapses of inflammatory bowel disease.

Contraindications—Bowel obstruction or perforation, or for prolonged periods.

Adverse effects—Cushingoid side-effects may occur with long-term glucocorticoid use (Ch. 10).

Therapeutic notes—Budesonide is locally acting and poorly absorbed, so has fewer systemic side-effects.

Aminosalicylates

Sulfasalazine, mesalazine and olsalazine are examples of aminosalicylates.

Mechanism of action—Sulfasalazine is broken down in the gut to the active component 5-aminosalicylate (5-ASA) and sulfapyridine which transports the drug to the colon. Mesalazine is 5-ASA and olsalazine is two molecules of 5-ASA. The mechanism of action of the active molecule 5-ASA is unknown, though is postulated to act by scavenging free radicals or interfering with cytokine networks.

Route of administration—Oral, rectal.

Indications—Maintenance therapy of inflammatory bowel conditions.

Contraindications—Aminosalicylates should not be given to people with salicylate hypersensitivity and renal impairment.

Adverse effects—Sulfapyridine is responsible for the majority of this drugs side-effects. Nausea, vomiting, headache and rashes. Blood disorders and oligospermia have been reported.

Immunosuppressives, cytotoxics and antibiotics

When steroids are needed to control symptoms, and side-effects are troublesome or potentially so, the immunosuppressant azathioprine (Ch. 10) is used as an adjunct to other therapies. In addition, cytotoxic drugs such as methotrexate (Ch. 12), anticytokine antibodies such as infliximab and certolizumab pegol (Ch. 10) and the antibiotic metronidazole (Ch. 11) have all been used to modulate the disease process with varying degrees of success.

Obesity

Obesity is becoming increasingly common in the West and is associated with many diseases such as cardiovascular disease, diabetes mellitus, gallstones and osteoarthritis.

Dietary restriction and an exercise programme should be explored prior to surgical or pharmacological intervention. The most widely used anti-obesity drugs act directly upon the gastrointestinal tract. There are also centrally acting appetite suppressants.

Drugs acting on the gastrointestinal tract

Orlistat and methylcellulose are examples of such anti-obesity drugs.

Mechanism of action—Orlistat is a pancreatitic lipase inhibitor, and reduces the breakdown and subsequent absorption of fat from the gut. Methylcellulose is believed to act as a bulk-forming agent, and reduces food intake by promoting early satiety (fullness).

Route of administration—Oral.

Adverse effects—Orlistat often results in oily, frequent stools, flatulence, abdominal and rectal pain. Methylcellulose may produce flatulence and abdominal distension.

Other anti-obesity drugs

The centrally acting appetite suppressant sibutramine is licensed for adjunctive management of obesity but for no more than 1 year's usage; weight loss may return after cessation. Numerous other drugs are being evaluated for their anti-obesity properties, including the endogenous mammalian peptide leptin, which appears to induce satiety and counteract the properties of another transmitter, neuropeptide Y, which is believed to promote feeding.

Anal disorders

Haemorrhoids, anal fissures and pruritus are commonly encountered problems. Bland ointments are the best treatment option, with careful attention to cleanliness. When necessary, topical preparations containing a local anaesthetic (Ch. 9) or corticosteroid (Ch. 10) may provide symptomatic relief. Perianal thrush can be treated with nystatin (Ch. 11). Haemorrhoids are often treated by injection with a sclerosant, commonly oily phenol.

Stoma care is simple, though requires a thoughtful, practical approach, and empathy with the patient. Details of specific stoma care options can be obtained from the *British National Formulary*.

THE PANCREAS AND GALL BLADDER

Pancreatic supplements

Pancreatic exocrine secretions contain important enzymes that break down proteins (trypsin, chymotrypsin), starch (amylase) and fats (lipase). These are essential for efficient digestion.

Pancreatin is an extract of pancreas containing protease, lipase and amylase, that is given by mouth to compensate for reduced or absent exocrine secretions in cystic fibrosis, and following pancreatectomy, total gastrectomy or chronic pancreatitis. Pancreatin is inactivated by gastric acid and so precautions must be taken to optimize delivery of the pancreatin to the duodenum.

Pancreatin preparations are best taken with food. Histamine H_2 antagonists (e.g. cimetidine) may be taken an hour before ingestion of the pancreatin to reduce gastric acid secretion, although acid-resistant (enterically coated formulations) are now available.

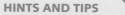

> **HINTS AND TIPS**
>
> Even though pancreatin contains peptides, which would normally be degraded in the stomach, these tablets are coated in an acid resistant layer, and the enzymes and proenzymes within them have endogenous resistance to both acid and proteases, and become active in the small intestine.

Gall bladder

Bile is secreted by the liver and is stored in the gall bladder. Bile contains cholesterol, phospholipids and bile salts. Bile salts are important for keeping cholesterol in solution. The formation of 'stones' in the bile (cholelithiasis) is relatively common and can result in blockage of the draining duct, with subsequent infection and inflammation (cholecystitis). Surgical removal of the gall bladder (cholecystectomy) has largely replaced the use of drugs in the management of symptomatic gallstones, although this is suitable for patients not treatable by other means.

The dissolution of small cholesterol stones is carried out by prolonged oral administration of the bile acid ursodeoxycholic acid.

Ursodeoxycholic acid

The bile salt ursodeoxycholic acid is administered orally, and handled by the body in the same fashion as endogenous bile salt. It works by:

- Decreasing secretion of cholesterol into the bile
- Decreasing cholesterol absorption from the intestine.

The net effect is a reduced cholesterol concentration in the bile and a tendency for the dissolution of existing stones.

Colestyramine

This orally administered anion-exchange resin binds bile acids in the gut and prevents their reabsorption and enterohepatic recirculation. It is used in the treatment of pruritus associated with partial biliary obstruction and primary biliary cirrhosis, and in hypercholesterolaemia.

BASIC CONCEPTS

Pain, which may be acute or chronic, is defined as an unpleasant sensory and emotional experience associated with actual or potential tissue damage. Pain is a subjective experience, as there are currently no means of accurately and objectively assessing the degree of pain a patient is experiencing.

An analgesic drug is one that effectively removes (or at least lessens) the sensation of pain. The principles of pain relief are:

1. Careful assessment
2. Diagnosis of the cause of the pain
3. Use of analgesics in accordance with the analgesic ladder (Fig. 9.1)
4. Regular review of the effectiveness of the prescribed drug.

Pain perception

Pain perception is best viewed as a three-stage process – activation of nociceptors, followed by the transmission and onward passage of pain information.

Activation of nociceptors in the peripheral tissues

Noxious thermal, chemical or mechanical stimuli can trigger the firing of primary afferent fibres (type C/Aδ), through the activation of nociceptors (pain-specific receptors) in the peripheral tissues (Fig. 9.2).

Transmission of pain information

Transmission of pain information from the periphery to the dorsal horn of the spinal cord is inhibited or amplified by a combination of local (spinal) neuronal circuits and descending tracts from higher brain centres. This constitutes the 'gate-control mechanism'. In the gate-control mechanism:

- The primary afferent fibres synapse in lamina I and II of the dorsal horn of the spinal cord.
- Transmitter peptides (substance P, calcitonin gene-related peptide, bradykinin, glutamate) and nitric oxide are involved in the ascending pain pathways, though the interactions are complex and have not yet been fully defined.

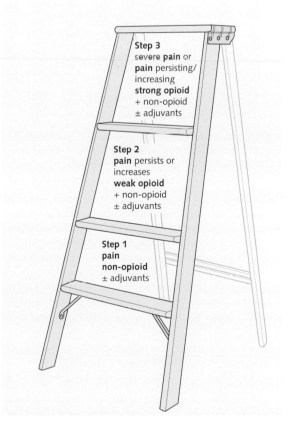

Step 3
severe **pain** or
pain persisting/
increasing
strong opioid
+ non-opioid
± adjuvants

Step 2
pain persists or
increases
weak opioid
+ non-opioid
± adjuvants

Step 1
pain
non-opioid
± adjuvants

Fig. 9.1 The World Health Organization (WHO) analgesic ladder for chronic pain.

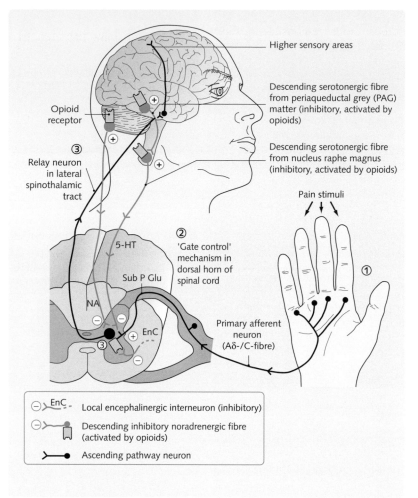

Fig. 9.2 Nociceptive pathways and sites of opioid action. (1) Activation of nociceptors in the peripheral tissues; (2) transmission of pain information; (3) onward passage of pain information to higher centres. (5-HT, 5-hydroxytryptamine (serotonin); Glu, glutamate; NA, noradrenaline; Sub P, substance P.)

- The activity of the dorsal horn relay neurons is modulated by several inhibitory inputs. These include: local inhibitory interneurons, which release opioid peptides; descending inhibitory noradrenergic fibres from the locus ceruleus area of the brainstem, which are activated by opioid peptides; and descending inhibitory serotonergic fibres from the nucleus raphe magnus and periaqueductal grey areas of the brainstem, which are also activated by opioid peptides (Fig. 9.2).

Onward passage of pain information

The onward passage of pain information is via the spinothalamic tract, to the higher centres of the brain. The higher centres of the brain coordinate the cognitive and emotional aspects of pain and control appropriate reactions. Opioid peptide release in both the spinal cord and the brainstem can reduce the activity of the dorsal horn relay neurons and cause analgesia (Fig. 9.2).

Opioid receptors

All opioids, whether endogenous peptides, naturally occurring drugs, or chemically synthesized drugs, interact with specific opioid receptors to produce their pharmacological effects.

Drugs interact with opioid receptors as either full agonists, partial agonists, mixed agonists (full agonists on one opioid receptor but partial agonists on another) or as antagonists. Opioid analgesics are agonists.

There are three major opioid receptor subtypes: μ, δ and κ. The existence of a fourth receptor(s) remains controversial.

Generally speaking:

- μ receptors are thought to be responsible for most of the analgesic effects of opioids and for some major adverse effects, e.g. respiratory depression. Most of the analgesic opioids in use are μ receptor agonists.
- δ receptors are probably more important in the periphery, but they may also contribute to analgesia.
- κ receptors contribute to analgesia at the spinal level, and may elicit sedation and dysphoria, but they produce relatively few adverse effects, and do not contribute to physical dependence.
- σ receptors are not selective opioid receptors, but they are the site of action of psychomimetic drugs, such as phencyclidine (PCP). They may account for the dysphoria produced by some opioids.

Opioid receptor activation has an inhibitory effect on synapses in the central nervous system (CNS) and in the gut (Fig. 9.3).

Secondary-messenger systems associated with opioid receptor activity include:

- μ/δ receptors, the activation of which causes hyperpolarization of a neuron by opening potassium channels and inhibiting calcium channels
- κ receptors, the activation of which inhibits calcium channels.

Activation of all opioid receptors by endogenous or exogenous opioids results in:

- Inhibition of the enzymes adenylase cyclase and thus a reduction in cAMP production
- Inhibition of voltage-gated calcium-channel opening
- Potassium-channel activation which causes hyperpolarization of the cell membrane.

Endogenous opioids

Physiologically, the CNS has its own 'endogenous opioids' that are the natural ligands for opioid receptors. There are three main families of endogenous opioid peptides occurring naturally in the CNS:

- Endorphins
- Dynorphins
- Enkephalins.

They are derived from three separate gene products (precursor molecules), but all possess homology at their amino end.

The expression and anatomical distribution of the products of these three precursor molecules within the CNS is varied, and each has a distinct range of affinities for the different types of opioid receptor (Fig. 9.4).

Though it is known that the endogenous opioids possess analgesic activity, their precise function is poorly defined. They are not used therapeutically.

COMMUNICATION

Mrs Moore is a 60-year-old patient with advanced breast cancer who is receiving chemotherapy. She suffers with bone pain due to metastases. She has been on several analgesics for the pain since its onset, including non-steroidal anti-inflammatory drugs (NSAIDs). NSAIDs were effective to start off with, however the pain sharply increased in severity over the following months and so a decision was made to give her co-proxamol. Co-proxamol is an example of a compound analgesic, containing dextropropoxyphene and paracetamol. Compound analgesics contain both

Fig. 9.3 Actions mediated by opioid receptor subtypes			
Action	**μ/δ**	**κ**	**σ**
Analgesia	Supraspinal and spinal	Spinal	—
Respiratory depression	Marked	Slight	—
Pupil	Constricts	—	Dilates
GIT mobility	Reduced (constipating)	—	—
Mood/effect	Euphoria inducing but also sedating	Dysphoria inducing mildly sedating	Marked dysphoric and psychomimetic actions
Physical dependence	+++	+	—
(GIT, gastrointestinal tract.)			

Fig. 9.4 Endogenous opioid peptides

Precursor molecules	Products	Relative opioid receptor affinity
Pro-opiomelanocortin (POMC)	Endorphins e.g. β-endorphin and other non-opioid peptides e.g. ACTH	μ
Proenkephalin	Enkephalins e.g. Leu^5 enkephalin, Met^5 enkephalin, extended Met^5 enkephalins	δ μ μ
Prodynorphin	Dynorphins e.g. dynorphin A	κ

(ACTH, adrenocorticotrophic hormone.)

an opioid and a non-opioid. Co-proxamol was more effective in controlling the pain and she was able to continue doing more of the daily activities she used to do, until now. She has increasingly been feeling the pain and is suffering terribly. Review of her pain management and symptoms is taken and she is put on regular morphine as part of her palliative care management.

OPIOID ANALGESIC DRUGS

Opioid analgesics are drugs, either naturally occurring (e.g. morphine) or chemically synthesized, that interact with specific opioid receptors to produce the pharmacological effect of analgesia.

Mechanism of action—Opioid analgesic drugs work by agonist action at opioid receptors (see above).

The sense of euphoria produced by strong opioids contributes to their analgesic activity by helping to reduce the anxiety and stress associated with pain. This effect also accounts for the illicit use of these drugs.

Route of administration—Oral, rectal, intravenous, intramuscular, transdermal and transmucosal (as lozenges).

Oral absorption is irregular and incomplete, necessitating larger doses; 70% is removed by first-pass hepatic metabolism. Fentanyl is available in a transdermal drug delivery system as a self-adhesive patch, which is changed every 72 hours. Transdermal fentanyl is particularly useful in patients prone to nausea, sedation or severe constipation with morphine. Morphine is the drug of choice for severe nociceptive pain.

Indications—Strong opioids (Fig. 9.5) are used in moderate to severe pain, particularly visceral, postoperative or cancer-related; in myocardial infarction and acute pulmonary oedema; and in perioperative analgesia (p. 146).

Weak opioids (Fig. 9.5) are used in the relief of 'mild to moderate' pain, as antitussives (Ch. 3) and as antidiarrhoeal agents (Ch. 8), taking advantage of these 'side-effects' of opioid analgesics.

Contraindications—Opioid analgesics should not be given to people in acute respiratory depression, with acute alcoholism, at risk of paralytic ileus, and with head injuries prior to neurological assessment (interferes with assessment of the level of consciousness).

Adverse effects—Opioid analgesics share many side-effects. These can be subdivided into central adverse actions and peripheral adverse actions.

Central adverse actions include the following:

- Drowsiness and sedation, in which initial excitement is followed by sedation and finally coma (on overdose)
- Reduction in sensitivity of the respiratory centre to carbon dioxide, leading to shallow and slow respiration
- Tolerance and dependence (Ch. 5)
- Suppression of cough, an effect exploited clinically in antitussives (Ch. 3)
- Vomiting due to stimulation of the chemoreceptor trigger zone (CTZ)
- Pupillary constriction due to stimulation of the parasympathetic third cranial nerve nucleus
- Hypotension and reduced cardiac output, which are partly due to reduced hypothalamic sympathetic outflow.

Peripheral adverse actions include the following:

- Constipation, is partly due to stimulation of cholinergic activity in gut wall ganglia which results in smooth wall spasm

Fig. 9.5 Opioid analgesics

Weak opioid analgesics	Strong opioid analgesics
Pentazocine Codeine Dihydrocodeine Dextropropoxyphene	Morphine Diamorphine Phenazocine Pethidine Buprenorphine Nalbuphine

- Contraction of smooth muscle in the sphincter of Oddi and in the ureters, which results in an increase in blood amylase and lipase due to pancreatic stasis
- Histamine release, which produces bronchospasm, flushing and arteriolar dilatation
- Lowered sympathetic discharge and direct arteriolar dilatation, which results in lowered cardiac output and hypotension.

Adverse effects of opioids tend to limit the dose that can be given, and the level of analgesia that can be maintained. The most serious of all these effects is respiratory depression, which is the most common cause of death from opioid overdose.

Constipation and nausea are also common problems and clinically it is common to co-administer laxatives and an antiemetic (Ch. 8).

Tolerance and dependence—Tolerance to opioid analgesics can be detected within 24–48 hours from the onset of administration, and it results in increased doses of the drug being needed to achieve the same clinical effect.

Dependence involves μ receptors and is both physical and psychological in nature and is discussed in Chapter 5. If physical dependence develops, it is characterized by a definite withdrawal syndrome following cessation of drug treatment. This syndrome comprises a complex mixture of irritable, and sometimes aggressive, behaviour combined with extremely unpleasant autonomic symptoms such as fever, sweating, yawning and pupillary dilatation. The withdrawal syndrome is relieved by the administration of μ receptor agonists, and worsened by the administration of μ receptor antagonists.

Psychological dependence of opioid analgesics is based on the positive reinforcement provided by euphoria.

In the clinical context, especially in terminal care, where tolerance and dependence can be monitored, they are not inevitably problematic. However, the fear of tolerance and dependence often leads to over-caution in the use of opioid analgesics, and inadequate pain control in some patients.

Therapeutic notes—Strong opioid analgesics include morphine, diamorphine (heroin), phenazocine, pethidine, buprenorphine and nalbuphine:

- **Morphine** remains the most valuable drug for severe pain relief, though it frequently causes nausea and vomiting. It is the drug of choice for severe pain in terminal care. Morphine is the standard against which other opioid analgesics are compared.
- **Diamorphine (heroin)** is twice as potent as morphine, owing to its greater penetration of the blood–brain barrier. It is metabolized to 6-acetylmorphine

and thence morphine in the body. Diamorphine causes less nausea and hypotension than morphine, but more euphoria.

- **Phenazocine** has a more prolonged action than morphine, and it can be administered sublingually. It can be useful in biliary colic as it has less of a tendency to increase biliary spasm than other opioids.
- **Pethidine** is more lipid soluble than morphine, and it has a rapid onset and short duration of action, making it useful in labour. Pethidine is equianalgesic compared with morphine, but it produces less constipation. Interaction with monoamine inhibitors is serious, causing fever, delirium and convulsions or respiratory depression.
- **Buprenorphine** has both agonist and antagonist actions at opioid receptors, and it may precipitate withdrawal symptoms in patients dependent on other opioids. It has a longer duration of action than morphine and its lipid solubility allows sublingual administration. Vomiting may be a problem. Unlike most opioid analgesics, the effects of buprenorphine are only partially antagonized by naloxone owing to its high-affinity attraction to opioid receptors.
- **Nalbuphine** is an agonist at κ receptors and an antagonist at μ receptors. It is equianalgesic compared with morphine, but it produces less nausea and vomiting. High doses cause dysphoria.

Weak opioid analgesics include pentazocine, codeine, dihydrocodeine and dextropropoxyphene:

- **Pentazocine** has both κ/σ receptor agonist and μ antagonist actions, and it may precipitate withdrawal symptoms in patients dependent on other opioids. Pentazocine is weak orally, but, by injection, it has a potency between that of morphine and codeine. It is not recommended because of the side-effects of thought disturbances and hallucinations, which probably are due to its action on σ receptors.
- **Codeine** has about one-twelfth of the analgesic potency of morphine. The incidence of nausea and constipation limit the dose and duration that can be used. Codeine is also used for its antitussive and antidiarrhoeal effects.
- **Dihydrocodeine** has an analgesic efficacy similar to that of codeine. It may cause dizziness and constipation.
- **Dextropropoxyphene** has an analgesic efficacy about half that of codeine (i.e. very mild), and so it is often combined with aspirin or paracetamol. Such mixtures can be dangerous in overdose, with dextropropoxyphene causing respiratory depression and acute heart failure and the paracetamol being hepatotoxic.

Opioid antagonists

Examples of opioid antagonists include naloxone and naltrexone.

Mechanism of action—These drugs act by specific antagonism at opioid receptors: μ, δ and κ receptors are blocked more or less equally. They block the actions of endogenous opioids as well as of morphine-like drugs.

Naloxone is short acting (half-life: 2–4 hours) while naltrexone is long acting (half-life: 10 hours).

Route of administration—Intravenous.

Indications—Opioid antagonists are given to reverse opioid-induced analgesia and respiratory depression rapidly, mainly after overdose, or to improve breathing in newborn babies who have been affected by opioids given to the mother.

Adverse effects—Precipitation of withdrawal in those with physical dependence on opioids. Reversal of analgesic effects of opiate agonist.

HEADACHE AND NEURALGIC PAIN

Headache

Headache is a very common presenting symptom, yet one which can be difficult to manage. The most common causes of headache include:

- Tension-type headache
- Migraine
- Headache associated with eye or sinus disease.

More sinister causes of headache (including meningitis and neoplasia) are less common, and these can often be confidently excluded by the history and by examination.

The pathophysiology underlying headache is unclear, though symptomatic relief is often obtained from NSAIDs and paracetamol (see p. 151). Some headaches are related to stress and anxiety, and these patients may benefit from antidepressant drugs (Ch. 5).

The management of migraine addresses the acute attacks or attempts to prevent migrainous episodes (prophylaxis) in those who experience frequent attacks. Drugs used for acute migrainous attacks:

- NSAIDs and paracetamol (see p. 151)
- Antiemetics (Ch. 8)
- Serotonin (5-HT$_1$) agonists.

Drugs used in migraine prophylaxis are:

- Antihistamine/serotonin (5-HT) antagonists
- β-Antagonists (Ch. 3)
- Tricyclic antidepressants (Ch. 5).

Serotonin (5-HT$_1$) agonists

Sumatriptan and rizatriptan are serotonin agonists.

Mechanism of action—Serotonin agonists are believed to reverse the dilatation of cerebral blood vessels in the acute attack, which may be responsible for some of the symptoms of migraine.

Route of administration—Oral, intranasal, subcutaneous.

Indications—Acute migrainous attacks.

Contraindications—Caution in coronary artery disease (may cause vasoconstriction of coronary vessels), hepatic impairment, pregnancy and breastfeeding.

Adverse effects—Sensations of tingling, heat, chest tightness.

Antihistamine/serotonin antagonists

Pizotifen is the main drug in this class.

Mechanism of action—Unlike the serotonin agonists, pizotifen appears to limit the initial pro-inflammatory and vascular changes which precede migrainous episodes.

Route of administration—Oral.

Indications—Prevention of vascular headache.

Contraindications—Cautions in urinary retention, angle-closure glaucoma, renal impairment, pregnancy, breastfeeding.

Adverse effects—Antimuscarinic effects, drowsiness, increased appetite.

> **HINTS AND TIPS**
>
> Headache is a common complaint, and more often than not it does not represent a sinister pathology. Analgesia will simply help control the symptoms so, if a patient frequently returns with pain, ensure to look for a treatable underlying cause.

Neuralgic pain

Neuralgic pain is classically nerve pain, in the distribution of a particular nerve or nerve root. The most common pathologies are sciatica, herpetic neuralgia and trigeminal neuralgia.

Neuralgia commonly occurs because of compression or entrapment of the nerve or nerve root, and definitive management relies on surgical release of the nerve.

Pharmacological options can be employed when surgery is ill advised, or ineffective, or as an adjunct. NSAIDs are not effective for neuralgic pain. Antidepressants, in particular amitriptyline, often have an 'analgesic' effect in neuralgic pain, and often at a dose lower than their antidepressant effect (Ch. 4).

The other main class of drug used orally in neuralgic pain are the antiepileptics, notably carbamazepine, phenytoin and more recently lamotrigine (Ch. 4). These potentially stabilize the neurons involved, and limit their activation.

Local anaesthesia of the nerve in question can provide relief for some patients, though nerve ablation with drugs or by surgical means can be performed to alleviate symptoms.

LOCAL ANAESTHESIA

Basic concepts

Local anaesthetics are drugs used to inhibit pain sensation. These drugs work by reversibly blocking nerve conduction.

Chemistry

All local anaesthetics have the same basic structure:

- An aromatic group (lipophilic end) linked to a basic side chain (hydrophilic end) by an ester or amide bond (Fig. 9.6)
- The basic side chain (usually a secondary or tertiary amine) is important because only the uncharged molecule can enter the nerve axoplasm.

Potency and duration of action are correlated with high lipid solubility.

Pharmacokinetics

Elimination of local anaesthetics depends on the nature of the chemical bond:

- Local anaesthetics with ester bonds are inactivated by plasma cholinesterases
- Local anaesthetics with amide bonds are degraded by N-dealkylation in the liver.

Metabolites can often be pharmacologically active.

Mechanism of block

Importance of pH and ionization

Local anaesthetics are weak bases ($pK_a = 8$–9). Only the uncharged form can penetrate lipid membranes; thus, quaternary ammonium compounds, which are fully protonated, must be injected directly into the nerve axon if they are to work.

The proportion of uncharged local anaesthetic is governed by the pH, the pK_a and the Henderson–Hasselbalch equation (Ch. 1):

$$B + H^+ = BH^+$$
$$pK_a = pH + \log[BH^+]/[B]$$

A local anaesthetic with a pK_a of 8.0 will be 10% uncharged at pH 7.0, 50% uncharged at pH 8.0, and 5% uncharged at pH 6.0.

Routes of block

The majority of local anaesthetics block by two routes (Fig. 9.7):

- The hydrophobic route, the uncharged form enters the membrane and blocks the channel from a site in the protein membrane interface.
- The hydrophilic route, the uncharged form crosses the membrane to the inside where the charged form blocks the channel. This pathway depends on the channel being open and, therefore, this type of block is use dependent. Use dependency is especially important in the antiarrhythmic action of local anaesthetics.
- Nerve block occurs when the number of non-inactivated channels (those unaffected by the drug) is insufficient to bring about depolarization to threshold.

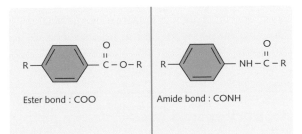

Fig. 9.6 General structure of ester- and amide-linked local anaesthetics.

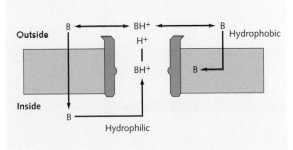

Fig. 9.7 Hydrophobic and hydrophilic routes of block for local anaesthesia.

Routes of administration

Surface anaesthesia

In surface anaesthesia, the local anaesthetic is applied directly to the mucous membranes, e.g. cornea, bronchial tree, oesophagus and genitourinary tract. The local anaesthetic, e.g. lidocaine, must be able to penetrate the tissues easily. For skin, tetracaine (amethocaine) is used to anaesthetize the skin prior to venepuncture, especially in children and anxious adults.

Problems occur when large areas, e.g. the bronchial tree, are anaesthetized.

Infiltration anaesthesia

Infiltration anaesthesia involves direct injection of a local anaesthetic into tissue. Often, a vasoconstrictor such as adrenaline is used with the local anaesthetic to prevent the spread of the local anaesthetic into the systemic circulation. Vasoconstrictors must never be used at extremities as ischaemia could result.

Intravenous regional anaesthesia (IVRA) involves the injection of the local anaesthetic distal to a cuff inflated above arterial pressure. It is important that the cuff is not released prematurely as this could cause the release of a potentially toxic bolus into the circulation. This type of local anaesthetic block is now seldom used.

Nerve block anaesthesia

In nerve block anaesthesia, local anaesthetic is injected close to the appropriate nerve trunk, e.g. the brachial plexus. The injection must be accurate in location.

Spinal and epidural anaesthesia

Spinal anaesthesia involves the injection of a local anaesthetic into the cerebrospinal fluid (CSF) in the subarachnoid space. A certain amount of spread can be controlled by increasing the specific gravity of the solution and tilting the patient.

In epidural anaesthesia, the local anaesthetic is injected into the space between the dura mater and the spinal cord.

In both spinal and epidural anaesthesia, the local anaesthetic acts by blocking mainly spinal roots, as opposed to the spinal cord itself. Problems arise from the block of preganglionic sympathetic fibres supplying the vasculature (causing vasodilatation) and the heart (causing bradycardia), both leading to hypotension. Rostral spread can lead to the blocking of intercostal and phrenic nerves and result in respiratory depression.

Unwanted effects

Unwanted effects of local anaesthetics are mainly associated with the spread of the drug into the systemic circulation. These include:

- Effects on the CNS, such as restlessness, tremor, confusion, agitation. At high doses, CNS depression can occur. Procaine is worse than lidocaine or prilocaine for causing CNS depression, and is seldom used. The exception is cocaine, which, owing to its monoamine-uptake blocking activity, produces euphoria.
- Respiratory depression.
- Possible effects on the cardiovascular system, including myocardial depression and vasodilatation.
- Visual disturbances and twitching.
- Severe toxicity causes convulsions and coma.

Properties and uses

Figure 9.8 shows the properties and uses of the main local anaesthetics, and Figure 9.9 lists other compounds that block sodium channels.

Fig. 9.8 Properties and uses of the main local anaesthetics

	Rate of onset	Duration	Tissue penetration	Chemistry	Common use
Cocaine	Rapid	Moderate	Rapid	Ester bond	ENT
Procaine	Moderate	Short	Slow	Ester bond	Little used, CNS effects
Tetracaine (amethocaine)	Slow	Long	Moderate	Ester bond	Topical, pre-venepuncture
Oxybuprocaine (benoxinate)	Rapid	Short	Rapid	Ester bond	Surface, ophthalmology
Benzocaine	Very slow	Very long	Rapid	Ester bond, no basic side chain	Surface ENT
Lidocaine (lignocaine)	Rapid	Moderate	Rapid	Amide bond	Widely used in all applications, EMLA
Prilocaine	Moderate	Moderate	Moderate	Amide bond	Many uses, IVRA, EMLA. Low toxicity
Bupivacaine	Slow	Long	Moderate	Amide bond	Epidural and spinal anaesthesia

(CNS, central nervous system; EMLA, eutectic mixture of local anaesthetics; ENT, ear, nose and throat; IVRA, intravenous regional anaesthetic.)

Fig. 9.9 Naturally occurring and synthetic sodium-channel blockers

Compound	Source	Type of block
Tetrodotoxin	Puffer fish	Outside only
Saxitoxin	Plankton	Outside only
μ-Conotoxins	Piscivorous marine snail	Affects inactivation
μ-Agatoxins	Funnel web spider	Affects inactivation
α-, β- and γ-toxins	Scorpions	Complex
QX314 and QX222	Synthetic, permanently charged local anaesthetics	Inside only (hydrophobic pathway)
Benzocaine	Synthetic, uncharged local anaesthetic	From within the membrane (hydrophilic pathway)
Local anaesthetics	Plant (cocaine), others synthetic	Inside and from within the membrane

GENERAL ANAESTHESIA

Basic concepts

General anaesthesia is the absence of sensation associated with a reversible loss of consciousness.

General anaesthetics are used as an adjunct to surgical procedures in order to render the patient unaware of, and unresponsive to, painful stimuli. Modern anaesthesia is characterized by the so-called balanced technique, in which drugs and anaesthetic agents are used specifically to produce:

- Analgesia
- Sleep/sedation
- Muscle relaxation and abolition of reflexes.

No one drug or anaesthetic agent can produce all these effects, and so a combination of agents is used in the three clinical stages of surgical general anaesthesia. The three stages are:

- Premedication
- Induction
- Maintenance.

Some may argue that a fourth stage exists, in which drugs are used to reverse the action of agents given in the previous three stages.

Premedication

Premedication is often given on the ward before the patient is taken to the operating theatre (Fig. 9.10), and it has four component aims:

- Relief from anxiety
- Reduction of parasympathetic bradycardia and secretions
- Analgesia
- Prevention of postoperative emesis.

Relief from anxiety

Oral benzodiazepines, e.g. diazepam and midazolam (p. 74), are most effective and they perform three useful functions:

- Relieve apprehension and anxiety before anaesthesia
- Lessen the amount of general anaesthetic required to achieve and to maintain unconsciousness
- Possibly, sedate postoperatively.

Reduction of parasympathetic bradycardia and secretions

Muscarinic antagonists, e.g. atropine and hyoscine (Ch. 4), are used to prevent salivation and bronchial secretions, and more importantly to protect the heart from arrhythmias, particularly bradycardia caused by some inhalation agents and neuromuscular blockers.

Analgesia

Opioid analgesics, e.g. fentanyl, are often given prior to an operation: although the patient is unconscious during surgery, adequate analgesia is important to stop physiological stress reactions to pain. NSAIDs are useful alternatives and adjuncts to opiates, though are likely to be inadequate for severe postoperative pain used alone.

Postoperative antiemesis

Drugs that provide postoperative antiemesis include metoclopramide and prochlorperazine. Nausea and vomiting are common after general anaesthesia, often because of the administration of opioid drugs peri- and postoperatively. Antiemetic drugs can be given with the premedication to inhibit this.

Induction

Intravenous agents (see Fig. 9.10) are used to produce a rapid induction of unconsciousness. Intravenous agents are preferred by patients, since injection lacks the menacing quality of having a mask placed over the face.

Prevention of acid aspiration in emergency and obstetric operations is crucial, and it relies on the administration of either an H_2-receptor antagonist or a proton pump inhibitor prior to induction (Ch. 8).

Maintenance

Inhalation anaesthetic agents (Fig. 9.10) are used to maintain a state of general anaesthesia after induction in most patients, though intravenous agents can be used via a continuous pump.

Fig. 9.10 General anaesthetic agents		
Premedication	**Induction/intravenous agents**	**Maintenance/ inhalation agents**
Relief from anxiety, e.g. diazepam, lorazepam	Barbiturates, e.g. thiopental	Nitrous oxide Halothane
Reduction of parasympathetic bradycardia and secretions, e.g. atropine, hyoscine	Non-barbiturates, e.g. propofol, ketamine	Enflurane Isoflurane Sevoflurane
Analgesia, e.g. NSAIDs, fentanyl		
Postoperative antiemesis, e.g. metoclopramide, prochlorperazine		
(NSAID, non-steroidal anti-inflammatory drug.)		

Anaesthetic agents

Anaesthetic agents depress all excitable tissues including central neurons, cardiac muscle and smooth and striated muscle. Different parts of the CNS have different sensitivities to anaesthetics, and the reticular activating system, which is responsible for consciousness, is among the most sensitive. Hence, it is possible to use anaesthetics at a concentration that produces unconsciousness without unduly depressing the cardiovascular or respiratory centres of the brain, or the myocardium. However, for the majority of anaesthetics the margin of safety is small.

Intravenous anaesthetics

Intravenous anaesthetics, e.g. thiopental, propofol and ketamine, are all CNS depressants. They produce anaesthesia by relatively selective depression of the reticular activating system of the brain. They may be used alone for short surgical procedures, but they are used mainly for the induction of anaesthesia, and, therefore, it is rapidity of onset that is the desirable feature.

Intravenous anaesthetics are all highly lipid-soluble agents and cross the blood–brain barrier rapidly; their rapid onset (<30 seconds) results from this rapid transfer into the brain, and high cerebral blood flow. Duration of action is short (minutes) and terminated by redistribution of the drug from the CNS into less well-perfused tissues (Fig. 9.11); drug metabolism is irrelevant to recovery.

Thiopental

Mechanism of action—Thiopental is a highly lipophilic member of the barbiturate group of CNS depressants that act to potentiate the inhibitory effect of GABA on the $GABA_A/Cl^-$ receptor channel complex.

Route of administration—Intravenous.

Indications—Rapid induction of general anaesthesia.

Contraindications—Thiopental should not be given to a patient with a previous allergy to it; porphyria.

Adverse effects—Respiratory depression, myocardial depression (bradycardia), vasodilatation, anaphylaxis. There is a risk of severe vasospasm if it is accidentally injected into an artery.

Therapeutic notes—Thiopental is a widely used induction agent, but it has no analgesic properties. It provides smooth and rapid (<30 seconds) induction but, owing to its narrow therapeutic margin, overdosage with consequent cardiorespiratory depression can occur. Thiopental is given as the sodium salt, which is unstable in solution and so it must be made up immediately before use.

Propofol

Mechanism of action—Propofol is similar to thiopental in its mechanism of action.

Route of administration—Intravenous.

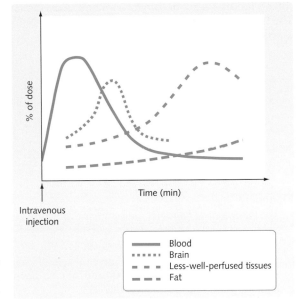

Fig. 9.11 Redistribution of intravenous anaesthetic agents to less well perfused tissues causes a short central duration of action. (Adapted from Rang HP, et al. *Pharmacology*, 7th Edn. Churchill Livingstone 2012.)

Indications—Induction or maintenance of general anaesthesia or sedation in intensive care units.

Contraindications—Propofol should not be given to patients with a previous allergy to it or sedation of ventilated children.

Adverse effects—Convulsions, anaphylaxis, and delayed recovery from anaesthesia have occasionally been reported as side-effects.

Therapeutic notes—Propofol is associated with rapid recovery without nausea or hangover, and it is very widely used. Propofol is the drug of choice if an intravenous agent is to be used to maintain anaesthesia by a continuous infusion.

COMMUNICATION

Dina is a 17-year-old student who presents to accident and emergency, looking very unwell and with severe pain in her right iliac fossa (lower right corner of her abdomen). Her mother told doctors that the pain had originally started around her belly button about a couple of hours ago and that she has vomited twice since. Examination reveals a tender abdomen with guarding. A computed tomography scan shows an inflamed appendix. She is rushed to theatre. Midazolam is given as sedation because she is rather anxious about the sudden forthcoming operation.

Hyoscine is given prior to the operation, since it dries bronchial and salivary secretions. Domperidone is also given beforehand for antiemesis. General anaesthesia is induced by propofol and maintained with isoflurane. The muscle relaxant rocuronium and the analgesic fentanyl (intravenous) are also given for the operation. Rocuronium is stopped before completion of the operation, but a small dose of neostigmine is required to fully reverse the effect of rocuronium.

Etomidate

Mechanism of action—The mechanism of action of etomidate is similar to that of thiopental.

Route of administration—Intravenous.

Indications—Rapid induction of general anaesthesia.

Contraindications—Etomidate should not be given to patients with a previous allergy to it.

Adverse effects—Extraneous muscle movement and pain on injection, possible adrenocortical suppression.

Therapeutic notes—Etomidate is an induction agent that gained favour over thiopental because of its larger therapeutic margin and faster metabolism leading to fewer hangover effects. Etomidate is more prone to causing extraneous muscle movement and pain on injection compared with other agents.

Ketamine

Mechanism of action—Ketamine produces full surgical anaesthesia but the form of the anaesthesia is known as dissociative anaesthesia, as the patient may remain conscious though amnesic and insensitive to pain. This effect is probably related to an action on *N*-methyl-D-aspartate (NMDA)-type glutamate receptors.

Ketamine is a derivative of the street drug PCP (angel dust).

Route of administration—Intravenous, intramuscular.

Indications—Ketamine is used in the induction and maintenance of anaesthesia, especially in children.

Contraindications—Ketamine should not be given to people with hypertension or psychosis.

Adverse effects—These include cardiovascular stimulation, tachycardia and raised arterial blood pressure, as well as transient psychotic sequelae such as vivid dreams and hallucinations.

Therapeutic notes—Ketamine is not often used as an induction agent, owing to the high incidence of dysphoria and hallucinations during recovery in adults. These effects are much less marked in children, and ketamine, in conjunction with a benzodiazepine, is often used for minor procedures in paediatrics.

Inhalation anaesthetics

Examples of inhalation anaesthetics include halothane, enflurane, isoflurane, sevoflurane and desflurane. Nitrous oxide also has anaesthetic properties.

Inhalation anaesthetics may be gases or volatile liquids. They are commonly used for the maintenance of anaesthesia after induction with an intravenous agent.

Mechanism of action—It is not known exactly how inhalation anaesthetic agents produce their effects. Unlike most drugs, inhalation anaesthetics do not all belong to one recognizable chemical class. The shape and electronic configuration of the molecule are evidently unimportant. A distinct anaesthetic 'receptor' is, therefore, unlikely; it would seem that the pharmacological action of inhalation anaesthetics is dependent on the physicochemical properties of the molecule.

Three theories of anaesthesia have received the most attention – the lipid, hydrate and protein theories.

The lipid theory arose because a close correlation was noticed between anaesthetic potency and lipid solubility. It has been suggested that anaesthetics dissolve in membrane lipid and affect its physical state by two possible mechanisms. These are:

- Volume expansion – which is supported by pressure reversal of anaesthesia, but qualitative inconsistencies exist
- Membrane fluidization – although the high concentrations required and weak effect of temperature make this difficult to accept.

The hydrate theory arose because anaesthetic molecules stabilize water molecules in their vicinity. It has been suggested that this alteration of the membrane accounts for the effects of anaesthetics.

Although there is some correlation between potency and the ability to form hydrates, anomalous compounds such as sulphur hexafluoride do not form hydrates, but they do have anaesthetic properties.

The protein theory arose because there is increasing evidence that anaesthetics may act by binding to discrete hydrophobic domains of membrane proteins. This would explain the 'cut-off' phenomenon and the stereoselectivity of anaesthetics, whereby the size of the domain excludes molecules above a certain size or that are the wrong shape. The protein theory is currently popular, but the nature of the target protein(s) in the CNS has not been identified. Possible targets include voltage-operated channels, receptor-operated channels, or secondary-messenger systems.

HINTS AND TIPS

Like the benzodiazepines and barbiturates, thiopental and propofol act via the $GABA_A/Cl^-$ receptor in causing CNS depression.

Pharmacokinetic aspects

The depth of anaesthesia produced by inhalation anaesthetics is directly related to the partial pressure (tension) of the agent in the arterial blood, as this determines the concentration of agent in the CNS. The concentration of anaesthetic in the blood is in turn determined by:

- The concentration of anaesthetic in the inspired gas (alveolar concentration)
- The solubility of the anaesthetic in blood (blood/gas partition coefficient)
- Cardiac output
- Alveolar ventilation.

Rapid induction and recovery are important properties of an anaesthetic agent, allowing flexible control over the arterial tension (and hence brain tension) and, therefore, the depth of anaesthesia. The speed at which induction of anaesthesia occurs is determined by two properties of the anaesthetic: its solubility in blood (blood/gas partition coefficient) and its solubility in fat (lipid solubility). Therefore:

- Agents of low blood solubility (e.g. nitrous oxide, enflurane) produce rapid induction and recovery because relatively small amounts are required to saturate the blood, and so the arterial tension (and hence brain tension) rises and falls quickly (Fig. 9.12).
- Agents of high blood solubility (e.g. halothane) have much slower induction and recovery times because much more anaesthetic solution is required before the arterial anaesthetic tension approaches that of the inspired gas (see Fig. 9.12).

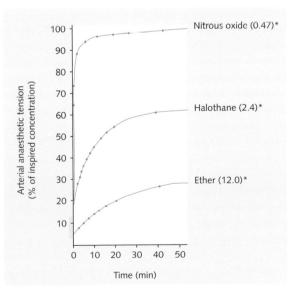

Fig. 9.12 Rate of equilibrium of inhalation anaesthetics in humans. (Adapted from Papper EM, Kitz R. *Uptake and Distribution of Anaesthetic Agents.* McGraw-Hill 1963.)

- Agents with high lipid solubility (e.g. ether) accumulate gradually in the body fat during prolonged anaesthesia, and so may produce a prolonged hangover if used for a long operation (see Fig. 9.12).

Nitrous oxide

Mechanism of action—See above.

Route of administration—Inhalation.

Indications—Nitrous oxide is used in the maintenance of anaesthesia (in combination with other agents), and for analgesia (50% mixture in oxygen: Entonox®).

Contraindications—Pneumothorax. Nitrous oxide diffuses into air containing closed spaces resulting in an increased pressure, in the case of pneumothorax, which may compromise breathing.

Adverse effects—Nitrous oxide was thought to be relatively free of side-effects – it has little effect on cardiovascular and respiratory systems – but the risk of bone marrow suppression is now a known factor.

Therapeutic notes—Nitrous oxide cannot produce surgical anaesthesia when administered alone, because of a lack of potency. It is commonly used as a non-flammable carrier gas for volatile agents, allowing their concentration to be reduced. As a 50% mixture in oxygen, nitrous oxide is a good analgesic, and it is used in childbirth and by paramedics.

Halothane

Mechanism of action—See above.

Route of administration—Inhalation.

Indications—Halothane is used in the maintenance of anaesthesia.

Contraindications—Halothane should not be given to people with a previous reaction to halothane or exposure to halothane in the previous 3 months.

Adverse effects—Like most volatile anaesthetics, halothane causes cardiorespiratory depression.

Respiratory depression results in elevated pCO_2 and perhaps ventricular arrhythmias. Halothane also depresses cardiac muscle fibres and may cause bradycardia. The result of this is a concentration-dependent hypotension.

The most significant toxic effect of halothane is severe hepatic necrosis, which occurs in 1 in 35 000 cases. Lesser degrees of liver damage may occur more frequently. The damage is caused by metabolites of the 20% of administered halothane that is biotransformed in the liver (80% of an administered dose is excreted by the lungs).

Therapeutic notes—Halothane is a halogenated hydrocarbon.

Enflurane

Mechanism of action—See above.

Route of administration—Inhalation.

Indications—Enflurane is used in the maintenance of anaesthesia.

Contraindications—Enflurane should not be given to people with epilepsy.

Adverse effects—Enflurane causes cardiorespiratory depression similar to that with halothane, although the incidence of arrhythmias is much lower than with halothane.

Enflurane undergoes only 2% metabolism in the liver, so it is much less likely than halothane to cause hepatotoxicity. The disadvantage of enflurane is that it may cause electroencephalogram (EEG) changes and muscle twitching, and special caution is needed in epileptic subjects.

Therapeutic notes—Enflurane is a volatile anaesthetic similar to, but less potent than, halothane, about twice the concentration being necessary for maintenance. Induction and recovery times are faster than for halothane.

Isoflurane

Mechanism of action—See above.

Route of administration—Inhalation.

Indications—It is used in the maintenance of anaesthesia.

Contraindications—Susceptibility to malignant hyperthermia.

Adverse effects—Isoflurane has actions similar to those of halothane, but it has fewer effects upon the cardiorespiratory system. Hypotension is caused by a dose-related decrease in systemic vascular resistance rather than a marked fall in cardiac output. Less hepatic metabolism (0.2%) occurs than with enflurane, so hepatotoxicity is even rarer.

Therapeutic notes—Isoflurane is an isomer of enflurane. It has a potency intermediate between that of halothane and enflurane.

Sevoflurane

Mechanism of action—See above.

Route of administration—Inhalation.

Indications—It is used both in gas induction and in the maintenance of anaesthesia.

Contraindications—Susceptibility to malignant hyperthermia.

Adverse effects—Similar to isoflurane.

Therapeutic notes—Sevoflurane is probably the most widely used inhalation agent.

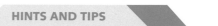

HINTS AND TIPS

Nitrous oxide is used as an adjunct to other inhaled agents, as it reduces the dose required to maintain anaesthesia, thus limiting side-effects and allowing more rapid recovery.

Use of neuromuscular blockers in anaesthesia

For some operations, e.g. intra-abdominal, complete relaxation of skeletal muscle is essential. Some general anaesthetic agents have significant neuromuscular blocking actions, but drugs that specifically block the neuromuscular junction are frequently employed, e.g. suxamethonium, rocuronium, vecuronium and atracurium (Ch. 4).

Inflammation, allergic diseases and immunosuppression

Objectives

After reading this chapter, you will:

* Understand the basic principles behind inflammation, allergies and immunosuppression
* Know the different drug classes used to treat these conditions and their mechanism of action
* Be aware of the indications, contraindications and adverse drug reactions.

INFLAMMATION

Inflammation describes the changes seen in response to tissue injury or insult including pain, redness, heat, swelling and loss of function. These changes occur because of dilatation of local blood vessels, which lead to increased permeability and increased receptiveness for leucocytes. This results in the accumulation of inflammatory cells at the site of injury. The main cells seen in an acute inflammatory response are neutrophils and macrophages. Lymphocytes, basophils and eosinophils also accumulate.

Inflammatory responses are produced and controlled by the interaction of a wide range of inflammatory mediators, some derived from leucocytes, some from the damaged tissues. Examples include:

* Histamine
* Kinins (bradykinin)
* Neuropeptides (substance-P, calcitonin gene-related peptide)
* Cytokines (e.g. interleukins (ILs))
* Arachidonic acid metabolites (eicosanoids).

Arachidonic acid metabolites: the eicosanoids

Of the inflammatory mediators mentioned above, the eicosanoids are of special importance because they are involved in the majority of inflammatory reactions and thus most anti-inflammatory therapy is based on the manipulation of their biosynthesis.

The eicosanoids are a family of polyunsaturated fatty acids formed from arachidonic acid. The biosynthetic pathway is shown in Figure 10.1. Arachidonic acid is derived mainly from phospholipids of cell membranes, from which it is mobilized by the action of the enzyme phospholipase A_2. Arachidonic acid is then further metabolized:

* By cyclooxygenase to produce the 'classic prostaglandins', thromboxane and prostacyclin, collectively known as the prostanoids
* By lipoxygenase to produce the leukotrienes

The actions of eicosanoids in inflammatory reactions are listed in Figure 10.2.

Anti-inflammatory drugs

The main drugs used for their broad-spectrum anti-inflammatory effects are:

* Non-steroidal anti-inflammatory drugs
* Steroidal anti-inflammatory drugs (glucocorticoids) (Ch. 6 and p. 154).

Both these classes of anti-inflammatory drug exert their effect by inhibiting the formation of eicosanoids (see Fig. 10.1).

In addition, a number of other drug classes have more restricted anti-inflammatory actions. These are:

* Disease-modifying antirheumatic drugs (DMARDs) (p. 155)
* Drugs used to treat gout (p. 156)
* Antihistamines (p. 162)
* Drugs used to treat skin disorders.

NSAIDs

NSAIDs all possess the ability to inhibit both forms of the enzyme cyclooxygenase (see Fig. 10.1), an action that is responsible for their pharmacological effects (see Fig. 10.4).

The first drugs of this type were the salicylates (e.g. aspirin), extracted from the bark of the willow tree. Subsequently, many synthetic and semi-synthetic NSAIDs have been created. Chemically and structurally heterogeneous, they are related through their common mechanism of action (Fig. 10.3).

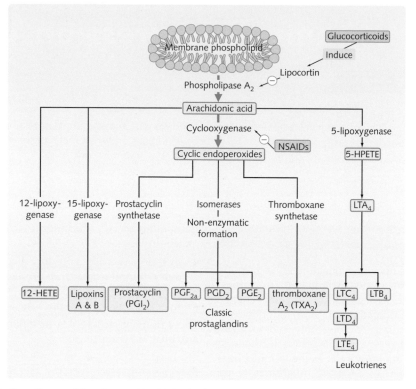

Fig. 10.1 Biosynthetic pathway of the eicosanoids. (HETE, hydroxyeicosatetraenoic acid; HPETE, hydroperoxyeicosatetraenoic acid; LT, leukotrienes; NSAID, non-steroidal anti-inflammatory drug; PG, prostaglandin.)

Fig. 10.2 Actions of the eicosanoids in the inflammatory reaction

Eicosanoid	Actions in inflammation
Prostanoids	
'Classic prostaglandins' e.g. PGD_2, PGE_2, PGF_2	Produce increased vasodilatation, vascular permeability and oedema in an inflammatory reaction; prostaglandins also sensitize nociceptive fibres to stimulation by other inflammatory mediators
Thromboxane A_2 (TXA_2)	Platelet aggregation and vasoconstriction
Prostacyclin (PGI_2)	Inhibition of platelet aggregation and vasodilatation
Leukotrienes	
E.g. LTB_4, LTC_4	Increase vascular permeability, promote leucocyte chemotaxis (and cause contraction of bronchial smooth muscle)

Mechanism of action—The main action of all the NSAIDs is inhibition of the enzyme cyclooxygenase. This enzyme is involved in the metabolism of arachidonic acid to form the prostanoids, i.e. the 'classic prostaglandins', prostacyclin and thromboxane A_2. Inhibition of cyclooxygenase can occur by several mechanisms:

- Irreversible inhibition – e.g. aspirin causes acetylation of the active site.
- Competitive inhibition – e.g. ibuprofen acts as a competitive substrate.
- Reversible, non-competitive inhibition – e.g. paracetamol has a free radical trapping action that interferes with the production of hydroperoxidases, which are believed to have an essential role in cyclooxygenase activity.

Cyclooxygenase exists in two enzyme isoforms:

- **COX-1:** Expressed in most tissues, especially platelets, gastric mucosa and renal vasculature, and involved in physiological cell signalling. Most adverse effects of NSAIDs are caused by inhibition of COX-1.
- **COX-2:** Induced at sites of inflammation and produces the prostanoids involved in inflammatory responses. Analgesic and anti-inflammatory effects of NSAIDs are largely due to inhibition of COX-2.

Fig. 10.3 Classes of non-steroidal anti-inflammatory drugs and comparison of their main actions

Chemical class	Examples	Analgesic	Antipyretic	Anti-inflammatory
Salicylic acids	Aspirin	+	+	+
Propionic acids	Ibuprofen Fenuprofen	+	+	+
Acetic acids	Indometacin	+	+	++
Oxicams	Piroxicam	+	+	++
Pyrazolones	Phenylbutazone	+/−	+	++
Fenemates	Mefenamic acid	+	+	+/−
para-Aminophenols	Paracetamol	+	+	−

COX-2-specific inhibitors have a reduced incidence of gastric side-effects. However, they are associated with an increased incidence of adverse cardiovascular events (such as myocardial infarction).

Clinical effects—NSAIDs work by the inhibition of cyclooxygenase and resulting inhibition of prostaglandin synthesis, producing three major clinical actions of potential therapeutic benefit: analgesia, an anti-inflammatory action and an antipyretic action (Fig. 10.4).

Not all NSAIDs possess these three actions to exactly the same extent, an example being the lack of anti-inflammatory activity possessed by paracetamol (see Fig. 10.3).

In addition aspirin has a pronounced effect on inhibiting platelet aggregation, due to reduced thromboxane synthesis. It is used in the primary and secondary prevention of cardiovascular and cerebrovascular events (Ch. 2).

Indications—NSAIDs are widely used for a variety of complaints. They are available on prescription and 'over the counter'. Their use includes musculoskeletal and joint diseases (strains, sprains, rheumatic problems, arthritis, gout, etc.), analgesia for mild to moderate pain relief and symptomatic relief in fever.

Contraindications—NSAIDs should not be given to people with gastrointestinal ulceration or bleeding, or a previous hypersensitivity to any NSAID. Caution

Fig. 10.4 Three major clinical actions of non-steroidal anti-inflammatory drugs (NSAIDs)

Clinical action	Mechanism of action
Analgesic action	The analgesic effect is largely a peripheral effect that is due to the inhibition of prostaglandin synthesis at the site of pain and inflammation Prostaglandins do not produce pain directly, but sensitize nociceptive fibre nerve endings to other inflammatory mediators (bradykinin, histamine, 5-HT), amplifying the basic pain message; prostaglandins of the E and F series are implicated in this sensitizing action Thus NSAIDs are most effective against pain where there is an inflammatory component A small component of the analgesic action of NSAIDs is a consequence of a central effect in reducing prostaglandin synthesis in the CNS; paracetamol especially works in this manner
Anti-inflammatory action	Prostaglandins produce increased vasodilatation, vascular permeability and oedema in an inflammatory reaction Inhibition of prostaglandin synthesis therefore reduces this part of the inflammatory reaction NSAIDs do not inhibit the numerous other mediators involved in an inflammatory reaction; thus inflammatory cell accumulation, for example, is not inhibited
Antipyretic action	During a fever leucocytes release inflammatory pyrogens (e.g. interleukin-1) as part of the immune response; these act on the thermoregulatory centre in the hypothalamus to cause an increase in body temperature This effect is believed to be mediated by an increase in hypothalamic prostaglandins (PGEs), the generation of which is inhibited by NSAIDs NSAIDs do not affect temperature under normal circumstances or in heat stroke

should be used in asthma and when renal function is impaired.

Adverse effects—Generalized adverse effects of NSAIDs are common, especially in the elderly and in chronic users, and mostly arise from the non-selective inhibition of COX-1 and COX-2 (Fig. 10.5).

Less commonly, liver disorders and bone marrow depression are seen. Other unwanted effects that are relatively specific to individual compounds are also seen (see below).

Therapeutic notes on individual NSAIDs

Salicylic acids, e.g. aspirin:

- Is cheap, and is still the drug of choice for many sorts of mild pain despite a relatively high incidence of gastrointestinal side-effects. It is also used for its antiplatelet action
- Produces tinnitus in toxic doses.

Propionic acids, e.g. ibuprofen:

- Has a low incidence of side-effects.

Acetic acids, e.g. indometacin:

- Is a highly potent inhibitor of COX that is effective but associated with a high incidence of side-effects.
- May cause neurological effects such as dizziness and confusion, as well as gastrointestinal upsets.

Oxicams, e.g. piroxicam:

- Is a potent drug widely used for chronic inflammatory conditions.
- Is given only once daily, but causes a relatively high incidence of gastrointestinal problems.

Pyrazolones, e.g. phenylbutazone:

- Is an extremely potent agent but can produce a fatal bone marrow aplasia. For this reason it is reserved for the treatment of intractable pain in ankylosing spondylitis.

Fenemates, e.g. mefenamic acid:

- Is a moderately potent drug
- Commonly causes gastrointestinal upsets and occasionally skin rashes.

para-**Aminophenols,** e.g. paracetamol:

- Is used as an analgesic and antipyretic but is not considered an anti-inflammatory drug.
- Is effective for pain, especially headaches, and fever. This is probably due to its mechanism of action in trapping free radicals and interfering with the production of hydroperoxidases, which are believed to have an essential role in cyclooxygenase activity. In areas of inflammation, phagocytic cells produce high levels of peroxide that swamp this effect. For more information see Chapter 9.

COX-2 specific inhibitors, e.g. lumiracoxib and celecoxib:

- Preferentially inhibit the inducible COX-2 enzyme, limiting COX-1-mediated side-effects observed with other, non-specific NSAIDs.

The COX-2 inhibitors are licensed in the UK for symptomatic relief in osteoarthritis and rheumatoid arthritis. They are contraindicated in inflammatory bowel disease, ischaemic heart disease or cerebrovascular disease.

Steroidal anti-inflammatory drugs (glucocorticoids)

There are two main groups of corticosteroids, the glucocorticoids and the mineralocorticoids. It is the glucocorticoids (such as cortisone and cortisol), which posses powerful anti-inflammatory actions that make them useful in several diseases, e.g. rheumatoid arthritis, inflammatory bowel conditions, bronchial asthma (see Ch. 3) and inflammatory conditions of the skin.

Their profound generalized inhibitory effects on inflammatory responses result from the effects of corticosteroids in altering the activity of certain

Fig. 10.5 General adverse effects of non-steroidal anti-inflammatory drugs (NSAIDs)

System	Adverse effect	Cause
GI	Dyspepsia, nausea, vomiting	Inhibition of the normal protective actions of prostaglandins on the gastric mucosa
	Ulcer formation and potential haemorrhage risk in chronic users	PGE_2 and PGI_2 normally inhibit gastric acid secretion, increase mucosal blood flow, and have a cytoprotective action
Renal	Renal damage/nephrotoxicity Renal failure can occur after years of chronic misuse	Inhibition of PGE_2- and PGI_2-mediated vasodilatation in the renal medulla and glomeruli
Other	Bronchospasm, skin rashes, other allergic-type reactions	Hypersensitivity reaction/allergy to drug

(GI, gastrointestinal; PC, prostaglandin.)

corticosteroid-responsive genes. The anti-inflammatory action results from:

- Reduced production of acute inflammatory mediators, especially the eicosanoids (see Fig. 10.1). Corticosteroids prevent the formation of arachidonic acid from membrane phospholipids by inducing the synthesis of a polypeptide called lipocortin. Lipocortin inhibits phospholipase A_2, the enzyme normally responsible for mobilizing arachidonic acid from cell membrane phospholipids, and thus inhibits the subsequent formation of both prostaglandins and leukotrienes.
- Reduced numbers and activity of circulating immunocompetent cells, neutrophils and macrophages.
- Decreased activity of macrophages and fibroblasts involved in the chronic stages of inflammation, leading to decreased inflammation and decreased healing. Glucocorticoids are discussed in detail in Ch. 6.

INFLAMMATORY DISEASES

Rheumatoid arthritis

DMARDs (disease modifying anti-rheumatic drugs)

DMARDs are a diverse group of agents that are mainly used in the treatment of rheumatoid arthritis, which is a chronic, progressive and destructive inflammatory disease of the joints (Fig. 10.6).

The mechanism of action of the DMARDs is often unclear – they appear to have a long-term depressive effect on the inflammatory response as well as possibly modulating other aspects of the immune system.

All DMARDs have a slow onset of action, with clinical improvement not becoming apparent until 4–6 months after the initiation of treatment. DMARDs

Fig. 10.6 Disease-modifying antirheumatic drugs (DMARDs)

Class	Example
Gold salts	Sodium aurothiomalate, auranofin
Penicillamine	Penicillamine
Antimalarials	Chloroquine, hydroxyquinine
Sulfasalazine	Sulfasalazine
Immunosuppressants	Cytotoxic drugs: methotrexate, azathioprine, ciclosporin

have been shown to improve symptoms and reduce disease activity. They are believed to slow erosive damage at joints.

DMARDs are generally indicated for use in severe, active, progressive rheumatoid arthritis when NSAIDs alone have proved inadequate. DMARDs are frequently used in combination with an NSAID and/or low-dose glucocorticoids.

Gold salts

Examples of gold salts include sodium aurothiomalate and auranofin.

Mechanism of action—The mechanism of action of gold salts is unknown – they may be taken up by, and inhibit, mononuclear macrophages, or may affect the production of free radicals.

Route of administration—Sodium aurothiomalate is given by intramuscular injection, and auranofin orally.

Adverse effects—Rashes, proteinuria, ulceration, diarrhoea, bone marrow suppression.

Therapeutic notes—Careful patient monitoring, including blood counts and urine analysis, is necessary. If any serious adverse effects develop, treatment must be stopped.

Penicillamine

Mechanism of action—The mechanism of action of penicillamine is unknown. It chelates metals and has immunomodulatory effects, including suppression of immunoglobulin production and effects on immune complexes. Penicillamine may also decrease synthesis of interleukin (IL).

Route of administration—Oral.

Adverse effects—Rashes, proteinuria, ulceration, gastrointestinal upsets, fever, transient loss of taste, bone marrow suppression.

Therapeutic notes—As for gold salts.

Antimalarials

Examples of antimalarials include chloroquine and hydroxychloroquine (Ch. 11).

Mechanism of action—The mechanism of antimalarials is unclear. They interfere with a wide variety of leucocyte functions, including IL-1 production by macrophages, lymphoproliferative responses and T-cell cytotoxic responses.

Route of administration—Oral.

Adverse effects—At the low doses currently recommended for antimalarials, toxicity is rare. The major adverse effect is retinal toxicity.

Therapeutic notes—People on antimalarials should have their vision monitored.

Sulfasalazine

Mechanism of action—Sulfasalazine is broken down in the gut into its two component molecules, 5-aminosalicylate (5-ASA) and sulfapyridine. The 5-ASA moiety is believed to be a free radical scavenger and responsible for most of this drug's antirheumatic effects.

Route of administration—Oral.

Adverse effects—Side-effects of sulfasalazine are mainly due to sulfapyridine; they are common, but rarely serious. These include nausea, vomiting, headache and rashes. Rarely, blood disorders and oligospermia are reported.

Therapeutic notes—People on sulfasalazine should have their blood counts monitored.

Immunosuppressants

Certain drugs with immunosuppressive actions have been shown to be effective in rheumatoid arthritis. These include azathioprine, ciclosporin and corticosteroids which may work by suppressing the autoimmune component of rheumatoid arthritis (p. 154).

> ### HINTS AND TIPS
>
> DMARDs are prescribed by a specialist. Patients taking these agents need regular blood tests to assess their renal and liver function, and to monitor their red and white blood cell counts.

Cytokine inhibitors

Cytokine inhibitors are also thought to retard destruction of joints caused by rheumatoid arthritis. They are usually used for highly active rheumatoid arthritis in those who have failed to respond to at least two standard DMARDs. The primary pro-inflammatory cytokines are tumour necrosis factor (TNF)-α and IL-1. Thus, their inflammatory role in diseases, such as rheumatoid arthritis can be reduced via cytokine inhibitors.

Monoclonal antibodies

Examples of monoclonal antibodies include adalimumab, tocilizumab and infliximab.

Mechanism of action—The monoclonal antibodies bind TNF-α, preventing its interaction with cell surface receptors and the subsequent proinflammatory events.

Indications—Moderate to severe rheumatoid arthritis, after DMARDs have not provided an adequate response.

Contraindications—Pregnancy, breastfeeding, severe infections, heart failure.

Route of administration—Subcutaneous injection.

Adverse effects—Tuberculosis, septicaemia, gastrointestinal disturbance, worsening heart failure, hypersensitivity reactions, blood disorders.

Interactions—Avoid concomitant use of live vaccines.

Therapeutic notes—Monitor for infections, discontinue if active tuberculosis is suspected.

Soluble TNF-α blocker

An example is etanercept.

Mechanism of action—Contains the ligand-binding component of the human TNF receptor. It, therefore, competes with the patient's own receptors, thereby acting like a sponge to remove most of the TNF-α molecules from the joints and blood.

Indications—Moderate to severe rheumatoid arthritis, after DMARDs have not provided an adequate response.

Contraindications—Pregnancy, breastfeeding, severe infections, heart failure.

Route of administration—Subcutaneous injection.

Adverse effects—Predisposition to infections, exacerbation of heart failure or demyelinating central nervous system (CNS) disorders, blood disorders.

Interactions—Avoid concomitant use of live vaccines.

Therapeutic notes—Monitor for infections.

> ### HINTS AND TIPS
>
> The -mab of adalimumab and infliximab stands for their being Monoclonal AntiBodies! The -rcept of etanercept is a useful clue to remember it is the soluble ReCEPTor for TNF-α!

> ### COMMUNICATION
>
> Mrs Arlington, a 50-year-old secretary, presented at her GP because of worsening pain in her left and right wrists and fingers, causing her increasing difficulty to type. Tender swelling is noted at those joints. A diagnosis of rheumatoid arthritis is made following X-ray showing erosions and blood tests showing that she is positive for IgM rheumatoid factor. Initially, she is given daily aspirin but is unable to tolerate it and returns 3 weeks later complaining of gastrointestinal pain. When planning alternative treatment, her hypertension and mild angina (cardiovascular risk factors) are taken into account. The aspirin is replaced by ibuprofen and she is given omeprazole (a proton pump inhibitor) to protect her stomach. This helps to begin with, however, 3 months later she presents with worsening symptoms. A diagnosis of progressive rheumatoid arthritis is made. The ibuprofen is replaced by prednisolone (a glucocorticoid) and she is put on the DMARD, sulfasalazine.

Gout

Gout is a condition in which uric acid (monosodium urate) crystals are deposited in tissues, especially in the joints, provoking an inflammatory response that manifests as an extremely painful acute arthritis. Uric acid crystallizes in the tissues when plasma urate levels are high, due to either excessive production or reduced renal excretion.

There are two treatment strategies for gout – treatment of an acute attack and prophylaxis against further attacks (Fig. 10.7).

Treatment of an acute attack

Non-steroidal anti-inflammatory drugs
At the onset of an acute attack of gout, NSAIDs are used for their general anti-inflammatory and analgesic effects (p. 151).

Aspirin and other salicylates are not used in gout as they inhibit uric acid excretion in the urine, exacerbating serum concentrations.

Colchicine
Mechanism of action—Colchicine helps in gouty arthritis by inhibiting the migration of leucocytes such as neutrophils into the inflamed joint. This effect is achieved as a result of the action of colchicine binding to tubulin, the protein monomer of microtubules, resulting in their depolymerization. The end result is that cytoskeletal movements and cell motility are severely inhibited.

The inhibition of microtubular function inhibits mitotic spindle formation, giving colchicine a cytotoxic effect on dividing cells. This cytotoxic effect is responsible for side-effects of colchicine.

Route of administration—Oral, rarely intravenously.

Adverse effects—Side-effects of colchicine include gastrointestinal toxicity, with nausea, vomiting and diarrhoea, occurring in 80% of people. Rarely, bone marrow suppression and renal failure occur.

Therapeutic notes—Colchicine is rapidly effective. It is given for the first 24 hours of an attack and then for no more than 7 days. Nausea and vomiting are common side-effects.

Prophylaxis against recurrent attacks

Preventative management of gout includes diet and lifestyle changes, as well as the use of drugs that reduce plasma uric acid concentration. These drugs should not be used during an acute attack, as they will initially worsen symptoms. NSAIDs or colchicine should be co-administered for the first 3 months of treatment, as initiation of prophylactic treatment may precipitate an acute attack.

Agents that reduce uric acid synthesis
Allopurinol and febuxostat (xanthine oxidase inhibitors) are examples of a drug that reduces uric acid synthesis.

Mechanism of action—Allopurinol inhibits the enzyme xanthine oxidase, which converts purines (from DNA breakdown) into uric acid, thus reducing uric acid production.

Route of administration—Oral

Adverse effects—Headaches, dyspepsia, diarrhoea, rash, drug interactions and acute exacerbation of gout initially. Rarely, life-threatening hypersensitivity occurs.

Therapeutic notes—Febuxostat is indicated in hyperuricaemia where urate deposition has occured (in the form of tophi or arthritis).

Agents that increase uric acid excretion
Uricosurics are drugs that increase uric acid excretion. Examples of uricosurics include sulfinpyrazone and probenecid.

Mechanism of action—Uricosurics compete with uric acid for reabsorption in the proximal tubules, preventing uric acid reabsorption and resulting in uricosuria.

Route of administration—Oral.

Adverse effects—Gastrointestinal upset, deposition of uric acid crystals in the kidney, interference with excretion of certain drugs, and acute exacerbation of gout initially.

Therapeutic notes—Uricosurics should not be used during an acute attack of gout. NSAIDs or colchicine should be co-administered for the first 3 months of treatment, as initiation of treatment may precipitate an acute attack.

Skin disorders

The most common skin diseases are eczema, acne, psoriasis, skin cancer (usually managed surgically), viral warts and urticaria.

Fig. 10.7 Drugs used in the treatment of gout	
Treatment of an acute attack	**Example**
NSAIDs	Indometacin
Immunosuppressive	Colchicine
Prophylaxis against recurrent attacks (reduction of plasma uric acid concentration)	
Agents that reduce uric acid synthesis	Allopurinol
Agents that increase uric acid excretion (Uricosurics)	Sulfinpyrazone, probenecid
(NSAID, non-steroidal anti-inflammatory drug.)	

Eczema (dermatitis)

Eczema is an inflammatory disease of the skin, defined by the presence of epidermal intercellular oedema or spongiosis. It can occur because of a number of factors, such as:

- Exogenous irritants and contact allergens
- Infections
- Atopy
- Drugs
- Certain environmental conditions such as low humidity and ultraviolet light.

Drugs used to treat eczema and their targets are shown in Figure 10.8.

Acne

Acne affects the pilosebaceous unit and occurs where these are numerous, such as on the face, back and chest. It is characterized by the presence of keratin plugs in the sebaceous duct openings, known as comedones. Other signs of worsening acne include inflammatory papules, pustules, nodules, cysts and scars.

Acne is stimulated by androgens, which is why it is related to puberty, and why the anti-androgen cyproterone is often used in females with acne (Ch. 6).

The drugs used to treat acne and their targets are shown in Figure 10.9.

Psoriasis

Psoriasis is a genetic skin disorder that manifests under certain conditions including stress, infection, damage from ultraviolet light, or trauma. In psoriasis, the turn-over rate of skin is eight times that of normal skin (7 days instead of 56 days). Psoriasis is characterized by:

- Thickened skin plaques
- Superficial scales

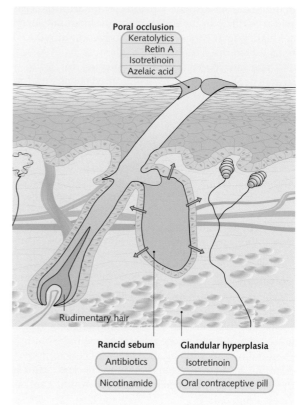

Fig. 10.9 Characteristics of acne and point of action of its drug treatment. (Redrawn from Page et al. 2006.)

- Dilated capillaries in the dermis (these might act to initiate psoriasis or as nourishment for hyperproliferating skin)
- An infiltrate of inflammatory cells, especially lymphocytes and neutrophils, in the epidermis and dermis, respectively.

Drugs used to treat psoriasis and their targets are shown in Figure 10.10.

Treatment of skin disorders

Corticosteroids

Examples of corticosteroids include clobetasol propionate, betamethasone, clobetasol butyrate and hydrocortisone (Fig. 10.11).

Mechanism of action—Corticosteroids suppress components of the inflammatory reaction (see Ch. 6 and Fig. 10.8).

Route of administration—Topically; orally, intradermally or intravenously in severe disease.

Indications—Corticosteroids are used for the relief of symptoms due to inflammatory conditions of the skin other than those due to infection, e.g. in eczema.

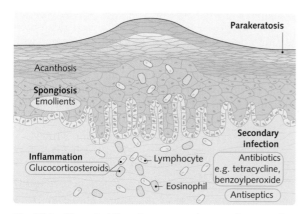

Fig. 10.8 Characteristics of eczema and point of action of its drug treatment. (Redrawn from Page et al. 2006.)

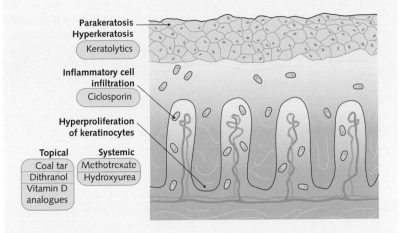

Fig. 10.10 Characteristics of psoriasis and point of action of its drug treatment. (Redrawn from Page et al. 2006.)

Fig. 10.11 Potency of some topical steroids (UK classification and nomenclature)		
Group	**Approved name**	**Proprietary name**
I (very potent)	Clobetasol propionate	Dermovate®
II (potent)	Betamethasone valerate 0.1% Beclometasone dipropionate Hydrocortisone 17-butyrate	Betnovate® Propaderm® Locoid®
III (moderately potent)	Clobetasone butyrate	Eumovate®
IV (mild)	Hydrocortisone 1% Hydrocortisone 2%	Various Various

Adapted from Graham-Brown et al. Mosby's Color Atlas and Text of Dermatology, 1st edn. 1998.

Contraindications—Rosacea, untreated skin infections.

Adverse effects—Most likely to occur with prolonged, or high dose therapy. Local – spread or worsening of infection, thinning of the skin, impaired wound healing, irreversible striae atrophicae. Systemic – immunosuppression, peptic ulceration, osteoporosis, hypertension, cataracts.

Therapeutic notes—Withdrawal of corticosteroids after high doses or prolonged use should be gradual (Ch. 6).

Dithranol

Dithranol is the most potent topical drug for the treatment of psoriasis.

Mechanism of action—Dithranol modifies keratinization, but the mechanism is unclear (see Fig. 10.10).

Route of administration—Topical.

Contraindications—Dithranol should not be given to people with hypersensitivity or acute and pustular psoriasis.

Adverse effects—Local skin irritation, staining of skin and hair.

Vitamin D analogues

Calcipotriol and tacalcitol are vitamin D analogue derivatives.

Vitamin D analogues are keratolytics, though also used in vitamin D deficiency related to gastrointestinal/biliary disease and renal failure (Ch. 8).

Mechanism of action—The exact mechanism of action is still unclear, but several effects of vitamin D analogues have been observed. These include inhibition of epidermal proliferation and induction of terminal keratinocyte differentiation (see Fig. 10.10).

The anti-inflammatory properties of vitamin D analogues include inhibition of T-cell proliferation and of cytokine release, decreased capacity of monocytes to stimulate T-cell proliferation and to stimulate lymphokine release from T cells, and inhibition of neutrophil accumulation in psoriatic skin.

Route of administration—Topical.

Indications—Psoriasis.

Contraindications—Vitamin D analogues should not be given to people with disorders of calcium metabolism. They should not be used on the face, as irritation may occur.

Adverse effects—Side-effects of vitamin D analogues include local irritation and dermatitis. High doses may affect calcium homoeostasis.

Tar preparations

Coal tar, made up of about 10 000 components, is a keratolytic that is more potent than salicylic acid. It also has anti-inflammatory and antipruritic properties.

Mechanism of action—Coal tar modifies keratinization, but the mechanism is unclear (see Fig. 10.10).

Route of administration—Topical.

Indications—Psoriasis and occasionally eczema.

Contraindications—Coal tar should not be given to people with acute or pustular psoriasis or in the presence of an infection. It should not be used on the face or on broken or inflamed skin.

Adverse effects—Skin irritation and acne-like eruptions, photosensitivity, staining of the skin and hair.

Salicylates

Salicylic acid is keratolytic at a concentration of 3–6%.

Mechanism of action—Salicylic acid causes desquamation via the solubilization of cell-surface proteins that maintain the integrity of the stratum corneum.

Route of administration—Topical.

Indications—Hyperkeratosis, eczema, psoriasis (combined with coal tar or dithranol preparations) and acne, wart and callus eradication.

Contraindications—Sensitivity to the drug, or broken or inflamed skin. High concentrations, such as those needed to treat warts, should not be given to people with diabetes mellitus or peripheral vascular disease, as ulceration may be induced.

Adverse effects—Side-effects of salicylic acid include anaphylactic shock in those sensitive to the drug, skin irritation and excessive drying, and systemic effects if used long term.

Emollients

Emollients are used to soothe and hydrate the skin. A simple preparation is aqueous cream, which is often as effective as more complex drugs.

Most creams are thin emollients, whereas a mixture of equal parts soft white paraffin and liquid paraffin is a thick emollient. Camphor, menthol and phenol preparations have antipruritic effects, whereas zinc- and titanium-based emollients have mild astringent (contracting) effects.

Mechanism of action—Emollients hydrate the skin and reduce transepidermal water loss.

Route of administration—Topical. Many emollients can be added to bath water.

Indications—Emollients are used for the long-term treatment of dry scaling disorders.

Contraindications—None.

Adverse effects—Some ingredients, such as lanolin or antibacterials, may induce an allergic reaction.

Therapeutic notes—The use of emollients lessens the need for topical steroids, therefore limiting potential side-effects.

Other drugs used in skin disease

Many other drugs are employed in the management of skin disease. Some of the more common drugs are summarized in Figure 10.12.

Preparations of drugs for use on skin

Drugs applied to the skin are delivered by a variety of vehicles such as ointments, creams, pastes, powders, aerosols, gels, lotions and tinctures. Factors affecting the choice of vehicle include:

- The solubility of the active drug
- The ability of the drug to penetrate the skin
- The stability of the drug–vehicle complex
- The ability of the vehicle to delay evaporation, this being greatest for ointments and least for tinctures.

Fig. 10.12 Other drugs used in skin disease, their indications and mechanisms of action

Drug	Indication	Mechanism of action
Benzoyl peroxide	Acne vulgaris	Antibacterial/keratolytic
Retinoids (vitamin A derivatives)	Psoriasis/acne	Keratolytic/cyto-inhibitory
Psoralen	Psoriasis	Mutates DNA/cytotoxic
Methotrexate	Psoriasis	Cytotoxic
Ciclosporin (cyclosporin)	Psoriasis	Immunosuppressant
Antibacterial, antiviral, antifungal	Skin infections/warts	Antimicrobial
Antiparasite preparations	Skin/hair infestations	Parasite toxins

From Graham-Brown et al. Mosby's Color Atlas and Text of Dermatology, 1st edn. 1998. By permission of Mosby.

ALLERGIC DISORDERS AND DRUG THERAPY

Allergic reactions occur when the immune system mounts an inappropriate response to an innocuous foreign substance.

Most common allergic disorders are caused by IgE-mediated type I immediate hypersensitivity reactions that occur in a previously sensitized person re-exposed to the sensitizing antigen. Type I immediate hypersensitivity reactions are also known as atopic disorders.

Patients with atopic diseases have an inherited predisposition to develop IgE antibodies to allergens that are normally innocuous and non-antigenic. These specific IgE antibodies become bound to high-affinity IgE receptors (FcεRI) on the surface of tissue mast cells and blood basophils. The cross-linking of this cell-surface-bound IgE by antigens (allergens), on subsequent exposure, induces degranulation and release of mediators such as histamine, leukotrienes and prostaglandins (Fig. 10.13).

The released vasoactive and inflammatory mediators produce many local and systemic effects, including vasodilatation, increased vascular permeability, smooth muscle contraction, oedema, glandular hypersecretion and inflammatory cell infiltration.

Depending on the site of this reaction and release of mediators, a variety of disorders can result (Fig. 10.14).

Drug therapy of allergic disorders

The most effective therapy in hypersensitivity reactions is avoidance of the offending antigen or environment. When this is not possible, drug therapy can be of use (Fig. 10.15).

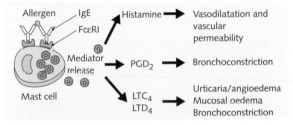
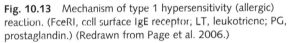

Fig. 10.13 Mechanism of type 1 hypersensitivity (allergic) reaction. (FcεRI, cell surface IgE receptor; LT, leukotriene; PG, prostaglandin.) (Redrawn from Page et al. 2006.)

> ### COMMUNICATION
>
> Adam, a 6-year-old boy, is rushed into accident and emergency with a blood pressure of 65/30 mmHg. He is clearly in distress, breathless and vomiting. Swollen lips and blisters around his mouth are also noted. His father tells the doctor that he had been fine previously and had just started having his lunch, peanut butter sandwiches. Suddenly he became severely unwell. The doctors acted quickly to diagnose anaphylactic shock. Adam is given oxygen and 250 µg adrenaline intramuscularly. Afterwards, he is also given chlorphenamine (H$_1$-receptor antagonist) and hydrocortisone to prevent relapse. He and his father are advised about the allergic reaction and taught to carry prefilled adrenaline syringes. Adam is also given a MedicAlert bracelet.

Fig. 10.14 Type I hypersensitivity/allergic disorders

Disorder	Site of reaction	Response	Common allergens
Anaphylaxis	Circulation	Oedema, circulatory collapse, death	Venoms Drugs
Allergic rhinitis/ hay fever	Nasal passages Conjunctiva	Irritation, oedema, mucosal hypersecretion	Pollen Dust
Asthma	Bronchioles	Bronchoconstriction, mucosal secretion, airway inflammation	Pollen Dust
Food allergy	GIT	Vomiting, diarrhoea, urticaria (hives)	Seafood Milk, etc.
Wheal and flare	Skin	Vasodilatation and oedema	Insect venom
(GIT, gastrointestinal tract.)			

Fig. 10.15 Drug therapy in allergic disorders

Disorder	Drugs used	Mechanism of action
Anaphylaxis	Adrenaline	Vasoconstriction (α_2) Bronchodilation (β_2)
	Antihistamines Glucocorticoids	Pro-inflammatory mediator antagonism Anti-inflammatory
Allergic rinitis/ hay fever	Antihistamines Mast-cell stabilizers Glucocorticoids Sympathomimetic vasoconstrictors	Pro-inflammatory mediator antagonism Inhibition of mast-cell degranulation Anti-inflammatory Decongestion of nasal mucosa
Asthma	See p. 48	See p. 48
Food allergies	Antihistamines	Pro-inflammatory mediator antagonism
Wheal and flare	Antihistamines	Pro-inflammatory mediator antagonism

Histamine and antihistamines

Histamine is a basic amine that is stored in mast cells and in circulating basophils; it is also found in the stomach and CNS. The effects of histamine are mediated by three different receptor types found on target cells (Fig. 10.16).

As the major chemical mediator released during an allergic reaction, histamine produces a number of effects, mainly via action on H_1-receptors. Therefore H_1 antagonists (antihistamines) are of potential benefit in the treatment of allergic disorders.

H_1-receptor antagonists: antihistamines

There are two types of H_1-receptor antagonists:

- **'Old' sedative types,** e.g. chlorphenamine and promethazine.
- **'New' non-sedative types,** e.g. cetirizine and loratadine.

Mechanism of action—Antagonism of histamine H_1-receptors (see Fig. 10.16). In the periphery, their action can inhibit allergic reactions where histamine is the main mediator involved.

The old-style antihistamines are able to cross the blood–brain barrier where both specific and non-specific actions in the CNS produce sedation and antiemetic effects.

Indications—The main use of H_1-receptor antagonists is in the treatment of seasonal allergic rhinitis (hay fever). They are also used for the treatment and prevention of allergic skin reactions such as urticarial rashes, pruritus and insect bites, and in the emergency treatment of anaphylactic shock.

The old-style H_1-receptor antagonists can also be used as mild hypnotics (Ch. 5), and to suppress nausea in motion sickness, owing to their actions on the CNS.

Route of administration—Oral, topical, transnasal. Intravenous chlorphenamine can be used in anaphylaxis.

Adverse effects—Old-style antihistamines produce quite pronounced sedation or fatigue, as well as anticholinergic effects such as dry mouth. The newer agents do not do this.

Fig. 10.16 Effects at histamine receptors

Histamine receptor	Effect
H_1	Responsible for most of the actions of histamine in a type I hypersensitivity reaction: - capillary and venous dilatation (producing 'flare' or systemic hypotension) - increased vascular permeability (producing 'wheal' or oedema) - contraction of smooth muscle (producing bronchial and gastrointestinal contraction)
H_2	Regulation of gastric acid secretion: - H_2-receptors respond to histamine secreted from the enterochromaffin-like cells that are adjacent to the parietal cell (see Ch. 10)
H_3	Involved in neurotransmission: - exact physiological role not clear (presynaptic inhibition of neurotransmitter release in the CNS and autonomic nervous system? Role in itch and pain perception?)

Rare hazardous arrhythmias are associated with a few H1-receptor antagonists (e.g. terfenadine), especially at high plasma levels or when in combination with imidazole antifungal agents or macrolide antibiotics (Ch. 11). Hypersensitivity reactions, especially to topically applied H1-receptor antagonists, may occur.

Mast-cell stabilizers, the anti-inflammatory glucocorticoids, and sympathomimetic decongestants are all used in allergy (see Ch. 3).

IMMUNOSUPPRESSANTS

HINTS AND TIPS

Immunosuppressant drugs are toxic agents, with adverse effects common, serious and frequently dose limiting.

Deliberate pharmacological suppression of the immune system is used in the following three main clinical areas:

- To suppress inappropriate autoimmune responses (e.g. systemic lupus erythematosus or rheumatoid arthritis), where the host immune system is 'attacking' host tissue
- To suppress host immune rejection responses to donor organ grafts or transplants
- To suppress donor immune responses against host antigens (prevention of graft versus host disease after bone marrow transplant (GVHD)).

The main pharmacological agents used for immunosuppression are:

- Calcineurin inhibitors
- Anti-proliferatives
- Glucocorticoids (Ch. 6).

Solid organ transplant patients require immunosuppression to prevent organ rejection. They are usually maintained on a corticosteroid combined with a calcineurin inhibitor (ciclosporin) or with an antiproliferative drug (azathioprine or mycophenolate mofetil), or with both.

COMMUNICATION

Mr Isaac, 40 years old, has diabetes. He develops end-stage renal failure due to diabetic nephropathy. He is able to receive a renal transplant. The operation is successful and he is started on ciclosporin, mycophenolate mofetil and prednisolone immunosuppression to prevent rejection. When he is discharged, he is also given co-trimoxazole (a mixture of the anti-bacterials, sulfamethoxazole and trimethoprim) and nystatin (anti-fungal) prophylactically. However, 2 months later, he develops an infection. Cytomegalovirus (CMV) is identified as the cause from his symptoms, chest X-ray and detection of CMV DNA by polymerase chain reaction test.

Mr Isaac is treated by two methods:

- A reduction in his immunosuppression (mycophenolate mofetil treatment is suspended). This is vital to allow a better immune response to clear the CMV. Close surveillance of graft function is important during this period.
- Specific anti-viral therapy (ganciclovir).

Mr Isaac responds to this therapy and his symptoms resolve after 6 days.

Calcineurin Inhibitors

The main drug in this class is ciclosporin.

Mechanism of action—Ciclosporin is a cyclic peptide, derived from fungi, that has powerful immunosuppressive activity. It has a selective inhibitory effect on T cells by inhibiting the T-cell receptor (TCR)-mediated signal-transduction pathway. It is believed to exert its actions after entering the T cell and preventing the transcription of specific genes (Fig. 10.17).

After entry into the T cell, ciclosporin specifically binds to its cytoplasmic binding protein, cyclophilin. This ciclosporin-cyclophilin complex then binds to a serine/threonine phosphatase called calcineurin, inhibiting its phosphatase activity. Calcineurin is normally activated when intracellular calcium ion levels rise following T-cell-receptor binding to the appropriate major histocompatibility complex: antigen complex. When calcineurin is active it dephosphorylates the cytoplasmic component of the nuclear factor of activated T cells (NF-ATc) into a form that migrates to the nucleus and induces transcription of genes such as IL-2 that are involved in T-cell activation.

Inhibition of calcineurin by the ciclosporin-cyclophilin complex therefore prevents the nuclear translocation of NF-ATc and the transcription of certain genes essential for the activation of T cells. Hence the production of IL-2 by T-helper cells, the maturation of cytotoxic T cells and the production of some other lymphokines, such as interferon-g, are all inhibited.

The overall action of ciclosporin is to suppress reversibly both cell-mediated and antibody-specific adaptive immune responses.

Indications—Ciclosporin is used for the prevention of graft and transplant rejection, and prevention of GVHD.

Route of administration—Oral, intravenous.

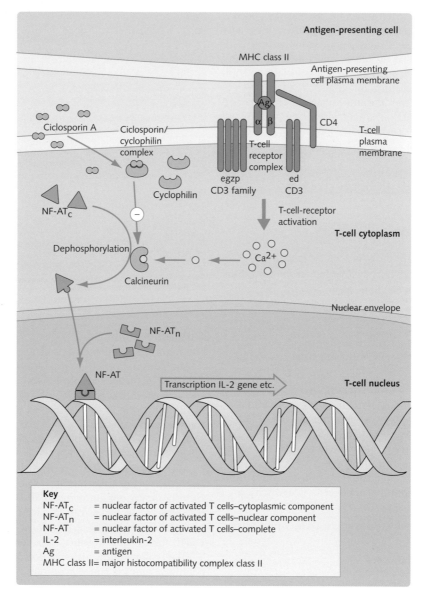

Fig. 10.17 Ciclosporin and T-cell suppression.

Adverse effects—Unlike most immunosuppressive agents, ciclosporin does not cause myelosuppression. It is markedly nephrotoxic to the proximal tubule of the kidney, and renal damage almost always occurs. This may be reversible or permanent. Hypertension occurs in 50% of people.

Less serious side-effects include mild hepatotoxicity, anorexia, lethargy, gastrointestinal upsets, hirsutism and gum hypertrophy.

Therapeutic notes—Ciclosporin is often used as part of a post-transplantation 'triple therapy' regimen with oral corticosteroids and azathioprine.

Anti-proliferatives

Azathioprine

Mechanism of action—Azathioprine is a prodrug that is converted into the active component 6-mercaptopurine in the liver. Mercaptopurine is a fraudulent purine nucleotide that impairs DNA synthesis, and has a cytotoxic action on dividing cells.

Indications—Azathioprine is used for the prevention of graft and transplant rejection, and autoimmune conditions when corticosteroid therapy alone is inadequate.

Route of administration—Oral, intravenous.

Adverse effects—Side-effects of azathioprine include bone marrow suppression, which can lead to leucopenia, thrombocytopenia and sometimes anaemia. This is often the dose-limiting side-effect.

Increased susceptibility to infections (often opportunistic pathogens), and to certain cancers (lymphomas) can occur. Common side-effects include gastrointestinal disturbances, nausea, vomiting and diarrhoea. Alopecia may be partial or complete, but is usually reversible.

Drug interaction with allopurinol necessitates lowering the dose of azathioprine.

Therapeutic notes—Azathioprine is used as part of a post-transplantation 'triple therapy' regimen with oral corticosteroids.

Mycophenolate mofetil

Mechanism of action—Mycophenolate mofetil is rapidly hydrolysed to mycophenolic acid, which is the active metabolite. Mycophenolic acid is a potent, uncompetitive and reversible inhibitor of iosine monophosphate dehydrogenase (IMPDH), and therefore, inhibits the pathway critical for T- and B-lymphocyte proliferation. It is selective because other cells are not solely reliant on this enzyme and so are able to maintain their rapid proliferation.

Indications—Prophylaxis of acute renal, cardiac or hepatic transplant rejection (in combination with ciclosporin and corticosteroids).

Contraindications—Pregnancy, those with hypersensitivity to the drug.

Route of administration—Oral, intravenous.

Adverse effects—Side-effects of mycophenolate mofetil include bone marrow suppression, which can lead to leucopenia, thrombocytopenia and sometimes anaemia. Increased susceptibility to infections (often opportunistic pathogens), and to certain cancers (lymphomas) can occur. Common side-effects include gastrointestinal disturbances, nausea, vomiting and diarrhoea. Alopecia may be partial or complete, but is usually reversible.

Glucocorticoids

The use of glucocorticoids as immunosuppressant agents involves both their anti-inflammatory actions and their effects on the immune system (Ch. 6).

Infectious diseases (11)

Objectives

After reading this chapter, you will:
- Have a basic understanding of bacterial, viral, fungal and parasitic infections
- Know how drugs act to defend against these infections
- Know the indications, contraindications and adverse drug effects associated with these drugs.

ANTIBACTERIAL DRUGS

Concepts of antibacterial chemotherapy

Bacteria are prokaryotic organisms. Some bacteria are pathogenic to humans and responsible for a number of medically important diseases.

The principal treatment of infections is with antibiotics. These antibacterial agents can be:
- bacteriostatic (i.e. they inhibit bacterial growth but do not kill the bacteria), or
- bactericidal (i.e. they kill bacteria).

Note that the distinction is not clear-cut as the ability of an antibacterial agent to inhibit or kill bacteria is partially dependent on its concentration. Also, the distinction is rarely of clinical significance, the exception being immunocompromised patients in whom bactericidal agents are necessary, as the host's immune system is not capable of final elimination of the bacteria.

Classification of antibiotics

There are three main ways of classifying antibiotics:
- Whether they are bactericidal or bacteriostatic
- By their site of action (Figs 11.1 and 11.2)
- By their chemical structure.

In this chapter, antibiotics have been described according to their site of action.

Antibiotic resistance

When an antibiotic is ineffective against a bacterium, that bacterium is said to be resistant. Resistance to antibiotics can be acquired or innate.

Innate resistance

Innate resistance is a long-standing characteristic of a particular species of bacteria. For instance, *Pseudomonas aeruginosa* has always been resistant to treatment with several antibiotics, including benzylpenicillin, vancomycin and fusidic acid.

Acquired resistance

Acquired resistance is when bacteria that were sensitive to an antibiotic become resistant. Biochemical mechanisms responsible for resistance to an antibiotic include:
- Production of enzymes that inactivate the drug
- Alteration of drug binding site
- Reduction in drug uptake and accumulation
- Development of altered metabolic pathways.

The major stimulus for the development of acquired resistance is the over use of antibiotics. Antibiotic use exerts selective pressure on bacteria to 'acquire' resistance to survive. Acquired resistance to antibiotics can develop in bacterial populations in many ways, although all involve genes that code for the resistance mechanism located either on the bacterial chromosome or on plasmids. The 'acquisition' of resistance by a bacterium can either be achieved de novo by spontaneous mutation, or by being transferred from another bacterium.

The development of clinical antibiotic drug resistance is a major problem imposing serious constraints on the medical treatment of many bacterial infections. Methicillin-resistant *Staphylococcus aureus* (MRSA) and some strains of *Mycobacteria tuberculosis* are examples of multidrug-resistant bacteria.

Prescribing antibiotics

Like most drugs, many antibiotics have side-effects. When prescribing antibiotics there are many considerations that determine which antibiotic to use, by which route, for how many days, etc. One should consider the following points when treating an infection:
- Identify the organism responsible for, or likely to be responsible for the symptoms
- Assess the severity of illness
- Previous antibiotic therapy
- Previous adverse/allergic response to antibiotics

167

Fig. 11.1 Sites of action of cytotoxic drugs that act on dividing cells

Site	Exploitable difference	Antibacterial drug
Peptidoglycan cell wall	Peptidoglycan cell walls are a uniquely prokaryotic feature not shared by eukaryotic (mammalian) cells. Drugs that act here are therefore very selective	Penicillins Cephalosporins Glycopeptides
Cytoplasmic membrane	Bacteria possess a plasma membrane within the wall which is a phospholipid bilayer, as in eukaryotes. However in bacteria the plasma membrane does not contain any sterols and this results in differential chemical behaviour that can be exploited	Polymyxins
Protein synthesis	The bacterial ribosome (50S+30S subunits) is sufficiently different from the mammalian ribosome (60S+40S subunits) that sites on the bacterial ribosome are good targets for drug action	Aminoglycosides Tetracyclines Chloramphenicol Macrolides Fusidic acid
Nucleic acids	The bacterial genome is in the form of a single circular strand of DNA plus ancillary plasmids unenclosed by a nuclear envelope, in contrast to the eukaryotic chromosomal arrangement within the nucleus. Drugs may interfere directly or indirectly with microbial DNA and RNA metabolism, replication and transcription	Antifolates Quinolones Rifampicin

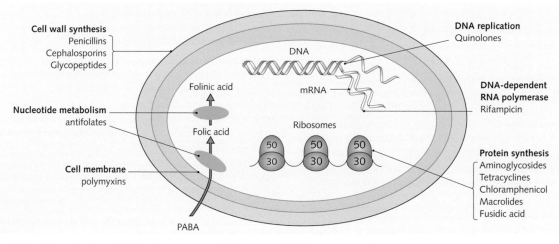

Fig. 11.2 Sites of action of different types of antibiotic agent. (PABA, para-aminobenzoic acid.)

- Other medications being taken and their possible interactions
- On-going medical considerations.

cefuroxime. The following day his temperature is noted to be 37.8°C and he reports general malaise and lethargy. The wound is still weeping with no improvement in appearance. MRSA is suspected and he is started on intravenous vancomycin.

Antibacterial drugs that inhibit cell wall synthesis

Penicillins

Examples of penicillins include benzylpenicillin, phenoxymethylpenicillin, flucloxacillin, amoxicillin and ampicillin.

Mechanism of action—Penicillins are bactericidal. Structurally they possess a thiazolidine ring connected to a β-lactam ring. The side chain from the β-lactam ring determines the unique pharmacological properties of the different penicillins.

Penicillins bind to penicillin-binding proteins on susceptible microorganisms. This interaction results in inhibition of peptide cross-linking within the microbial cell wall, and indirect activation of autolytic enzymes. The combined result is lysis (see Fig. 11.2).

Spectrum of activity—Penicillins exhibit considerable diversity in their spectrum of activity (Fig. 11.3).

Benzylpenicillin is active against aerobic Gram-positive and Gram-negative cocci and many anaerobic organisms. Many staphylococci are now resistant to benzylpenicillin. Flucloxacillin is used against penicillin-resistant staphylococci as it is not inactivated by their β-lactamase. Phenoxymethylpenicillin is similar to benzylpenicillin but less active. Amoxicillin and ampicillin are broad-spectrum penicillins.

Route of administration—Benzylpenicillin must be administered parenterally as it is inactivated when given orally. Phenoxymethylpenicillin, flucloxacillin, amoxicillin and ampicillin are active when given orally. Consult the *British National Formulary (BNF)* for parenteral routes.

Contraindications—Known hypersensitivity to penicillins or cephalosporins.

Adverse effects—Generally very specific and safe antibiotics. Hypersensitivity reactions are the main adverse effect, including rashes (common) and anaphylaxis (rare). Neurotoxicity occurs at excessively high cerebrospinal fluid (CSF) concentrations. Diarrhoea is common, owing to disturbance of normal colonic flora.

Therapeutic notes—Resistance to penicillins is often due to production of β-lactamase by some microorganisms, which hydrolyses the β-lactam ring. This resistance gene is located in a plasmid and is transferable. Flucloxacillin is resistant to β-lactamase.

Cephalosporins

The cephalosporins comprise a large group of drugs. The three main subgroups include:

- First-generation drugs, e.g. cefadroxil (oral) and cefradine (parenteral).

Fig. 11.3 Drugs of choice and alternatives for selected common bacterial pathogens

Bacterium	Drug(s) of choice	Alternatives	Comments
Streptococcus species	Penicillin	First-generation cephalosporins Erythromycin Clindamycin Vancomycin	A few strains are penicillin resistant, especially some *S. Pneumoniae* Erythromycin is only for mild infections Vancomycin is only for serious infections
Enterococcus species	Penicillin or ampicillin plus gentamicin	Vancomycin plus gentamicin	There are some strains for which streptomycin is synergistic but gentamicin is not Some strains are resistant to synergy with any aminoglycoside
Staphylococcus species	Antistaphylococcal penicillin, e.g. flucloxacillin	First-generation cephalosporins Vancomycin	Vancomycin is required for methicillin-resistant strains Rifampicin is occasionally used to eradicate the nasal carriage state
Neisseria meningitidis	Penicillin	Chloramphenicol Third-generation cephalosporins	Rare strains are penicillin resistant
Neisseria gonorrhoeae	Cefixime	Ciprofloxacin Third-generation cephalosporins	Some strains are fluoroquinolone resistant (especially in Asia)

(Continued)

Fig. 11.3 Drugs of choice and alternatives for selected common bacterial pathogens—Cont'd

Bacterium	Drug(s) of choice	Alternatives	Comments
Bordetella pertussis	Erythromycin	Trimethoprim with sulfamethoxazole	
Haemophilus influenzae	Aminopenicillin (ampicillin, amoxicillin)	Cefuroxime Third-generation cephalosporins Chloramphenicol	Approximately 30% are aminopenicillin-resistant: aminopenicillins should not be used empirically in serious infections until susceptibility results are available Rifampicin is used to eradicate the nasal carriage state
Enterobacteria in urine	Trimethoprim with sulfamethoxazole	Ciprofloxacin Gentamicin Nitrofurantoin	β-lactams are less effective than trimethoprim with sulfamethoxazole or fluoroquinolones for the treatment of urinary tract infection
Enterobacteria in cerebrospinal fluid	Third-generation cephalosporin	Trimethoprim with sulfamethoxazole	In neonates only, aminoglycosides are equivalent to third- generation cephalosporins Experience with trimethoprim with sulfamethoxazole in meningitis is limited
Enterobacteria elsewhere (blood, lung, etc.)	Gentamicin Third-generation cephalosporins Ciprofloxacin	Trimethoprim with sulfamethoxazole	Two-drug therapy is sometimes used in serious infection Monotherapy with a third-generation cephalosporin should be avoided if the pathogen is *Enterobacter cloacae, E. aerogenes, Serratia marcescens* or *Citrobacter freundii*
Pseudomonas aeruginosa	Antipseudomonal penicillin plus aminoglycoside	Ceftazidime Ciprofloxacin	Two-drug therapy recommended except for urinary tract infection
Bacteroides fragilis	Metronidazole or clindamycin	Imipenem Penicillin β-lactamase inhibitors	*B. fragilis* is usually involved in polymicrobial infections; therefore another antibiotic active against Enterobacteriaceae is often required
Mycoplasma penumoniae	Macrolides, e.g. erythromycin	Tetracycline	Although tetracyclines are as effective as macrolides, the latter are recommended because of better activity against *Pneumococcus*, which can mimic this infection
Chlamydia trachomatis	Tetracycline	Azithromycin Erythromycin	Azithromycin is the only therapy effective in a single dose Erythromycin is used in pregnancy
Rickettsial species	Tetracycline	Chloramphenicol	
Listeria monocytogenes	Ampicillin plus gentamicin	Vancomycin plus gentamicin	
Legionella species	Erythromycin	Tetracycline	Rifampicin is occasionally used as a second agent in severe cases
Clostridium difficile	Metronidazole	Vancomycin (oral)	
Mycobacterium tuberculosis	Isoniazid plus rifampicin plus pyrazinamide plus ethambutol	Streptomycin Fluoroquinolones Cycloserine Clarithromycin Capreomycin	Directly observed therapy is recommended Isoniazid is used alone for preventive therapy
Mycobacterium leprae	Dapsone plus rifampicin ± clofazimine	Clarithromycin	Thalidomide is useful for erythema nodosum leprosum

- Second-generation drugs, e.g. cefuroxime (oral) and cefamandole (parenteral).
- Third-generation drugs, e.g. cefixime (oral) and cefotaxime (parenteral).

Mechanism of action—Cephalosporins are bactericidal. They are β-lactam-containing antibiotics and inhibit bacterial cell wall synthesis in a manner similar to the penicillins. Structurally cephalosporins possess a dihydrothiazine ring connected to the β-lactam ring that makes them more resistant to hydrolysis by β-lactamases than are the penicillins.

Spectrum of activity—The cephalosporins are broad-spectrum antibiotics that are second-choice agents for many infections (see Fig. 11.3).

Route of administration—Oral, intravenous, intramuscular. Consult the *BNF*.

Contraindications—Known hypersensitivity to cephalosporins or penicillins.

Adverse effects—Side-effects of the cephalosporins include hypersensitivity reactions, which occur in a similar and cross-reacting fashion to the penicillins. Diarrhoea is common, owing to disturbance of normal colonic flora. Nausea and vomiting may also occur.

Therapeutic notes—The cephalosporins can be inactivated by the β-lactamase enzyme, though the later-generation drugs are more resistant to hydrolysis.

Glycopeptides

Vancomycin and teicoplanin are the classical glycopeptides.

Mechanism of action—Glycopeptides are bactericidal. They inhibit peptidoglycan synthesis, with possible effects on RNA synthesis (see Fig. 11.2).

Spectrum of activity—Vancomycin is active only against aerobic and anaerobic Gram-positive bacteria. Glycopeptides are reserved for resistant staphylococcal infections and *Clostridium difficile* in antibiotic-associated pseudomembranous colitis (see Fig. 11.3).

Route of administration—Glycopeptides are usually administered intravenously as they are not well absorbed orally. Oral administration is reserved for when a local gastrointestinal tract effect is required, e.g. in colitis.

Adverse effects—Side-effects of glycopeptides include ototoxicity and nephrotoxicity at high plasma levels, and fever, rashes and local phlebitis at the site of infection.

Therapeutic notes—Acquired resistance to vancomycin is rare, but reports of vancomycin-resistant enterococci are becoming more common.

Monobactam and carbapenems

Aztreonam is a monobactam antibiotic, which is less likely to cause hypersensitivity reactions in penicillin-sensitive patients. Carbapenems have the broadest spectrum of activity of all the β-lactams and include ertapenem, imipenem (used with cilastatin to increase duration of action) and meropenem. Both groups contain β-lactam rings, though they are resistant to many β-lactamases. For indications, spectrum of activity and adverse effects consult the *BNF*.

Antibacterial drugs that inhibit bacterial nucleic acids

Antibacterial drugs that inhibit bacterial nucleic acids include (Fig. 11.2):

- The antifolates, which affect DNA metabolism
- The quinolones, which affect DNA replication and packaging
- Rifampicin, which affects transcription (p. 174).

Antifolates

Examples of antifolates include the sulphonamides (e.g. sulfadiazine) and trimethoprim.

Mechanism of action—Folate is an essential co-factor in the synthesis of purines and hence of DNA. Bacteria, unlike mammals, must synthesize their own folate from *para*-aminobenzoic acid (Fig. 11.2). This pathway can be inhibited at two points: the sulphonamides inhibit dihydrofolate synthetase, and are bacteriostatic while trimethoprim inhibits dihydrofolate reductase and are bacteriostatic.

Spectrum of activity—The sulphonamides are used for 'simple' urinary tract infections (UTIs). Trimethoprim and co-trimoxazole (trimethoprim and sulfamethoxazole) are used for UTIs and respiratory tract infections (see Fig. 11.3).

Route of administration—Oral, intravenous.

Contraindications—Pregnant women – as there is a theoretical teratogenic risk with antifolates. Neonates – as bilirubin displacement can damage the neonatal brain (kernicterus).

Adverse effects—Nausea, vomiting and hypersensitivity reactions, e.g. rashes, fever, Stevens–Johnson syndrome. The sulphonamides are relatively insoluble and can cause crystalluria, while trimethoprim can cause myelosuppression/agranulocytosis.

Therapeutic notes—Antifolates are often used in combined preparations as they have synergistic effects. Resistance is common and is due to the production of enzymes that have reduced affinity for the drugs. Resistance can be acquired on plasmids in Gram-negative bacteria.

Quinolones

Ciprofloxacin and nalidixic acid are quinolones.

Mechanism of action—Quinolones are bactericidal. They act by inhibiting prokaryotic DNA gyrase. This enzyme packages DNA into supercoils and is essential for DNA replication and repair (see Fig. 11.2).

Spectrum of activity—Ciprofloxacin has a broad spectrum of activity, while nalidixic acid is more narrowly active against Gram-negative organisms (see Fig. 11.3).

Route of administration—Oral, intravenous. Ciprofloxacin is so well absorbed orally that intravenous administration is rarely required unless the patient is unable to tolerate oral medication.

Contraindications—Quinolones should not be given with theophylline as theophylline toxicity may be precipitated.

Adverse effects—Gastrointestinal upset. Rarely, hypersensitivity and central nervous system (CNS) disturbances occur.

Antibacterial drugs that inhibit protein synthesis

Antibacterial drugs that inhibit protein synthesis include:

- Aminoglycosides
- Tetracyclines
- Chloramphenicol
- Macrolides
- Lincosamides
- Fusidic acid.

The site of action of these drugs is summarized in Figure 11.4.

Aminoglycosides

Examples of aminoglycosides include gentamicin, streptomycin, netilmicin and amikacin.

Mechanism of action—Aminoglycosides are bactericidal. They bind irreversibly to the 30S portion of the bacterial ribosome. This inhibits the translation of mRNA to protein and causes more frequent misreading of the prokaryotic genetic code (see Fig. 11.4).

Spectrum of activity—Aminoglycosides have a broad spectrum of activity but with low activity against anaerobes, streptococci and pneumococci (see Fig. 11.3). Streptomycin is used against *Mycobacterium tuberculosis* (p. 174).

Route of administration—Parenteral only.

Contraindications—Acute neuromuscular blockade can occur if an aminoglycoside is used in combination with anaesthesia or other neuromuscular blockers.

Adverse effects—Dose-related ototoxicity and nephrotoxicity at high plasma levels.

Therapeutic notes—Resistance to aminoglycosides is increasing and is primarily due to plasmid-borne genes encoding degradative enzymes.

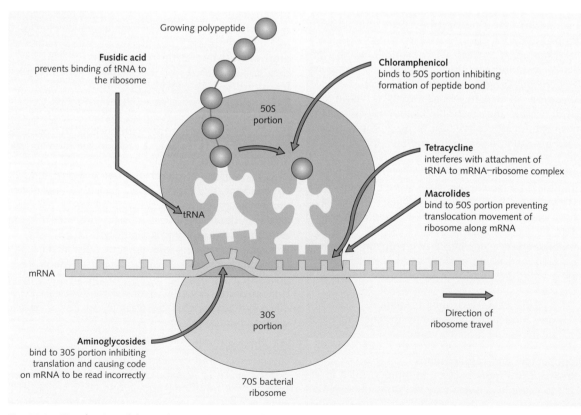

Fig. 11.4   Site of action of the antibiotics which inhibit bacterial protein synthesis.

Tetracyclines

Examples of tetracyclines include tetracycline, minocycline, doxycycline.

Mechanism of action—Tetracyclines are bacteriostatic. They work by selective uptake into bacterial cells due to active bacterial transport systems not possessed by mammalian cells. The tetracycline then binds reversibly to the 30S subunit of the bacterial ribosome, interfering with the attachment of tRNA to the mRNA ribosome complex (see Fig. 11.4).

Spectrum of activity—Tetracyclines have broad-spectrum activity against Gram-positive and Gram-negative bacteria, as well as intracellular pathogens (see Fig. 11.3).

Route of administration—Oral, intravenous. Oral absorption is incomplete and can be impaired by calcium (e.g. milk), and magnesium or aluminium salts (e.g. antacids).

Contraindications—Tetracyclines should not be given to children or pregnant women.

Adverse effects—Gastrointestinal disturbances which are common after oral administration. In children, tetracyclines depress bone growth, and produce permanent discolouration of teeth.

Therapeutic notes—Resistance to tetracyclines is slow to develop, but is now widespread. In the majority of cases, resistance is due to decreased uptake of the drug, and is plasmid borne.

Chloramphenicol

Mechanism of action—Chloramphenicol is both bactericidal and bacteriostatic, depending on the bacterial species. It reversibly binds to the 50S subunit of the bacterial ribosome, inhibiting the formation of peptide bonds (see Fig. 11.4).

Spectrum of activity—Chloramphenicol has a broad spectrum of activity against many Gram-positive cocci and Gram-negative organisms (see Fig. 11.3). Because of its toxicity, it is reserved for life-threatening infections, especially typhoid fever and meningitis.

Route of administration—Oral, intravenous.

Contraindications—Chloramphenicol should not be given to pregnant women or neonates.

Adverse effects—Myelosuppression, reversible anaemia. Neutropenia and thrombocytopenia may occur during chronic administration. Fatal aplastic anaemia is rare.

Neonates cannot metabolize chloramphenicol and 'grey baby syndrome' may develop, which comprises pallor, abdominal distension, vomiting and collapse.

Therapeutic notes—Resistance to chloramphenicol is due to a plasmid-borne gene encoding an enzyme that inactivates the drug by acetylation. Blood monitoring is necessary.

Macrolides

Erythromycin, clarithromycin and azithromycin are examples of macrolides.

Mechanism of action—Macrolides are bacteriostatic/bactericidal. They reversibly bind to the 50S subunit of the bacterial ribosome, preventing the translocation movement of the ribosome along mRNA (see Fig. 11.3).

Spectrum of activity—Erythromycin is effective against most Gram-positive bacteria and spirochaetes. Clarithromycin is active against *Haemophilus influenzae*, *Mycobacterium avium cellulare* and *Helicobacter pylori*.

Route of administration—Oral, intravenous.

Adverse effects—Side-effects of erythromycin include gastrointestinal disturbance, which is common after oral administration. Liver damage and jaundice can occur after chronic administration.

Therapeutic notes—Resistance to erythromycin results from a mutation of the binding site on the 50S subunit. Erythromycin has a similar spectrum of activity to penicillin and is an effective alternative in penicillin-sensitive patients. Azithromycin can be given as a one-off dose for uncomplicated chlamydial infections of the genital tract.

Fusidic acid

Mechanism of action—Fusidic acid is a steroid that prevents binding of tRNA to the ribosome (Fig. 11.4).

Spectrum of activity—Fusidic acid has a narrow spectrum of activity, particularly against Gram-positive bacteria (see Fig. 11.3).

Route of administration—Oral, intravenous.

Adverse effects—Gastrointestinal disturbance. Skin eruptions and jaundice may occur.

Therapeutic notes—Resistance to fusidic acid can occur via mutation or by plasmid-borne mechanisms.

Lincosamides

Clindamycin is a lincosamide.

Mechanism of action—Similar to the macrolides.

Spectrum of activity—Clindamycin is active against Gram-positive cocci, including penicillin-resistant staphylococci, and many anaerobes.

Route of administration—Oral, parenteral.

Adverse effects—Antibiotic-associated (pseudomembranous) colitis; greater risk than for other antibiotics.

Therapeutic notes—Clindamycin is used for staphylococcal joint and bone infections.

Miscellaneous antibacterials

Other antibacterial drugs include:

* Metronidazole
* Nitrofurantoin
* Bacitracin
* Polymyxins.

Metronidazole and tinidazole

Mechanism of action—Metronidazole is bactericidal. It is metabolized to an intermediate that inhibits bacterial DNA synthesis and degrades existing DNA.

Its selectivity is due to the fact that the intermediate toxic metabolite is not produced in mammalian cells.

Spectrum of activity—Metronidazole is antiprotozoal (p. 183) and has antibacterial activity against anaerobic bacteria (see Fig. 11.3).

Route of administration—Oral, rectal, intravenous, topical.

Contraindications—Metronidazole should not be given to pregnant women.

Adverse effects—Mild headache, gastrointestinal disturbance. Adverse drug reactions occur with alcohol.

Therapeutic notes—Acquired resistance to metronidazole is rare. Tinidazole is similar to metronidazole but has a longer duration of action.

Nitrofurantoin

Mechanism of action—The mechanism of action of nitrofurantoin is uncertain though it possibly interferes with bacterial DNA metabolism.

Spectrum of activity—Nitrofurantoin is active against Gram-positive bacteria and *Escherichia coli* (see Fig. 11.3).

Route of administration—Oral; it reaches high therapeutic concentrations in the urine.

Adverse effects—Gastrointestinal disturbance. Pulmonary complications can occur with chronic therapy.

Therapeutic notes—Rarely, chromosomal resistance to nitrofurantoin can occur.

Bacitracin

Mechanism of action—Bacitracin is a natural antibiotic, isolated from *Bacillus subtilis*, that inhibits bacterial cell wall formation.

Spectrum of activity—Bacitracin is similar in its spectrum of activity to penicillin (see Fig. 11.3).

Route of administration—Topical.

Adverse effects—Well tolerated when used topically. Serious nephrotoxicity can occur if it is used systemically

Therapeutic notes—Bacitracin is much less likely to cause hypersensitivity reactions than penicillin. Acquired resistance is rare.

Polymyxins

Colistin is an example of a polymyxin, though this class is seldom prescribed due to its toxicity

Mechanism of action—Polymyxins are bactericidal. They are peptides that interact with phospholipids on the outer plasma cell membranes of Gram-negative bacteria, disrupting their structure. This disruption destroys the bacteria's osmotic barrier, leading to lysis (Fig. 11.2).

Spectrum of activity—Polymyxins are active only against Gram-negative bacteria including *Pseudomonas aeruginosa* (see Fig. 11.3).

Route of administration—Intravenous, intramuscular, inhalation. Oral polymyxins are given to sterilise the bowel in neutropenic patients.

Adverse effects—Perioral and peripheral, paraesthesia, vertigo, nephrotoxicity, neurotoxicity

Therapeutic notes—Resistance to polymyxins is rare.

Antimycobacterial drugs

The mycobacteria are slow-growing intracellular bacilli that cause tuberculosis (*Mycobacterium tuberculosis*) and leprosy (*Mycobacterium leprae*) in humans.

Mycobacteria differ in their structure and lifestyle from Gram-positive and Gram-negative bacteria and are treated with different drugs.

Antituberculosis therapy

The first-line drugs used in the treatment of tuberculosis are:

- **Isoniazid:** Inhibits the production of mycolic acid, a component of the cell wall unique to mycobacteria, and is bactericidal against growing organisms. Taken orally it penetrates tuberculous lesions well. Adverse effects occur in about 5% of patients and include peripheral neuropathy, hepatotoxicity and autoimmune phenomena. Resistance is rare in developed countries, but not in less-developed areas.
- **Rifampicin:** Inhibits DNA-dependent RNA polymerase, causing a bactericidal effect. It is a potent drug, active orally. Adverse effects are infrequent but can be serious, e.g. hepatotoxicity and 'toxic syndromes'. Orange discoloration of the urine is a common side-effect. There are many drug interactions, and resistance can develop rapidly.
- **Ethambutol:** Is bacteriostatic. The mechanism of action is uncertain, involving impaired synthesis of the mycobacterial cell wall. Ethambutol is administered orally. Adverse effects are uncommon but reversible optic neuritis may occur. Resistance often develops.
- **Pyrazinamide:** Its mechanism of action is uncertain but may involve metabolism of drug within *Mycobacteria tuberculosis* to produce a toxic product, pyrazinoic acid, which works as a bacteriostatic agent in the low pH environment of the phagolysosome. It is active orally. Adverse effects are hepatotoxicity and raised plasma urate levels that can lead to gout. Resistance can develop rapidly.

The second-line drugs used for tuberculosis infections when first-line drugs have been discontinued owing to resistance or adverse effects are:

- **Capreomycin:** A peptide drug given intramuscularly. It can cause ototoxicity and kidney damage.
- **Cycloserine:** A broad-spectrum drug that inhibits peptidoglycan synthesis. This drug is administered orally, and can cause CNS toxicity.
- **New macrolides**, e.g. azithromycin and clarithromycin.
- **Quinolones**, e.g. ciprofloxacin.

To reduce the emergence of resistant organisms, compound drug therapy is used to treat tuberculosis, involving:

- An initial phase, designed to reduce the bacterial population as quickly as possible and prevent emergence of drug-resistance, lasts about two months and consists of three drugs: isoniazid, rifampicin and pyrazinamide. Ethambutol is added where there may be resistance to isoniazid (e.g. those who have previously been treated for tuberculosis or the immunocompromised).
- Continuation phase of four months consisting of two drugs: isoniazid and rifampicin. Longer treatment regimens may be needed for patients with meningitis or bone/joint involvement.

Anti-leprosy therapy
- Tuberculoid leprosy is treated with dapsone and rifampicin for 6 months.
- Lepromatous leprosy is treated with dapsone, rifampicin and clofazimine for up to 2 years.

Dapsone resembles sulphonamides chemically and may inhibit folate synthesis in a similar way. It is active orally. Adverse effects are numerous, and some fatal. Consult the *BNF*.

Clofazimine is a chemically complex dye that accumulates in macrophages, possibly acting on mycobacterial DNA. As a dye, clofazimine can discolour the skin and urine red. Other adverse effects are numerous. It is active orally.

> **HINTS AND TIPS**
>
> Grouping of antibacterial drugs by their mechanism of action rather than chemical structure is easier, more important and more relevant to your understanding.

ANTIVIRAL DRUGS

Concepts of viral infection

Viruses are obligate intracellular parasites that lack independent metabolism and can only replicate within the host cells they enter and infect. A virus particle, or virion, consists essentially of DNA or RNA enclosed in a protein coat (capsid). In addition, certain viruses may possess a lipoprotein envelope and replicative enzymes (Fig. 11.5).

Viruses are classified largely according to the architecture of the virion and the nature of their genetic material. Viral nucleic acid may be single stranded (ss) or double stranded (ds) (Fig. 11.6).

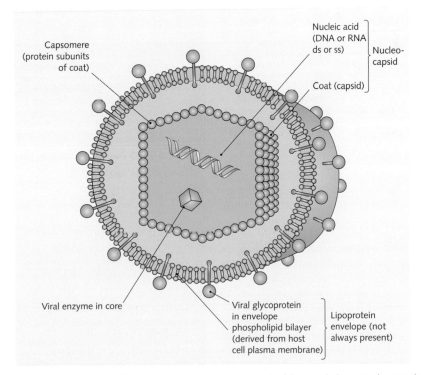

Fig. 11.5   Diagrammatic representation of the components of a virion. ds, double stranded; ss, single stranded.

Fig. 11.6 Classification of selected medically important viruses and the diseases they cause

Family	ss/ds	Viruses	Diseases
DNA viruses			
Herpes viruses	ds	Herpes simplex (HSV)* Varicella zoster (VZV)* Cytomegalovirus (CMV)* Epstein-Barr virus (EBV)*	Cold sores, genital herpes Chickenpox, shingles Cytomegalic disease Infectious mononucleosis
Poxviruses	ds	Variola	Smallpox
Adenoviruses	ds	Adenoviruses	Acute respiratory disease
Hepadnaviruses	ds	Hepatitis B	Hepatitis
Papovaviruses	ds	Papilloma	Warts
Parvoviruses	ss	B19	Erythema infectiosum
RNA viruses			
Orthomyxoviruses	ss	Influenza A* and B*	Influenza
Paramyxoviruses	ss	Measles virus Mumps virus Parainfluenza Respiratory syncytial*	Measles Mumps Respiratory infection Respiratory infection
Coronaviruses	ss	Coronavirus	Respiratory infection
Rhabdoviruses	ss	Rabies virus	Rabies
Picornaviruses	ss	Enteroviruses Rhinoviruses Hepatitis A	Meningitis Colds Hepatitis
Calciviruses	ss	Norwalk virus	Gastroenteritis
Togaviruses	ss	Alphaviruses Rubivirus	Encephalitis, haemorrhagic fevers Rubella
Reoviruses	ds	Rotavirus	Gastroenteritis
Arenavirus	ss	Lymphocytic choriomeningitis Lassavirus*	Meningitis Lassa fever
Retroviruses	ss	HIV I, II*	AIDS

*viruses for which effective chemotherapy exists. ds, double stranded; ss, single stranded.

Antiviral agents

Because viruses have an intracellular replication cycle and share many of the metabolic processes of the host cell, it has proved extremely difficult to find drugs that are selectively toxic to them. In addition, by the time a viral infection becomes detectable clinically, the viral replication process tends to be very far advanced, making chemotherapeutic intervention difficult. All current antiviral agents are virustatic rather than virucidal and thus rely upon host immunocompetence for a complete clinical cure.

Nevertheless, antiviral chemotherapy is clinically effective against some viral diseases (identified with an asterisk in Fig. 11.6). The viruses include:

- Herpesviruses (herpes simplex virus (HSV), varicella zoster virus (VZV) and cytomegalovirus (CMV))
- Influenza viruses A and more recently B
- Respiratory syncytial virus, arenaviruses
- HIV-1.

The selective inhibition of these viruses by drugs depends on either:

- Inhibition of unique steps in the viral replication pathways, such as adsorption of the virion to the cell receptor, penetration, uncoating, assembly and release.
- Preferential inhibition of steps shared with the host cell, which include transcription and translation.

In addition to chemotherapy, immune-based therapies, such as the use of immunoglobulins and cytokines in viral infection, are also mentioned below.

Inhibition of attachment to or penetration of host cells

Amantadine

Mechanism of action—Amantadine blocks a primitive ion channel in the viral membrane (named M_2) preventing fusion of a virion to host cell membranes, and inhibits the release of newly synthesised viruses from the host cell (Fig. 11.7).

Route of administration—Oral.

Indications—Amantadine is used for the prophylaxis and treatment of acute influenza A in groups at risk. It is not effective against influenza B.

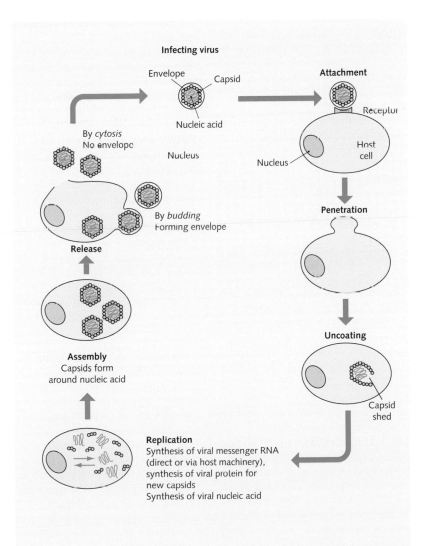

Fig. 11.7   Stages in the infection of a host's cell and replication of a virus. Several thousand virus particles may be formed from each cell. (Reproduced with permission from Mims et al. *Medical Microbiology*, 2nd edn. Mosby, 1998.)

Adverse effects—Some patients (5–10%) report non-serious dizziness, slurred speech and insomnia. Neurological side-effects and renal failure can occur at high concentrations.

Therapeutic notes—Resistance has been reported in 25–50% of patients. Amantadine is not used widely due to problems with resistance, its narrow spectrum of activity and because influenza vaccines are often preferred.

Neuraminidase inhibitors

Zanamivir belongs to the neuraminidase inhibitor class of drugs.

Mechanism of action—Zanamivir inhibits the release of newly synthesised viruses from the host cell by inhibiting the enzyme (neuraminidase) which is responsible for cleaving the peptide links between virus and host.

Route of administration—Zanamivir is delivered by inhalation, though its sister drug oseltamivir may be given orally.

Indications—Treatment of influenza A or B virus within 48 hours after onset of symptoms when influenza is endemic in the community.

Contraindications—Breastfeeding.

Adverse effects—Gastrointestinal disturbances.

Immunoglobulins

Examples of immunoglobulins include human normal immunoglobulin (HNIg/gamma globulin) and specific immunoglobulins, e.g. hepatitis B (HBIg), rabies (RIg), varicella zoster (VZIg) and cytomegalovirus (CMVIg) immunoglobulins.

Mechanism of action—Immunoglobulins bind specifically to antigenic determinants on the outside of virions. By specifically binding to a virus, the immunoglobulins may neutralize it by coating the virus and preventing its attachment and entry into host cells.

HNIg is prepared from pooled plasma of ∼1000 donors and contains antibodies to measles, mumps, varicella and hepatitis A.

Specific immunoglobulins are prepared by pooling the plasma of selected donors with high levels of the antibody required.

Route of administration—Intramuscular, though immunoglobulins can be given intravenously.

Indications—HNIg is administered for the protection of susceptible contacts against hepatitis A, measles, mumps and rubella. Specific immunoglobulins may attenuate or prevent hepatitis and rabies following known exposure, and before the onset of signs and symptoms, e.g. following exposure to a rabid animal. VZIg and CMVIg are indicated for prophylactic use to prevent chickenpox, and cytomegalic disease in immunosuppressed patients at risk.

Contraindications—Immunoglobulins should not be given to people with known antibody against IgA.

Adverse effects—Malaise, chills, fever and (rarely) anaphylaxis.

Therapeutic notes—Protection with immunoglobulins is immediate and lasts several weeks. HNIg may interfere with vaccinations for 3 months.

Inhibition of nucleic acid replication

Aciclovir and related drugs

Aciclovir, famciclovir and valaciclovir are all closely related anti-viral drugs.

Mechanism of action—Aciclovir and related drugs are characterized by their selective phosphorylation in herpes-infected cells. This takes place by a viral thymidine kinase rather than host kinase, as a first step.

Phosphorylation yields a triphosphate nucleotide that inhibits viral DNA polymerase and viral DNA synthesis.

These drugs are selectively toxic to infected cells because, in the absence of viral thymidine kinase, the host kinase activates only a small amount of the drug. In addition, the DNA polymerase of herpes virus has a much higher affinity for the activated drug than has cellular DNA polymerase (Fig. 11.7).

Route of administration—Topical, oral, parenteral.

Indications—Aciclovir and related drugs are used for the prophylaxis and treatment of herpes simplex and varicella zoster virus infections, superficial and systemic, particularly in the immunocompromised.

Adverse effects—Side-effects are minimal. Rarely, renal impairment and encephalopathy occur.

Therapeutic notes—The herpes genome in latent (non-replicating) cells is not affected by aciclovir therapy and so recurrence of infection after cessation of treatment is to be expected.

CMV is resistant to aciclovir because its genome does not encode thymidine kinase.

Ganciclovir

Mechanism of action—Ganciclovir is a synthetic nucleoside analogue, structurally related to aciclovir. It also requires conversion to the triphosphate nucleotide form, though by a different kinase. Ganciclovir acts as a substrate for viral DNA polymerase and as a chain terminator aborting virus replication.

Route of administration—Oral, intravenous.

Indications—While as active as aciclovir against HSV and VZV, ganciclovir is reserved for the treatment of severe CMV infections in immunocompromised people, owing to its side-effects.

Adverse effects—Reversible neutropenia in 40% of patients. There is occasional rash, nausea and encephalopathy.

Therapeutic notes—Maintenance therapy with ganciclovir at a reduced dose may be necessary to prevent recurrence of CMV.

Ribavirin (tribavirin)

Mechanism of action—Ribavirin is a nucleoside analogue that selectively interferes with viral nucleic acid synthesis in a manner similar to aciclovir.

Route of administration—For respiratory syncytial virus (RSV) by inhalation; for Lassa virus intravenously.

Indications—Severe respiratory syncytial virus bronchiolitis in infants. Lassa fever.

Adverse effects—Reticulocytosis, respiratory depression.

Therapeutic notes—The necessity of aerosol administration for RSV limits the usefulness of this effective drug.

Nucleoside analogue reverse transcriptase inhibitors

Examples of nucleoside reverse transcriptase inhibitors include zidovudine (AZT), and the newer drugs, abacavir, didanosine (ddI), lamivudine (3TC), stavudine (d4T) and zalcitabine (ddC).

Mechanism of action—These nucleotide analogues all require intracellular conversion to the corresponding triphosphate nucleotide for activation. The active triphosphates competitively inhibit reverse transcriptase, and cause termination of DNA chain elongation once incorporated. Affinity for viral reverse transcriptase is 100 times that for host DNA polymerase (Fig. 11.8, site 3).

Route of administration—Oral.

Indications—Nucleoside reverse transcriptase inhibitors are used for the management of asymptomatic and symptomatic HIV infections, and the prevention of maternal fetal HIV transmission.

Adverse effects—Side-effects of AZT are uncommon at the recommended low dosage in patients with asymptomatic or mild HIV infections, but more common in acquired immune deficiency syndrome (AIDS) patients on higher dosage regimens.

Toxicity to human myeloid and erythroid progenitor cells commonly causes anaemia and neutropenia, i.e. bone marrow suppression. Other common side-effects include nausea, insomnia, headaches and myalgia.

The major dose-limiting effects of ddI are pancreatitis and peripheral neuropathy, and of ddC and d4T, peripheral neuropathy.

Therapeutic notes—Drug resistance evolves to all the current nucleoside reverse transcriptase inhibitors by the development of mutations in reverse transcriptase, although the kinetics of resistance development varies for the different drugs (e.g. 6–18 months for AZT). Combined therapies may have a place in increasing efficacy synergistically and reducing emergence of resistant strains.

Non-nucleoside reverse transcriptase inhibitors

Efavirenz and nevirapine are examples of drugs within this class.

Mechanism of action—Efavirenz and nevirapine both bind to reverse transcriptase near the catalytic site, leading to a conformational change that inactivates this enzyme.

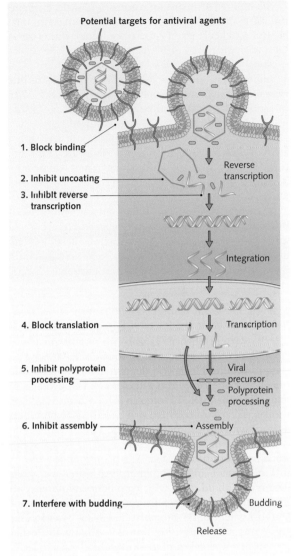

Potential targets for antiviral agents

1. Block binding
2. Inhibit uncoating
3. Inhibit reverse transcription
4. Block translation
5. Inhibit polyprotein processing
6. Inhibit assembly
7. Interfere with budding

Reverse transcription
Integration
Transcription
Viral precursor Polyprotein processing
Assembly
Budding
Release

Fig. 11.8 The HIV replicative cycle and potential sites of antiviral drug action.

Route of administration—Oral.

Contraindications—Breastfeeding.

Adverse effects—Generally well tolerated. Rash, dizziness and headache may occur.

Therapeutic notes—Resistance can develop quickly when subtherapeutic doses are employed.

Inhibition of post-translational events

Protease inhibitors

Examples of protease inhibitors include saquinavir, and the newer drugs, ritonavir, indinavir, nelfinavir and amprenavir.

Mechanism of action—Protease inhibitors prevents the virus-specific protease of HIV cleaving the inert polyprotein product of translation into various structural and functional proteins (see Fig. 11.8, site 5).

Route of administration—Oral.

Indications—Protease inhibitors are used for the management of asymptomatic and symptomatic HIV infections, in combination with nucleoside reverse transcriptase inhibitors.

Adverse effects—Protease inhibitors are well tolerated. Nausea, vomiting and diarrhoea are common. In addition, indinavir and ritonavir may cause taste disturbances, and saquinavir may cause buccal and mucosal ulceration.

Therapeutic notes—Combination treatment between protease inhibitors and nucleoside reverse transcriptase inhibitors produces additive antiviral effects and reduces the incidence of resistance. Such combination therapy is termed highly active antiretroviral therapy (HAART).

Immunomodulators

Interferons

Mechanism of action—Interferons (IFNs) are endogenous cytokines with antiviral activity, that are normally produced by leucocytes and other cells in response to viral infection. Three major classes have been identified (α, β and γ) and have been shown to have immunoregulatory and antiproliferative effects.

The mechanism of the antiviral effect of IFN varies for different viruses and cells. IFNs have been shown to bind to cell-surface receptors and signal a cascade of events that interfere with viral penetration, uncoating, synthesis, or methylation of mRNA, translation of viral protein, viral assembly and viral release (see Fig. 11.7). IFNs induce enzymes in the host cell that inhibit the translation of viral mRNA.

The relatively recent production of IFNs in large quantities by cell culture and recombinant DNA technology has allowed their evaluation and prescription as antiviral agents.

Route of administration—Intravenous, intramuscular.

Indications—The exact role of interferons (IFNs) in the treatment of viral infections remains unclear. They have a wide spectrum of activity and have been shown to be effective in the treatment of chronic hepatitis (B and C) among others.

Adverse effects—Influenza-like syndrome with fatigue, fever, myalgia, nausea and diarrhoea is the commonest side-effect. Chronic administration can cause bone marrow depression and neurological effects.

Therapeutic notes—The role of IFNs remains to be clearly established. Their usefulness has been limited by the need for repeated injections and dose-limiting adverse effects.

Drugs used in HIV infection

Infection with the human immunodeficiency virus (HIV) ultimately results in progression to the acquired immunodeficiency syndrome (AIDS). There are currently no drugs which can prevent this progression, though there are numerous agents on the market and in clinical trials which delay the rate of progression.

There are a variety of potential sites for antiviral drug action in the HIV-1 replicative cycle (see Fig. 11.8). The four main classes of drug used in the treatment of HIV have already been discussed, but consist of:

- Nucleoside reverse transcriptase inhibitors, e.g. zidovudine, prevent DNA chain elongation and have a competitive inhibitory effect on reverse transcriptase (see Fig. 11.8, site 3).
- Non-nucleoside reverse transcriptase inhibitors, e.g. nevirapine, inactivate reverse transcriptase (see Fig. 11.8, site 3).
- Protease inhibitors, e.g. ritonavir, prevent viral assembly and budding (see Fig. 11.8, site 5).
- Fusion inhibitors, e.g. enfuvirtide, prevent cell infection by preventing fusion of the HIV virus with the host cell (see Fig 11.8, site 1).

Recently licensed drugs include Raltegravir, a HIV-1 integrase inhibitor that may be used to treat HIV-1 which is either resistant to other drugs or to treat patients showing viral replication. Maraviroc has similar indications but blocks the interaction between HIV-1 and the chemokine receptor CCR5 on host cells.

COMMUNICATION

Dr Hiroshimi, a 28-year-old man, presents with a 3-week history of persistent flu-like symptoms. He denies any foreign travel but he admits having unprotected sexual intercourse, last summer, with a number of homosexual men. On examination his temperature is 39°C. He is counselled for the possibility of HIV and wished to have a HIV test.

Two years on his CD4+ T-lymphocyte count is found to be low and his viral count raised. A decision is made to commence highly active anti-retroviral therapy (HAART), consisting of zidovudine, lamivudine and nevirapine.

He continued to have regular follow-ups. Then years later he is found to have a sore and painful throat. On examination he has whitish velvety plaques on the mucous membranes of the mouth and tongue. The pattern on the tongue is distinctive of oral candidiasis. He is given nystatin (antifungal) mouthwash and a chance to re-discuss his anti-retroviral therapy.

Future anti-HIV drug therapy

A number of strategies are being pursued in research laboratories across the world in the quest for effective drugs to treat HIV infection. These strategies include:

- Drugs which interrupt HIV binding to host cells, notably the gp120 envelope protein
- Drugs designed specifically to 'smother' and prevent its entry into cells
- Antisense oligonucleotides to complement specific portions of the viral genome and inhibit transcription and replication.

ANTIFUNGAL DRUGS

Concepts of fungal infection

Fungi are members of a kingdom of eukaryotic organisms that live as saprophytes or parasites. A few species of fungi are pathogenic to humans. Fungal infections are termed mycoses and may be superficial, affecting the skin, nails, hair, mucous membranes, or systemic, affecting deep tissues and organs.

Three main groups of fungi cause disease in humans (Fig. 11.9). Fungal pathogenicity results from mycotoxin production, allergenicity/inflammatory reactions and tissue invasion. Opportunistic fungal infections are important causes of disease in the immunosuppressed.

Antifungal drugs

There are four main classes of antifungal drugs:

- Polyene macrolides
- Imidazole antifungals
- Triazole antifungals
- Other antifungals.

The sites of action of the antifungal drugs are summarized in Figure 11.10.

Polyene macrolides

Examples of polyene macrolides include amphotericin B and nystatin.

Mechanism of action—Polyene macrolides bind to ergosterol in the fungal cell membrane, forming pores through which cell constituents are lost. This results in fatal damage (Fig. 11.11). These drugs are selectively toxic because in human cells the major sterol is cholesterol, not ergosterol.

Route of administration—Amphotericin B is administered topically and intravenously. Nystatin is too toxic for intravenous use. It is not absorbed orally at all and so is applied topically as a cream or vaginal pessaries, or tablets sucked so as to deliver the drug via the oral membranes.

Indications—Amphotericin is a broad-spectrum antifungal used in potentially fatal systemic infections. Nystatin is used to suppress candidiasis (thrush) on the skin and mucous membranes (oral and vaginal).

Adverse effects—Fever, chills and nausea. Long-term therapy invariably causes renal damage. Nystatin may cause oral sensitization.

Therapeutic notes—Creatinine clearance must be monitored during amphotericin therapy to exclude renal damage. Resistance can develop in vivo to amphotericin, but not to nystatin.

Imidazoles

Examples of imidazoles include clotrimazole, miconazole and ketoconazole.

Mechanism of action—Imidazoles have a broad spectrum of activity. They inhibit fungal lipid (especially ergosterol) synthesis in cell membranes. Interference with fungal oxidative enzymes results in the accumulation of 14α-methyl sterols, which may disrupt the

Fig. 11.9 Main groups of fungi causing disease in humans			
Fungal class	Form	Example	Disease caused
Moulds	Filamentous branching mycelia	Dermatophytes, e.g. *Tinea* spp. *Aspergillus fumigatus*	Athlete's foot, ringworm and other superficial mycoses. Pulmonary or disseminated aspergillosis
True yeasts	Unicellular (round or oval)	*Cryptococcus neoformans*	Cryptococcal meningitis and lung infections in the immunocompromised
Yeast-like fungi	Similar to yeasts but can also form long (non-branching) filaments	*Candida albicans*	Oral and vaginal thrush, endocarditis and septicaemias

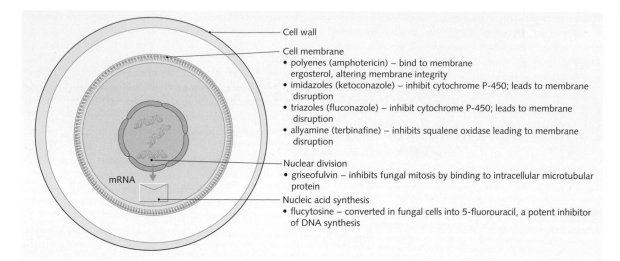

Fig. 11.10 Sites of action of antifungal drugs.

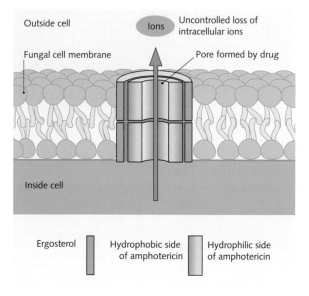

Fig. 11.11 Mechanism of action of polyene antifungal agents.

packing of acyl chains of phospholipids, inhibiting growth and interfering with membrane-bound enzyme systems.

Route of administration—Intravenous, topical. Ketoconazole is given orally as, unlike the other imidazoles, it is well absorbed by this route.

Indications—Candidiasis and dermatophyte mycoses. Miconazole can also be used intravenously as an alternative to amphotericin in disseminated mycoses. Because ketoconazole is active orally, it can be used for systemic mycoses.

Adverse effects—Topical use of imidazoles tends to be unproblematic. Intravenous miconazole is often limited by side-effects of nausea, faintness and haematological disorders. Oral ketoconazole can cause serious hepatotoxicity and adreno-suppression.

Therapeutic notes—Resistance rarely develops to imidazoles.

Triazoles

Examples of triazoles include fluconazole and itraconazole.

Mechanism of action—Triazoles are similar to imidazoles (see above), although they have greater selectivity against fungi and cause fewer endocrinological problems.

Route of administration—Oral.

Indications—Fluconazole can be used for a wide range of systemic and superficial infections, including cryptococcal meningitis, as it reaches the cerebrospinal fluid in high concentrations. Itraconazole is similarly indicated, although unlike fluconazole, it can be used against *Aspergillus*.

Adverse effects—Nausea, diarrhoea and rashes. Itraconazole is well tolerated, though nausea, headaches and abdominal pain can occur, but should not be given to patients with liver damage.

Therapeutic notes—Resistance rarely develops to the triazoles.

Other antifungals

Allylamines

Terbinafine is an example of an allylamine.

Mechanism of action—Terbinafine prevents ergosterol synthesis by inhibiting the enzyme squalene oxidase, resulting in squalene accumulation, which leads to membrane disruption and cell death. It is lipophilic and penetrates superficial tissues well, including the nails.

Route of administration—Oral, topical.

Indications—Terbinafine has been recently introduced against dermatophyte infections including ringworm, where oral therapy is appropriate because of the site and severity of extent of infection.

Adverse effects—Mild nausea, abdominal pain, skin reactions. Loss of taste has been reported.

Therapeutic notes—Resistance rarely develops. Initial trials with terbinafine show impressive clinical and mycological cure rates.

Flucytosine

Mechanism of action—Flucytosine is imported into fungal, but not human, cells, where it is converted into 5-fluorouracil, a potent inhibitor of DNA synthesis.

Route of administration—Intravenous.

Indications—Flucytosine is most active against yeasts, and is indicated for use in systemic candidiasis and as an adjunct to amphotericin in cryptococcal meningitis.

Adverse effects—Nausea and vomiting are common. Rare side-effects include hepatotoxicity, hair loss and bone-marrow suppression.

Therapeutic notes—Weekly blood counts of patients on flucytosine are necessary to monitor bone marrow suppression.

Griseofulvin

Mechanism of action—The action of griseofulvin is not fully established, but it probably interferes with microtubule formation or nucleic acid synthesis and polymerization. It is selectively concentrated in keratin and therefore is suitable for treating dermatophyte mycoses.

Route of administration—Oral.

Indications—Griseofulvin is the drug of choice for widespread or intractable dermatophyte infections, where topical therapy has failed.

Adverse effects—Hypersensitivity reactions, headaches, rashes, photosensitivity

Therapeutic notes—Because griseofulvin is fungistatic rather than fungicidal, treatment regimens are long, amounting to several weeks or months. Griseofulvin is more effective for skin than nail infections.

> **HINTS AND TIPS**
>
> Superficial mycoses (e.g. athlete's foot/thrush) are common and usually easily treated with topical drugs that have few adverse effects. Deep mycoses are rare (except in the immunocompromised), serious and may be fatal despite therapy with systemic drugs, which often have adverse effects.

ANTIPROTOZOAL DRUGS

Concepts of protozoal infection

Protozoa are members of a phylum of unicellular organisms, some of which are parasitic pathogens in humans, causing several diseases of medical and global importance. Parasitic protozoa replicate within the host's body and are usually divided into four subphyla according to their type of locomotion (Fig. 11.12).

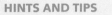

Fig. 11.12 Classification of medically important protozoan species causing disease in humans

Subphyla	Defining characteristics	Medically important species	Disease
Amoebae (sarcodina)	Amoeboid movement with pseudopods	*Entamoeba histolytica*	Amoebiasis (amoebic dysentery)
Flagellates (mastigophora)	Flagella that produces a whip-like movement	*Giardia lamblia* *Trichomonas vaginalis* *Leishmania* spp. *Trypanosoma* spp.	Giardiasis Trichomonal vaginitis Leishmaniasis Trypanosomiasis (sleeping sickness and Chagas' disease)
Cilates (ciliophora)	Cilia beat to produce movement	—	—
Sporozoans (sporozoa)	No locomotor organs in adult stage	Plasmodium spp.	Malaria

Malaria

Malaria is responsible for 2 million deaths per year and 200 million people worldwide are infected. Malaria is caused by four species of plasmodial parasites that are transmitted by female anopheline mosquitoes.

Antimalarial drugs target different phases of the life cycle of the malarial parasite (Fig. 11.13). This life cycle proceeds as follows:

- When an infected mosquito feeds on a human it injects sporozoites into the bloodstream from its salivary glands.
- The sporozoites rapidly penetrate the liver where they transform and grow into tissue schizonts containing large numbers of merozoites. In the case of *Plasmodium vivax* and *P. ovale*, some schizonts remain dormant in the liver for years (hypnozoites), before rupturing to cause a relapse.
- The large tissue schizonts rupture after 5–20 days, releasing thousands of merozoites that invade circulating red blood cells (RBCs), and multiply inside the cell.
- The host's RBCs rupture, leading to the release of more merozoites. These then invade and destroy more RBCs. This cycle of invasion/destruction causes the episodic chills and fever that characterize malaria.

- Some merozoites develop into gametocytes. If these are taken up by a feeding mosquito, the insect becomes infected, thus completing the cycle.

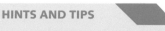

The clinical features and severity of malaria depend upon the species of parasite and the immunological status of the person infected. Clinically significant malaria is less common in adults who have always lived in endemic areas, as partial immunity develops.

The four types of plasmodium causing malaria are:

- *P. falciparum:* Widespread and causes malignant tertian (fever every third day) malaria. There is no exo-erythrocytic stage, so that, if the erythrocytic forms are eradicated, relapses do not occur.
- *P. vivax:* Widespread and causes benign, tertian relapsing malaria. Exo-erythrocytic forms may persist in the liver for years and cause relapses.
- *P. malariae:* Rare and causes benign quartan (fever every fourth day) malaria. There is no

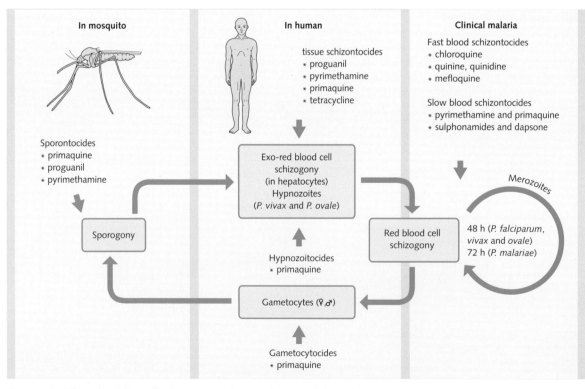

Fig. 11.13 Life cycle of the malarial parasite and point of action of chemotherapeutic agents.

exo-erythrocytic stage, so that, if the erythrocytic forms are eradicated, relapses do not occur.

- *P. ovale:* Mainly African and causes a rare form of benign relapsing malaria. Exo-erythrocytic forms may persist in the liver for years and cause relapses.

Approaches to antimalarial chemotherapy

Antimalarial drugs are usually classified in terms of their action against different stages of the parasite (see Fig. 11.13). They are used to protect against or cure malaria or to prevent transmission.

Prophylactic use
The aim of prophylactic use is to prevent the occurrence of infection in a previously healthy individual who is at potential exposure risk.

Suppressive prophylaxis involves the use of blood schizonticides to prevent acute attacks; causal prophylaxis involves the use of tissue schizonticides or drugs against the sporozoite to prevent the parasite becoming established in the liver.

Curative (therapeutic use)
Antimalarial drugs can be used curatively (therapeutically) against an established infection.

Suppressive treatment aims to control acute attacks, usually with blood schizonticides; radical treatment aims to kill dormant liver forms, usually with a hypnozonticide, to prevent relapsing malaria.

Antimalarial drugs

4-aminoquinolines
Chloroquine is an example of a 4-aminoquinoline.

Mechanism of action—Chloroquine is a rapidly acting blood schizonticide (see Fig. 11.13). It is concentrated 100-fold in erythrocytes that contain plasmodial parasites; this occurs because ferriprotoporphyrin IX, a degradation product of haemoglobin digestion by the parasites, acts as a chloroquine receptor. It is unclear how the high chloroquine concentrations kill the parasites; possibly, the digestion of haemoglobin is inhibited.

Route of administration—Oral. In severe falciparum malaria infections, injections or infusions can be used.

Indications—Suppressive chemoprophylaxis and treatment of susceptible strains of plasmodium.

Adverse effects—Nausea, vomiting, headache, rashes and, rarely, neurological effects.

Therapeutic notes—Chloroquine is considered safe for use in pregnant women. It rapidly controls fever (24–48 hours) but cannot produce a lasting radical cure in *P. vivax* and *P. ovale* strain infections, as it does not affect hypnozoites.

In most areas, *P. falciparum* is resistant to chloroquine, necessitating combination chemoprophylaxis with antifolates (see later).

Quinoline-methanols
Examples of quinoline-methanols include quinine and mefloquine.

Mechanism of action—Quinoline-methanols are rapidly acting blood schizonticides (see Fig. 11.13). It is not precisely known how the quinoline-methanols work but, like chloroquine, they are known to bind to a product of haemoglobin digestion.

Route of administration—Quinine is administered orally or by rate-controlled infusion in severe cases. Mefloquine is only given orally.

Indications—Quinine is the drug of choice for treating the acute clinical attack of falciparum malaria resistant to chloroquine. Mefloquine is effective against all malarial species including multidrug-resistant *P. falciparum*, and can also be used for chemoprophylaxis.

Adverse effects—Quinine may cause tinnitus, headache, nausea, blurring of vision, hypoglycaemia and, rarely, blood disorders. Overdose results in profound hypotension due to peripheral vasodilatation and myocardial depression (see Ch. 2). Quinine is safe in pregnancy.

Mefloquine may cause nausea, vomiting, gastrointestinal disturbance and postural hypotension. Rarely, acute neuropathic conditions may occur. Mefloquine may cause fetal abnormalities.

Therapeutic notes—The quinoline-methanols are used in combination therapy with other agents such as the sulphonamides or tetracyclines.

Antifolates
Examples of antifolates include type 1 drugs, e.g. sulphonamides and dapsone, and type 2 drugs, e.g. pyrimethamine and proguanil. Both types are useful.

Mechanism of action—Antifolates are slow-acting (in comparison with chloroquine, quinine and mefloquine) blood schizonticides, tissue schizonticides and sporonticides. These drugs inhibit the formation of folate compounds and thus inhibit DNA synthesis and cell division. All growing stages of the malarial parasite are affected.

The sulphonamides and dapsone are known as type 1 antifolate drugs. They compete with *para*-aminobenzoic acid for the enzyme dihydropteroate synthetase, which is found only in the parasites.

Proguanil and pyrimethamine are known as type 2 antifolate drugs. They selectively inhibit malarial dihydrofolate reductase.

These two groups of drugs act on the same pathway but at different points; they are used in combination as their synergistic blockade is more powerful than any one drug acting alone.

Route of administration—Oral.

Indications—Antifolates are used in combination for the causal chemoprophylaxis of malaria, or in combination with quinine for the treatment of acute chloroquine-resistant malaria.

Adverse effects—Antifolates have almost no side-effects if used in therapeutic doses. In toxic doses, type 2 antifolates can inhibit mammalian dihydrofolate reductase and cause a megaloblastic anaemia. Skin rashes occasionally occur.

Therapeutic notes—Common chemoprophylactic combinations include chloroquine plus pyrimethamine with a sulphonamide or dapsone.

8-aminoquinolines

Primaquine is an example of an 8-aminoquinoline.

Mechanism of action—Primaquine is an hypno-zonicide and gametocide. It is unclear how the drug works, but it may cause oxidative damage to the parasite. It is effective against the non-growing stages of malaria, i.e. hypnozoites and gametocytes (see Fig. 11.13).

Route of administration—Oral.

Indications—Primaquine is used for the radical cure of relapsing malarias (*P. ovale* and *P. vivax*) and prevention of transmission of *P. falciparum*.

Contraindications—Pregnancy.

Adverse effects—Nausea, vomiting, bone marrow depression. Intravenous haemolysis can occur in people with glucose 6-phosphate deficiency.

Therapeutic notes—Primaquine is usually used in combination with chloroquine. Resistance is rare.

Artemisinin

Artemisinin is given with the antimalarial lumefantrine, since together they are much more effective than either drug given individually. There is a synergistic effect.

Mechanism of action—A peroxide (trioxane) structure is responsible for its blood schizontocide activity against plasmodium, including multiresistant stains of *P. falciparum*.

Route of administration—Oral.

Indications—Treatment of uncomplicated falciparum malaria.

Contraindications—Breastfeeding, congestive heart failure, congenital Q-T interval prolongation, arrhythmias.

Adverse effects—Nausea, vomiting, abdominal pain, diarrhoea, dizziness, arthralgia, myalgia.

COMMUNICATION

Mr Mallory, a 25-year-old student, presents with a 4-day history of high fever (40°C), general malaise, feeling intensely cold and shaking followed by profuse sweating. He denies any homosexual contacts, unprotected sexual intercourse or intravenous drug use. He returned from Nigeria 3 weeks ago and was completing his proguanil with atovaquone malarial prophylaxis treatment. On examination he looked unwell. His pulse was 98 beats per minutes with a blood pressure of 132/72 mmHg. There are no heart murmurs. There are no enlarged lymph nodes.

Blood tests reveal raised bilirubin with normal liver enzymes, mild anaemia and a low platelet count. Light microscopy of a Giemsa-stained blood smear shows approximately 1% of red blood cells are infected with *Plasmodium* parasite.

He is kept well hydrated and treated with oral quinine for 7 days, after which his fever resolves and he starts to improve.

Treatment of other protozoal infections

Amoebiasis

Amoebic dysentery is caused by infection with *Entamoeba histolytica*, which is ingested in a cystic form. Dysentery results from invasion of the intestinal wall by the parasite. Occasionally, the organism encysts in the liver, forming abscesses.

Metronidazole (p. 174) is the drug of choice for acute invasive amoebic dysentery, it kills the trophozoites though has no activity against the cyst forms. Diloxanide and tinidazole are also used to treat amoebiasis.

Giardiasis

Giardiasis is a bowel infection caused by the flagellate *Giardia lamblia*. Infection follows ingestion of contaminated water or food and involves flatulence and diarrhoea.

Metronidazole (p. 174) is the drug of choice for giardiasis.

Trichomonas vaginitis

Trichomonas vaginitis is caused by the flagellate *Trichomonas vaginalis*. It is a sexually transmitted inflammatory condition of the female vagina and, occasionally, male urethra.

Metronidazole is the drug of choice for trichomonas vaginitis.

Trypanosomiasis and leishmaniasis

Trypanosomiasis

African trypanosomiasis (sleeping sickness) and South American trypanosomiasis (Chagas' disease) are caused by species of flagellate trypanosome.

Insect vectors introduce the parasites into the human host, where they reproduce, causing bouts of parasitaemia and fever. Toxins released cause damage to organs. The CNS is affected in sleeping sickness, and the heart, liver, spleen, bone and intestine in Chagas' disease.

The drug suramin kills the African trypanosomiasis parasite, possibly related to an ability to reversibly inhibit a number of enzymes (in the host and parasite). However, it does not penetrate into the CNS and thus its use is restricted to early trypanosomiasis.

Melarsoprol is used to treat the late CNS form of African trypanosomiasis. It may act by inactivating pyruvate kinase, a critical enzyme in the metabolism of trypanosomes.

Nifurtimox and benznidazole are used to treat acute American trypanosomiasis, although their role in the chronic phase is still unclear. Superoxide and other reactive oxygen species are generated from the drugs, but it is unknown if this is part of the mechanism of action.

Leishmaniasis

Leishmania species are flagellated parasites that are transmitted by a sandfly vector, assuming a non-flagellated intracellular form that resides within macrophages on infecting humans. Clinical infections range from simple, resolving cutaneous infections to systemic 'visceral' forms with hepatomegaly, splenomegaly, anaemia and fever.

Leishmaniasis can usually be treated with stibogluconate, a trivalent antimonial compound that reacts with thiol groups and reduces adenosine triphosphate (ATP) production in the parasite.

HINTS AND TIPS

The prophylaxis and treatment of trypanosomiasis and leishmaniasis are difficult and of variable efficacy. The drugs used are generally toxic and dangerous, making specialized knowledge essential.

Pneumocystis pneumonia

Pneumocystis pneumonia is most often associated with HIV infection, and is now considered an AIDS-defining illness. The infective agent *Pneumocystis jiroveci* (previously called *Pneumocystis carinii*) is not truly a protozoa, though it has similarities with both protozoa and fungi, and remains difficult to classify.

Signs and symptoms of *Pneumocystis jiroveci* pneumonia are similar to other pneumonias, but culture is not possible, and the microorganism must be visualised on direct microscopy.

High-dose oral or parenteral co-trimoxazole (trimethoprim and sulfamethoxazole) is the drug of choice, with parenteral pentamidine as an alternative.

ANTHELMINTIC DRUGS

HINTS AND TIPS

All the anthelmintic drugs described in this chapter are administered orally.

Concepts of helminthic infection

Helminth is derived from the Greek *helmins*, meaning worm. Anthelmintic drugs are therefore medicines acting against parasitic worms.

The three groups of helminths that parasitize humans are:

- Cestoda (tapeworms)
- Nematoda (roundworms)
- Trematoda (flukes).

Figure 11.14 lists medically important helminth infections and the main drugs used in their treatment.

The anthelmintic drugs

To be effective, an anthelmintic drug must be able to penetrate the cuticle of the worm, or gain access to its alimentary tract, so that it may exert its pharmacological effect on the physiology of the worm.

Anthelmintic drugs act on parasitic worms by a number of mechanisms. These include:

- Damaging or killing the worm directly
- Paralysing the worm
- Damaging the cuticle of the worm so that host defences, such as digestion and immune rejection, can affect the worm
- Interfering with worm metabolism.

Because there is great diversity across the different helminth classes, drugs highly effective against one species of worm are often ineffectual against another species.

Niclosamide

Mechanism of action—Niclosamide, a salicylamide derivative, is the most used drug for tapeworm infestations. It blocks glucose uptake at high concentrations, irreversibly damaging the scolex (attachment end) of the tapeworm, leading to the release and expulsion of the tapeworm. It is a safe, selective drug since very little is absorbed from the gastrointestinal tract.

Route of administration—Oral.
Indications—Tapeworm infestation (see Fig. 11.14).
Adverse effects—Mild gastrointestinal disturbance.
Therapeutic notes—Patients are fasted before treatment with niclosamide. Purgatives to expel the dead worm segments (proglottides) can be used, but are probably unnecessary since the worm may be digested after the effects of the drug.

Praziquantel

Mechanism of action—Praziquantel increases the permeability of the helminth plasma membrane to calcium. At low concentrations this causes contraction and spastic paralysis and, at higher concentrations, vesiculation and vacuolization damage is caused to the tegument of the worm.

Route of administration—Oral.

Fig. 11.14 Classification of medically important helminth infections and the main drugs in their treatment

	Helminth species	Drugs used in treatment
Cestodes		
Beef tapeworm	*Taenia saginata*	Niclosamide, praziquantel
Pork tapeworm	*Taenia solium*	Niclosamide, praziquantel
Fish tapeworm	*Diphyllobothrium latum*	Niclosamide, praziquantel
Hydatid tapeworm	*Echinococcus granulosus*	Albendazole
Nematodes		
Intestinal species		
Common round worms	*Ascaris lumbricoides*	Mebendazole, piperazine
Threadworms/pin worms	*Enterobius vermicularis*	Mebendazole, piperazine
Threadworms (USA)	*Strongyloides stercoralis*	Thiabendazole, albendazole
Whipworms	*Trichuris trichiura*	Mebandazole
Hookworms	*Necator americanus*	Mebendazole
	Ankylostoma duodenale	Mebendazole
Tissue species		
Trichinella	*Trichinella spiralis*	Thiabendazole
Guinea worm	*Dracunculus medinesis*	Metronidazole*
Filariaroidea	*Wucheria bancrofti*	Diethylcarbamazine
	Loa loa	Diethylcarbamazine
	Brugia malayi	Diethylcarbamazine
	Onchocerca volvulus	Ivermectin
Trematodes		
Blood flukes/schistosomes	*Schistosoma japonicum*	Praziquantel
	Schistosoma mansoni	Praziquantel
	Schistosoma haematobium	Praziquantel

*see p. 187.

Indications—Praziquantel is the drug of choice for all schistosome infections (see Fig. 11.14), and for cysticercosis (a rare cestode condition caused by encystation of larvae of the tapeworm *Taenia solium* in human organs).

Adverse effects—Mild gastrointestinal disturbance, and headache and dizziness may occur shortly after administration.

Therapeutic notes—Praziquantel should be taken after meals three times a day for 2 days only.

Piperazine

Mechanism of action—Piperazine is a reversible neuromuscular blocker that causes a flaccid paralysis in worms, leading to their expulsion by gastrointestinal peristalsis. It has very little effect on the host.

Route of administration—Oral.

Indications—Piperazine is used for roundworm and threadworm gastrointestinal infestation.

Adverse effects—Gastrointestinal disturbance, and neurotoxic effects (dizziness) may occur.

Therapeutic notes—A single dose of piperazine is usually effective for treating roundworm infection; threadworm infestation may require a longer course (7 days).

Benzimidazoles

Examples of benzimidazoles include mebendazole, thiabendazole and albendazole.

Mechanism of action—Benzimidazoles bind with high affinity to a site on tubulin dimers, thus preventing the polymerization of microtubules. Subsequent depolymerization leads to complete breakdown of the microtubule.

The selectivity of benzimidazoles arises because they are 250–400 times more potent in helminth than in mammalian tissue. The process takes time to have effect, and the worm may not be expelled for days.

Route of administration—Oral.

Indications—Benzimidazoles are used in the treatment of hydatid disease, and many nematode infestations (see Fig. 11.14).

Contraindications—Benzimidazoles should not be given to pregnant women as they are teratogenic and embryotoxic.

Adverse effects—Occasional gastrointestinal disturbance. Thiabendazole causes more frequent gastrointestinal disturbance, headache and dizziness. Serious hepatotoxicity rarely occurs.

Therapeutic notes—Dosage regimens of benzimidazoles range from a single dose for pinworm infestation to multiple doses for up to 5 days for trichinosis.

Diethylcarbamazine

Mechanism of action—It is not clear exactly how diethylcarbamazine exerts its filaricidal effect. It has been suggested that it damages or modifies the parasites in such a way as to make them more susceptible to host immune defences.

Diethylcarbamazine kills both microfilariae in the peripheral circulation and adult worms in the lymphatics.

Route of administration—Oral.

Indications—Diethylcarbamazine is the drug of choice for lymphatic filariasis caused by *Wucheria bancrofti, Loa loa* and *Brugia malayi* (see Fig. 11.14).

Adverse effects—Gastrointestinal disturbance, headache, lassitude.

Material from the damaged and dead worms causes allergic side-effects, including skin reactions, lymph gland enlargement, dizziness and tachycardia, lasting from 3 to 7 days.

Therapeutic notes—To minimize the dangerous sudden release of dead worm material, the initial dose of diethylcarbamazine is started low and then increased and maintained for 21 days.

Ivermectin

Mechanism of action—Ivermectin immobilizes the tapeworm *Onchocerca volvulus* by causing tonic paralysis of the peripheral muscle system. It does this by potentiating the effect of γ-aminobutyric acid at the worm's neuromuscular junction.

Route of administration—Oral.

Indications—Ivermectin is the drug of choice for *Onchocerca volvulus*, which causes river blindness and may be the most effective drug for chronic *Strongyloides* infection (see Fig. 11.14).

Adverse effects—Ocular irritation, transient electrocardiographic changes and somnolence. An immediate immune reaction to dead microfilariae (Mazzotti reaction) can be severe.

Levamisole

Mechanism of action—Levamisole stimulates nicotinic receptors at the neuromuscular junction and results in a spastic paralysis, which causes faecal worm expulsion.

Route of administration—Oral.

Indications—Treatment of choice for *Ascaris lumbricoides* round worm infection (see Fig. 11.14).

Adverse effects—Mild nausea and vomiting

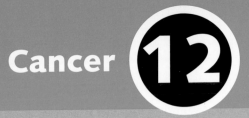

Cancer 12

● **Objectives**

After reading this chapter, you will:
• Have a good understanding of cancer and the cell cycle
• Know the different classes of drugs that are used to treat cancer and how their mechanisms of action result in beneficial and adverse effects.

CONCEPTS OF CANCER CHEMOTHERAPY

Cancer

Cancers are malignant neoplasms (new growths). Despite their variability, cancers share the characteristics of:

• Uncontrolled proliferation
• Local invasiveness
• Tendency to spread (metastasis)
• Changes in some aspects of original cell morphology/retention of other characteristics.

Cancers account for 20–25% of deaths in the Western world; attempts to cure or palliate cancer use three principal methods: surgery, radiotherapy and chemotherapy. These methods are not mutually exclusive, often being used in combination, e.g. adjuvant chemotherapy after surgical removal of a tumour.

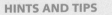

HINTS AND TIPS

Adjuvant chemotherapy is given after successful treatment of a cancer, where no remaining disease is found, for prophylaxis against re-occurrence.

Chemotherapy

Cancer chemotherapy is the use of drugs to inhibit the rate of growth of, or to kill, cancerous cells while having minimal effects on non-neoplastic host cells.

In a fashion similar to antimicrobial chemotherapy, the ideal anti-cancer drugs target malignant cells in preference to non-malignant cells. This is achieved by exploiting the molecular differences between them.

COMMUNICATION

Mr Collins is a 60-year-old delivery man, who presents with a 6-week history of passage of fresh blood from his anus and diarrhoea (he is normally slightly constipated). He also admits to low appetite, significant weight loss and feeling fatigued. He is referred for investigative colonoscopy, which reveals an abnormal growth in the descending colon. A biopsy reveals adenocarcinoma of the colon. Staging CT scans show no other areas of disease. He is managed by surgical resection of the tumour. Following this he undergoes adjuvant chemotherapy consisting of six cycles of 5-fluorouracil.

The most striking difference between cancerous and non-cancerous cells is their accelerated rate of cell division. This remains the main target for therapeutic intervention at present, though newer drugs are being developed which recognize other molecular differences.

The chemotherapeutic techniques currently used include:

• Cytotoxic therapy – which is the main approach
• Endocrine therapy
• Immunotherapy.

Cancers differ in their sensitivity to chemotherapy, from the very sensitive (e.g. lymphomas, testicular carcinomas) where complete clinical cures can be achieved, to the resistant (generally solid tumours, e.g. colorectal, squamous cell bronchial carcinoma).

A diagnosis of cancer carries a significant social and emotional impact. Hair loss and sickness are more often the initial concern for patients, rather than other potentially serious side-effects of chemotherapy. Nausea and vomiting should be taken seriously in cancer management, as these can have a devastating impact on quality of life; antiemetic drugs are discussed in Chapter 8.

CYTOTOXIC CHEMOTHERAPY

Mechanisms of action

Most cytotoxic drugs affect DNA synthesis. They can be classified according to their site of action on the process of DNA synthesis within the cancer cell (Fig. 12.1).

Cytotoxic drugs are therefore most active against actively cycling/proliferating cells, both normal and malignant, and least active against non-dividing cells.

Some drugs are only effective at killing cycling cells during specific parts of the cell cycle. These are known as phase-specific drugs (Fig. 12.2). Other drugs are cyto-toxic towards cycling cells throughout the cell cycle (e.g. alkylating agents) and are known as cycle-specific drugs.

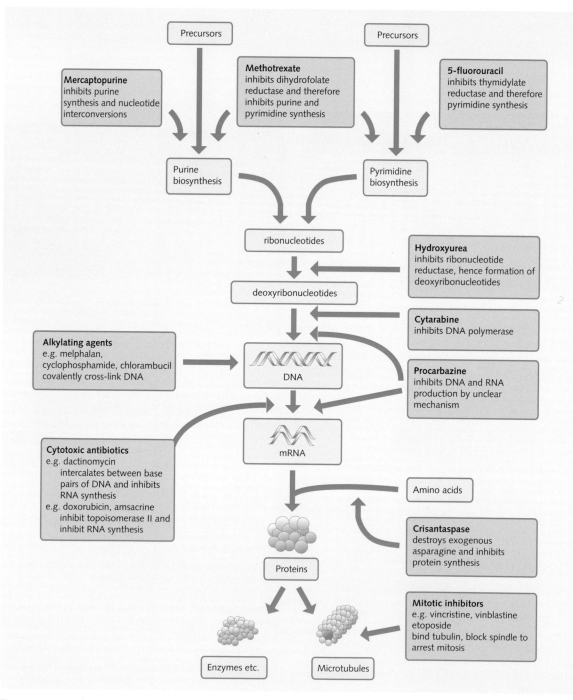

Fig. 12.1   Sites of action of cytotoxic drugs that act on dividing cells.

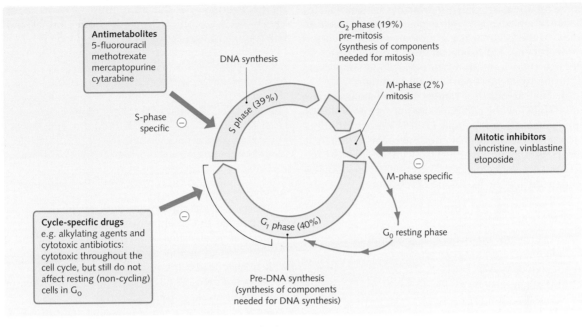

Fig. 12.2 Cell cycle and point of action of phase-specific drugs.

Selectivity

Cytotoxic drugs are not specifically toxic to cancer cells, and the selectivity they show is marginal at best.

Cytotoxic drugs affect all dividing tissues, both normal and malignant, and thus are likely to have general toxic side-effects (see Fig. 12.4). The side-effects of cytotoxic drugs are most often related to the inhibition of division of non-cancerous host cells, namely in the gut, in the bone marrow and in the reproductive and immune systems.

Relative selectivity can occur with some cancers because:

- In malignant tumours a higher proportion of cells are undergoing proliferation than in normal proliferating tissues
- Normal cells seem to recover from chemotherapeutic inhibition faster than some cancer cells
- Synchronized cell cycling may leave cytotoxic drugs vulnerable in discrete periods.

Knowledge of these principles and knowing that cytotoxic drugs kill a constant fraction, not a constant number, of cells, lays down the foundation for chemotherapeutic dosing schedules (Fig. 12.3).

Resistance to cytotoxic drugs

Genetic resistance to cytotoxic drugs can be inherent to the cancer cell line or acquired during the course of chemotherapy, as a result of selection imposed by the chemotherapeutic agent.

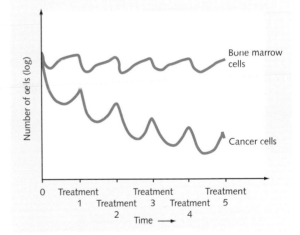

Fig. 12.3 Theoretical anticancer cytotoxic dosing schedule, allowing recovery of normal tissues.

Mechanisms of genetic resistance to cytotoxic drugs

The mechanisms of genetic resistance to cytotoxic drugs include:

- Abnormal transport
- Decreased cellular retention
- Increased cellular inactivation (binding/metabolism)
- Altered target protein
- Enhanced repair of DNA
- Altered processing.

Some tumours are relatively resistant to chemotherapy because they exist in so-called 'pharmacological sanctuaries'. These occur when a tumour is in a privileged compartment, e.g. inside the blood–brain barrier, or in large solid tumours when poor blood supply and diffusion limit the penetration of the drug.

In clinical practice, cancers may be treated more successfully with combinations of cytotoxic drugs simultaneously, for example FEC (5-flourouracil, epirubicin and cyclophosphamide) for breast cancer. The theory is that multiple attacks with cytotoxic agents acting at different biochemical sites will increase efficacy while reducing the likelihood of resistance.

Cytotoxic agents

Cytotoxic agents, the major group of anticancer drugs, include the:

- Alkylating agents
- Antimetabolites
- Cytotoxic antibiotics
- Mitotic inhibitors
- Platinum compounds
- Miscellaneous agents.

COMMUNICATION

Mrs Overton, 58 years old, presents to her GP following increasing vague abdominal pain and discomfort for the past 4 months and abdominal distension for the past 1 month. She is referred to accident and emergency and admitted. A CT scan is done and an ascitic drain inserted, from which a sample of the fluid is sent to cytology. CT shows ovarian and omental masses. Cytological examination of ascitic fluid indicates adenocarcinoma.

Laparotomy is done allowing peritoneal biopsy which shows ovarian malignancy. Mrs Overton's management includes removal of her uterus, ovaries and omentum. After surgery she is started on a 6-month course of carboplatin and paclitaxel.

Alkylating agents

Examples of alkylating agents include melphalan, cyclophosphamide and chlorambucil.

Mechanism of action—Alkylating agents act via a reactive alkyl group that reacts to form covalent bonds with nucleic acids. There follows either cross-linking of the two strands of DNA, preventing replication, or DNA strand breakage (see Fig. 12.1).

Route of administration—Melphalan and cyclophosphamide orally and intravenously; chlorambucil orally.

Indications—Melphalan is used in myeloma and in some solid tumours. Cyclophosphamide is used to treat a variety of leukaemias, and lymphomas, and some solid tumours. Chlorambucil is used for leukaemias, lymphomas and ovarian cancers.

Adverse effects—Generalized cytotoxicity is common with alkylating agents (Fig. 12.4). A urinary metabolite of cyclophosphamide, acrolein, may cause serious haemorrhagic cystitis.

Damage to gametogenesis and the development of secondary acute non-lymphocytic leukaemias is a particular problem with these alkylating agents.

Fig. 12.4 General adverse effects of cytotoxic drugs	
Site	**Effects**
Bone marrow	Myelosuppression can lead to leucopenia, thrombocytopenia and sometimes anaemia, this is often the dose-limiting side-effect; there is a high risk of haemorrhage, immunosuppression and infection as a result
Gastrointestinal tract	Inhibition of mucosal cell division may produce anorexia, ulceration or diarrhoea; nausea and vomiting are common, especially with alkylating agents and cisplatin
Skin	Loss of hair (alopecia) may be partial or complete but is usually reversible
Wounds	Impaired wound healing results from cell reproduction inhibition
Reproductive system	Sterility, teratogenesis and mutagenicity are all possible
Secondary cancers	Many cytotoxic drugs are carcinogenic, additionally the immunosuppression resulting from myelosuppression may reduce immune surveillance of emerging dysplastic cells, leading to an increased risk of development of some cancers after chemotherapy

Therapeutic notes—Extensive clinical experience is available with alkylating agents.

Antimetabolites

Examples of antimetabolites include the folic acid antagonists (e.g. methotrexate), antipyrimidines (e.g. fluorouracil and cytarabine) and antipurines (e.g. mercaptopurine).

Mechanism of action—Antimetabolites are analogues of normal metabolites and act by competition, replacing the natural metabolite and then subverting cellular processes (see Fig. 12.1).

Methotrexate competitively antagonizes dihydrofolate reductase and prevents the regeneration of intermediates (tetrahydrofolate) essential for the synthesis of purine and thymidylate, thus inhibiting the synthesis of DNA. Fluorouracil is converted into a fraudulent pyrimidine nucleotide, fluorodeoxyuridine monophosphate, that inhibits thymidylate synthetase, impairing DNA synthesis. Cytarabine is converted intracellularly to a triphosphate form that inhibits DNA polymerase. Mercaptopurine is converted into a fraudulent purine nucleotide that impairs DNA synthesis.

Route of administration—Methotrexate is administered orally, intravenously, intramuscularly and intrathecally. Fluorouracil is usually given intravenously, although it can be given orally and topically. Cytarabine is given subcutaneously intravenously and intrathecally; mercaptopurine is given orally.

Indications—Methotrexate is used for acute lymphoblastic leukaemia, and non Hodgkin's lymphoma. Fluorouracil is used for solid tumours and some malignant skin conditions. Cytarabine is used for acute myeloblastic leukaemia. Mercaptopurine is used as maintenance therapy for acute leukaemias.

Adverse effects—A common side-effect of antimetabolites is generalized cytotoxicity (see Fig. 12.4).

Therapeutic notes—Methotrexate should not be given to people with significant hepatic or renal impairment.

Cytotoxic antibiotics

Dactinomycin (actinomycin D), bleomycin and doxorubicin are examples of cytotoxic antibiotics.

Mechanism of action—Cytotoxic antibiotics act by various means.

Dactinomycin prevents transcription by interfering with RNA polymerase. Doxorubicin inhibits transcription and DNA replication by inhibiting topoisomerase II. Bleomycin acts to fragment DNA chains.

Route of administration—Intravenous. Doxorubicin can be given intravesically for bladder cancer.

Indications—Dactinomycin is principally used in paediatric cancers. Doxorubicin is used for acute leukaemias, lymphomas and a variety of solid tumours. Bleomycin is used for lymphomas and certain solid tumours.

Adverse effects—Generalized cytotoxicity (see Fig. 12.4). Doxorubicin produces dose-dependent cardiotoxicity, due to irreversible free radical damage to the myocardium. Bleomycin may cause pulmonary fibrosis.

Mitotic inhibitors

Examples of mitotic inhibitors include the vinca alkaloids, vincristine, vinblastine and vinorelbine, ixabepilone and etoposide.

Mechanism of action—Mitotic inhibitors act by binding tubulin and inhibiting the polymerization of microtubules which is necessary to form the mitotic spindle. This prevents mitosis, and arrests dividing cells at metaphase (see Fig. 12.1).

Route of administration—The vinca alkaloids are administered intravenously, and etoposide orally or intravenously.

Indications—Mitotic inhibitors are used for acute leukaemias, lymphomas and some solid tumours.

Adverse effects—Side-effects of mitotic inhibitors result from the fact that tubulin polymerization is relatively indiscriminate, inhibiting other cellular processes that involve microtubules, as well as cell division.

Generalized cytotoxicity occurs (Fig. 12.4), except that vincristine is unusual in producing little or no bone marrow suppression.

Neurological and neuromuscular effects occur, especially with vincristine, and include peripheral neuropathy leading to paraesthesia, loss of reflexes and weakness. Recovery from these effects occurs but is slow.

Therapeutic notes—Intrathecal administration of vinca alkaloids is contraindicated as it is usually fatal. Ixabepilone, an epithilone, is not lisenced for use in metastatic breast cancer after conventional therapy has failed.

COMMUNICATION

Mr Bishop is a 66-year-old painter, who presents to his GP with 4-month history of increasing shortness of breath and significant weight loss, with a 2-week history of fresh blood haemoptysis four to five times per day. The patient also complains of lethargy, breathlessness on lying down and increasing pain in his spine. Mr Bishop has smoked 20 cigarettes per day for the past 50 years. On examination, breath sounds are absent and there is stony dullness to percussion. He also has right axillary lymphadenopathy.

Mr Bishop is referred for urgent investigation. Chest X-ray reveals a large pleural effusion on the right. Aspiration of the pleural effusion shows malignant cells. Tissue obtained at bronchoscopy confirms squamous cell carcinoma of the bronchus. Staging scans show liver and bone metastases. His management includes cisplatin and vinorelbine chemotherapy.

Platinum compounds

Cisplatin (first-generation drug), carboplatin (second generation), and lastly oxaliplatin (third generation).

Mechanism of action—Cross linking of DNA subunits, thus inhibiting DNA synthesis, transcription and function. They can act in any cell cycle.

Indications—Cisplatin is mainly used for lung, cervical, bladder, testicular and ovarian cancers (although carboplatin is preferred for ovarian cancer). Carboplatin is mainly used for advanced ovarian and lung cancer (particularly small cell type). Oxaliplatin is used in combination with 5-flourouracil and folinic acid to treat metastatic colorectal cancer and as colon cancer adjuvant treatment.

Contraindications—Pregnancy breastfeeding.

Route of administration—Intravenous.

Adverse effects—Cisplatin may cause nausea, vomiting, nephrotoxicity ototoxicity peripheral neuropathy, hypomagnesaemia, myelosuppression. Carboplatin has the same adverse effects as cisplatin but all to a lesser extent, with the exception of greater myelosuppression. Oxaliplatin may cause neurotoxicity, gastrointestinal disturbances, myelosuppression.

Multikinase inhibitors

Multikinase inhibitors (pazopanib, sunitinib, sorafenib, imatinib) are used, for example, in advanced renal cell carcinoma. They inhibit vascular endothelial growth factor and platelet derived growth factor. If, in advanced renal cell carcinoma multikinase inhibitors are not affective, mTOR (mammalian target of rapamycin) kinase inhibitors (e.g. everolimus, temsirolimus) can be considered.

Miscellaneous agents

Several chemotherapeutic cytotoxic agents do not fall into any of the aforementioned groups.

Procarbazine

Mechanism of action—Procarbazine is a methylhydrazine derivative with monoamine oxidase inhibitor actions and cytotoxicity. It inhibits DNA and RNA synthesis by a mechanism that is unclear (see Fig. 12.1).

Route of administration—Oral.

Indication—Procarbazine is the first-line drug for lymphomas such as Hodgkin's.

Adverse effects—Generalized cytotoxicity (see Fig. 12.4). It causes an adverse reaction in combination with alcohol.

Therapeutic notes—Procarbazine forms part of MOPP (mechlorethamine [chlormethine], vincristine, procarbazine and prednisone) therapy for Hodgkin's lymphoma.

Hydroxyurea

Mechanism of action—Hydroxyurea causes the inhibition of ribonucleotide reductase and hence the formation of deoxyribonucleotides (Fig. 12.1).

Route of administration—Oral.

Indications—Hydroxyurea is used for chronic myeloid leukaemia. Polycythemia rubra vera.

Adverse effects—Generalized cytotoxicity (see Fig. 12.4).

Crisantaspase

Mechanism of action—Some tumour cells lose the ability to synthesize asparagine, requiring an exogenous source of the substance to grow; normal host cells can synthesize their own. Crisantaspase is a preparation of bacterial asparaginase that breaks down any circulating asparagine, hence inhibiting the growth of some cancers, namely acute lymphoblastic leukaemia (see Fig. 12.1).

Route of administration—Intramuscular, subcutaneous.

Indication—Acute lymphoblastic leukaemia.

Adverse effects—The most serious side-effects of crisantaspase include severe toxicity to the liver and pancreas. CNS depression and anaphylaxis are also risks.

Therapeutic notes—Regular testing of patients given crisantaspase is necessary to monitor organ functions.

Many other anti-cancer agents are used in the management of malignant tumours, including: mTOR kinase inhibitors (temsirolimus, everolimus), amsacrine, altretamine, dacarbazine, mitotane, pentostatin, taxanes, thalidomide, topoisomerase I inhibitors, and tretinoin. Detailed information on these can be gained from the *British National Formulary (BNF)* or specialist textbooks.

ENDOCRINE THERAPY

Hormones and antihormones

The growth of some cancers is hormone dependent. Growth of such tumours can be inhibited by surgical removal of the source of the driving hormone, such as the gonads, adrenals or pituitary. Increasingly, however, administration of hormones or antihormones is preferred.

Endocrine therapy can cause side-effects, the nature of which can normally be deduced from the physiological effects of the hormone being given or antagonized. Endocrine therapy generally has the advantage that it has far fewer serious adverse effects than cytotoxic therapy.

Hormones used in endocrine therapy include:

- Adrenocortical steroids (Ch. 6), e.g. prednisolone, which inhibit the growth of cancers of the lymphoid tissues and blood. In addition they are used to treat some of the complications of the cancer (e.g. oedema).
- Oestrogen antagonists, e.g. tamoxifen, which are competitive inhibitors at oestrogen receptors. Inhibition of the stimulatory effects of oestrogen suppresses the division of breast cancer cells. Tamoxifen is indicated for use in postmenopausal women with metastatic disease.
- Oestrogens (Ch. 6), e.g. diethylstilbestrol, which have an antiandrogenic effect and can be used to suppress androgen-dependent prostatic cancers.
- Progesterones (Ch. 6), which inhibit endometrial cancer and carcinomas of the prostate and breast.
- Androgen antagonists, e.g. flutamide, which inhibit androgen-dependent prostatic cancers. Gonadotrophin-releasing hormone (GnRH) analogues have a similar effect as they inhibit GnRH release via negative feedback.

IMMUNOTHERAPY

Immunotherapy of cancer is derived from the fact that bacterial infections sometimes provoked the regression of cancer, i.e. indirect immunostimulation. Approaches of immunotherapy include:

- The use of tumour-specific monoclonal antibodies to target drugs specifically to cancerous cells; the so called 'magic-bullet' approach (see below).
- The use of vaccines e.g. bacille Calmette Guérin (BCG) to provide non-specific immunostimulation.
- The use of specific vaccines prepared using tumour cells from similar cancers, in an attempt to raise an adaptive immune response against the cancer. An example of autologous cellular immunotherapy is Sipuleucel-T, the first approved 'cancer vaccine' for metastatic prostate cancer. It is hoped more immunotherapy for solid cancers will be produced.
- Immunostimulation using drugs, e.g. levamisole.
- The use of cytokines to regulate the immune response so as to favourably target the cancer. Cytokines used include interferon a, interleukin (IL)-2, and tumour necrosis factor.
- The use of recombinant colony-stimulating factors to reduce the level and duration of neutropenia after cytotoxic chemotherapy.
- Recombinant human granulocyte colony-stimulating factor (rh-G-CSF; filgrastim) and granulocyte-macrophage colony-stimulating factor (GM-CSF; molgramostim) promote the development of their respective haemopoietic stem cells in the marrow. Their use to raise white blood cell counts after cytotoxic chemotherapy is effective, although this has not been shown to alter overall survival rates.

Monoclonal antibodies

Examples are: rituximab, alemtuzumab, cetuximab, trastuzumab, ofatumumab

Mechanism of action—Monoclonal antibodies recognize the pattern of proteins that are found on the surface of the cancer cell and lock onto them. It can then either trigger the body's immune system to destroy the cell or it may be attached to a cancer drug or radioactive substance, which can target the selected cells.

Indications—Some haematological malignancies.

- Trastuzumab is licensed for metastatic breast cancer in patients with tumours overexpressing human epidermal growth factor 2 (HER2) receptor.
- Cetuximab in combination with irinotecan, is licensed for metastatic colorectal cancers overexpressing epidermal growth factor receptors.

Contraindications—Severe dyspnoea at rest, breastfeeding.

Route of administration—Intravenous.

Adverse effects—Hypersensitivity reactions, chills, fevers, cardiotoxicity, hypotension, gastrointestinal symptoms, airway obstruction, aches and pains.

Antibody Directed Enzyme Pro-drug Therapy (ADEPT) uses monoclonal antibodies to carry enzymes directly to the cancer cells. A cytotoxic pro-drug is then administered, which is only activated in cells with the enzyme, thus resulting in treatment targeting cancer cells but not normal cells.

THE FUTURE

There are many drugs that may be potential candidates as anticancer agents and many are being tested in ongoing trials across the world. The most promising areas appear to be monoclonal antibodies, antisense oligonucleotides, inhibitors of enzymes responsible for cell invasiveness and metastasis, and agents which interfere with tumour angiogenesis (formation of new blood vessels).

It is believed that modulation of the host's immune system will become part of cancer therapy in the future, in addition to novel methods of drug delivery, including liposomes and viral vectors.

SELF-ASSESSMENT

Best of fives (BOFs)

Indicate which one of the five possible answers is correct:

Chapter 1 Introduction to pharmacology

1. In which phase of drug development can all the patients be prescribed the drug?
   a. Preclinical
   b. Phase 1
   c. Phase 2
   d. Phase 3
   e. Phase 4

2. What is the plasma pH?
   a. 7.4
   b. 8.0
   c. 2.0
   d. 7.0
   e. 6.0

3. Which one of the following is a generic name of a drug?
   a. Syntometrine®
   b. Paracetamol
   c. Calpol®
   d. N-acetyl-p-aminophenol
   e. Proguanil hydrochloride

4. Which one of these is a type of G-protein linked receptor?
   a. Nicotinic acetylcholine receptor
   b. Insulin receptor
   c. β-Adrenergic receptor
   d. Steroid receptor
   e. PGF receptor

5. What is the symbol for the dissociation constant?
   a. Kc
   b. Ka
   c. Ke
   d. Kd
   e. Kb

6. What is the most direct route of drug administration?
   a. Intravenous
   b. Intramuscular
   c. Per rectum
   d. Subcutaneous
   e. Per oral

7. Which drug can cause enzyme inhibition?
   a. Rifampicin
   b. Phenytoin
   c. Corticosteroids
   d. Ethanol
   e. Phenobarbital

Chapter 2 Cardiovascular system

1. Depolarization occurs in which phase of the cardiac action potential?
   a. Phase 0
   b. Phase 1
   c. Phase 2
   d. Phase 3
   e. Phase 4

2. What is the resting membrane potential of nodal cells?
   a. 60 mv
   b. −40 mv
   c. 40 mv
   d. −60 mv
   e. −85 mv

3. Which one of these is a cardiac glycoside?
   a. Propanolol
   b. Milrinone
   c. Hydralazine
   d. Disopyramide
   e. Digoxin

4. What class of anti-arrhythmics are β-adrenoceptor antagonists?
   a. Class Ia
   b. Class Ib
   c. Class II
   d. Class III
   e. Class IV

5. ACE inhibitors are contraindicated in which one of the following?
   a. Asthma
   b. Aortic Stenosis
   c. Hypertension
   d. Diabetes
   e. Eczema

6. Which causes a decrease in heart rate?
   a. β-Blockers
   b. Caffeine
   c. Adrenaline
   d. Shock
   e. Phaeochromocytoma

7. What part of the heart pumps deoxygenated blood to the lungs?
   a. Pulmonary vein
   b. Aorta
   c. Superior vena cava
   d. Pulmonary artery
   e. Inferior vena cava

Chapter 3 Respiratory system

1. What type of hypersensitivity occurs in an asthma attack?
   a. Type 1
   b. Type 2
   c. Type 3
   d. Type 4
   e. Type 5

2. At what stage should long term oxygen therapy be considered in the treatment of COPD?
   a. Stage 0
   b. Stage 1
   c. Stage 2
   d. Stage 3
   e. Stage 4

3. Which is not part of the upper respiratory tract?
   a. Nasopharynx
   b. Epiglottis
   c. Larynx
   d. Trachea
   e. Bronchioles

4. Which one is not a bronchodilator used in asthma?
   a. β_2-Agonists
   b. Glucocorticoids
   c. Leukotreine antagonists
   d. Xanthines
   e. Ipratropium bromide

5. What is the first line drug used in the relief of an asthma attack?
   a. Glucocorticoid
   b. Aminophylline
   c. Short acting β_2-agonist
   d. Ipratropium bromide
   e. Long acting β_2-agonist

6. What percentage of oxygen should be given in a severe asthma attack?
   a. 10%
   b. 20%
   c. 50%
   d. 75%
   e. 100%

7. Which one is a common side effect of β_2-agonists?
   a. Tremor
   b. Ankle oedema
   c. Oral candidiasis

   d. Bradycardia
   e. Weight gain

Chapter 4 Peripheral nervous system

1. Which drug is a depolarizing blocker of postsynaptic receptors at the NMJ?
   a. Pancuronium
   b. Suxamethonium
   c. Gallamine
   d. Vecuronium
   e. Atracurium

2. Which adrenoceptor agonist is used first line in anaphylactic shock?
   a. Noradrenaline
   b. Clonidine
   c. Adrenaline
   d. Dobutamine
   e. Salbutamol

3. Which drug is not an adrenoceptor antagonist?
   a. Labetolol
   b. Phentolamine
   c. Prazosin
   d. Propanolol
   e. Isoprenaline

4. Which parasympathetic muscarinic receptor is found principally in the heart?
   a. M_1
   b. M_2
   c. M_3
   d. M_4
   e. M_5

5. Which parasympathetic muscarinic receptor is principally found in the eye?
   a. M_1
   b. M_2
   c. M_3
   d. M_4
   e. M_5

6. Which drug is not a muscarinic agonist?
   a. Carbachol
   b. Metacholine
   c. Muscarine
   d. Pilocarpine
   e. Atropine

7. Which muscarinic antagonist may be used as a bronchodilator?
   a. Ipratropium
   b. Hyoscine
   c. Cyclopentolate
   d. Tropicamide
   e. Pirenzepine

Chapter 5 Central nervous system

1. Which part of the brain is responsible for vision?
   a. Parietal lobe
   b. Occipital lobe
   c. Frontal lobe
   d. Temporal lobe
   e. Cerebellum

2. Which is not a common symptom of Parkinson's disease?
   a. Shuffling gait
   b. Blank expression
   c. Speech impairment
   d. Intention tremor
   e. Bradykinesia

3. Which drug is not used in the treatment of Parkinson's disease?
   a. Dopamine agonists
   b. MAO_B inhibitors
   c. Amantadine
   d. COMT inhibitors
   e. Dopamine antagonists

4. Citalopram belongs to which category of antidepressant?
   a. SSRIs
   b. TCAs
   c. SNRIs
   d. MAOIs
   e. RIMAs

5. In which condition are TCAs not contraindicated?
   a. Recent myocardial infarction
   b. Manic phase
   c. Asthma
   d. Severe liver disease
   e. Epilepsy

6. Which drug is a typical antipsychotic?
   a. Clozapine
   b. Haloperidol
   c. Pimozide
   d. Risperidone
   e. Olanzapine

7. Which is not a common side effect of dopamine antagonists?
   a. Amenorrhoea
   b. Sedation
   c. Weight loss
   d. Dystonia
   e. Parkinsonism

Chapter 6 Endocrine and reproductive systems

1. Which drug is not usually given for people with osteoporosis?
   a. Calcium salts
   b. Calcitonin
   c. Vitamin D
   d. HRT
   e. Bisphosphonates

2. Which contraceptive should not be given to breastfeeding women?
   a. COCP
   b. POP
   c. Implant
   d. Depo injection
   e. Mirena coil

3. Which is not a symptom of hyperthyroidism?
   a. Tachycardia
   b. Increased appetite
   c. Tremor
   d. Increased temperature
   e. Weight gain

4. Which is not a mineralcorticoid?
   a. Prednisolone
   b. Fludrocortisone
   c. Dexamethasone
   d. Beclometasone
   e. Hydrocortisone

5. Which is used to control type 1 diabetes?
   a. Insulin
   b. Metformin
   c. Acarbose
   d. Thiazolidinediones
   e. Dietary control only

6. Which side effect is not caused by prolonged steroid use?
   a. Osteoporosis
   b. Weight gain
   c. Hypoglycaemia
   d. Muscle wasting
   e. Thinning of skin

7. Which drug is used to postpone premature labour?
   a. Oxytocin
   b. Prostaglandin E
   c. Ergometrine
   d. Salbutamol
   e. Gosereline

Chapter 7 Kidney and urinary system

1. Which part of the nephron is the main site of potassium secretion?
   a. Glomerulus
   b. Proximal tubule
   c. Juxtaglomerulus apparatus
   d. Loop of Henle
   e. Distal convuluted tubule

2. What type of drug is furosemide?
   a. α-Blocker
   b. Potassium sparing diuretic
   c. Loop diuretic
   d. Osmotic diuretic
   e. Thiazide diuretic

3. Thiazide diuretics can cause which one of the following?
   a. Hyperkalaemia
   b. Hyperuricaemia
   c. Hypernatraemia
   d. Hypomagnesaemia
   e. Hypocalcaemia

4. Sildenafil is used in the treament of which condition?
   a. Erectile dysfunction
   b. Stress incontinence
   c. Urinary retention
   d. Hypertension
   e. Heart failure

5. What should acute urinary retention be treated with?
   a. Antimuscarinic
   b. Anti-androgens
   c. Parasympathomimetics
   d. Urethral catheterization
   e. α-Blocker

6. **Oxybutinin does not cause which side effect?**
   a. Dry mouth
   b. Hypoglycaemia
   c. Constipation
   d. Blurred vision
   e. Nausea

7. What percentage of sodium is reabsorbed in the kidney?
   a. 0%
   b. 25%
   c. 50%
   d. 75%
   e. 99%

Chapter 8 Gastrointestinal system

1. In the stomach, hydrochloric acid is secreted by which cells?
   a. Peptic cells
   b. Parietal cells
   c. Mucus-secreting cells
   d. Paracrine cells
   e. G cells

2. H pylori is present in what percentage of patients with peptic ulcers?
   a. 25%
   b. 50%
   c. 75%
   d. 90%
   e. 100%

3. Which is not an anti-emetic?
   a. Ipecacuanha
   b. Cyclizine
   c. Prochlorperazine
   d. Domperidone
   e. Ondansetron

4. Which drug is not contraindicated for use in a patient with bowel obstruction?
   a. Glucocorticoids
   b. Stimulant laxatives
   c. Faecal softeners
   d. Osmotic laxatives
   e. Bulk forming laxatives

5. Which is the first line treatment for obesity?
   a. Sibutramine
   b. Orlistat
   c. Gastric banding
   d. Methylcellulose
   e. Diet and exercise

6. By which route should ursodeoxycholic acid be administered?
   a. Per rectum
   b. Per oral
   c. Intravenous
   d. Intramuscular
   e. Subcutaneously

7. Which enzyme breaks down starch?
   a. Chymotrypsin
   b. Protease
   c. Amylase
   d. Lipase
   e. Trypsin

Chapter 9 Pain and anaesthesia

1. Which opioid is considered a strong (step 3) analgesic?
   a. Morphine
   b. Codeine
   c. Dihydrocodeine
   d. Pentazocine
   e. Dextropropoxyphene

2. Which is the least affective route of administering opioid analgesics?
   a. Intramuscular
   b. Transdermal
   c. Per oral
   d. Per rectum
   e. Intravenously

3. Which of the following is naloxone used for?
   a. General anaesthetic
   b. Local anaesthetic
   c. Neuralgic pain relief
   d. Headache
   e. Opioid overdose

4. In the treatment of neuralgic pain, which drug provides some pain relief?
   a. Morphine
   b. Amitryptiline
   c. Paracetamol
   d. Codeine
   e. Aspirin

5. Which drug is used in the prophylaxis of migraine?
   a. NSAIDs
   b. Paracetamol
   c. Antiemetics
   d. Serotonin antagonists
   e. Serotonin agonists

6. Which drug is used as an induction anaesthetic?
   a. Propofol
   b. Nitrous oxide
   c. Halothane
   d. Enflurane
   e. Isoflurane

7. Which is the most rapid acting local anaesthetic?
   a. Benzocaine
   b. Bupivacaine
   c. Tetracaine
   d. Procaine
   e. Lignocaine

Chapter 10 Inflammation, allergic diseases and immunosuppression

1. Which is not an inflammatory mediator?
   a. Histamine
   b. Gastrin
   c. Bradykinin
   d. Interleukins
   e. Substance P

2. Which NSAID does not have an anti-inflammatory action?
   a. Aspirin
   b. Indomethacin
   c. Paracetamol
   d. Phenylbutazone
   e. Ibuprofen

3. Which class of DMARDs does chloroquine belong to?
   a. Gold salts
   b. Penicillamine
   c. Sulfasalazine
   d. Antimalarials
   e. Immunosuppresants

4. Which drug is most commonly used in the treatment of acute gout?
   a. Indomethacin
   b. Colchicine
   c. Allopurinol
   d. Sulfinpyrazone
   e. Probenecid

5. Which drug is commonly used as a prophylaxis against gout?
   a. Indomethacin
   b. Colchicine
   c. Allopurinol
   d. Sulfinpyrazone
   e. Probenecid

6. Which topical steroid is most potent?
   a. Hydrocortisone 2%
   b. Clobetasol propionate
   c. Betametasone valerate 0.1%
   d. Clobetasol butyrate
   e. Hydrocortisone 1%

7. Which drug is not used as a treatment for psoriasis?
   a. Retinoids
   b. Psoralen
   c. Methotrexate
   d. Cyclosporin
   e. Ketokonazole

Chapter 11 Infectious diseases

1. Which antibacterial drug affects the cytoplasmic membrane of bacteria?
   a. Aminoglycosides
   b. Tetracyclines
   c. Penicillins
   d. Cephalosporins
   e. Polymyxins

2. Which antibiotic is bacteriostatic?
   a. Flucloxacillin
   b. Cefuroxime
   c. Tetracycline
   d. Ciprofloxacin
   e. Vancomycin

3. Which antibiotic is used first line in the treatment of streptococcus?
   a. Cefixime
   b. Penicilline
   c. Erythromycin
   d. Trimethoprim
   e. Gentamicin

4. Which drug is not used in the treatment of tuberculosis?
   a. Tetracycline
   b. Rifampicin
   c. Isoniazid
   d. Pyrazinamide
   e. Ethambutol

5. Which virus is double stranded?
   a. Parvovirus
   b. Orthomyxovirus
   c. Rhabdovirus
   d. Herpes virus
   e. Retrovirus

6. What drug is used first line to treat the herpes virus causing cold sores?
   a. Ganciclovir
   b. Nevirapine
   c. Aciclovir
   d. Zidovudine
   e. Ribavirin

7. What drug is used to treat candidiasis?
   a. Griseofulvin
   b. Clotrimazole
   c. Allylamine
   d. Salbutamol
   e. Flucytosine

Chapter 12 Cancer

1. Which cytotoxic drug is an alkylating agent?
   a. Methotrexate
   b. Cyclophosphamide
   c. Danctinomycin
   d. Vinblastine
   e. Cisplatin

2. What phase of cell cycle is affected most by cytotoxic drugs?
   a. G_0
   b. G_1
   c. G_2
   d. S
   e. M

3. Methotrexate affects which phase of the cell cycle?
   a. G_0
   b. G_1
   c. G_2
   d. S
   e. M

4. Which drug is an oestrogen antagonist?
   a. Tamoxifen
   b. Diethylstilbestrol
   c. Flutamide
   d. Rituximab
   e. Prednisolone

5. Which monoclonal antibody is liscenced for use in HER2 breast cancer?
   a. Alemtuzumab
   b. Rituximab
   c. Trastuzumab
   d. Cetuximab
   e. Bevacizumab

6. Which is not a common side effect of chemotherapy?
   a. Sterility
   b. Nausea
   c. Alopecia
   d. Thrombocytophilia
   e. Impaired wound healing

7. Which drug is an antimetabolite?
   a. 5-Fluorouracil
   b. Vincristine
   c. Cyclophosphamide
   d. Etoposide
   e. Bleomycin

Extended-matching questions (EMQs)

For each scenario described below choose the *single* most likely option from the list of options.

Each option may be used once, more than once or not at all.

1. G-protein linked receptors

A. Activation of phospholipase C

B. Activation of guanylyl cyclase on the membrane of endothelial cells

C. Fast synaptic neurotransmission

D. Phosphorylation of tyrosine residues

E. Activation of protein kinase C

F. Inactivation of protein kinase C

G. Malignancy

H. Inactivation of adenylyl cyclase

I. Activation of adenylyl cyclase

J. None of the above

Instruction: Match one of the options listed above to the lead-in given below.

1. DAG and IP_3 cause

2. Bradykinin causes

3. Cholera causes

4. Pertussis causes

5. DAG and IP_3 production follows

2. Pharmacokinetics

A. Redistribution

B. Reduction

C. Absorption

D. Oxidation

E. Phase 2 metabolism

F. Phase 1 metabolism

G. First-pass metabolism

H. Hydrolysis

I. Creatinine clearance

J. Dithranol

Instruction: Match one of the options listed above to the descriptions given below.

1. The drug is often one taken orally, absorbed through the intestinal wall, goes directly to the liver through the portal venous system and gets metabolized there before reaching the target organ.

2. The drug is oxidised, reduced or hydrolysed resulting in an increase in polarity of the drug and provision of a site for further reactions.

3. The drug is conjugated, resulting in it becoming more hydrophilic and thus more readily excretable.

4. Warfarin, the anticoagulant, is inactivated in this way to result in the transformation of a ketone group into a hydroxyl group

5. Drugs leave the circulation and enter tissues perfused by blood.

3. Emergency and nervous system drugs

A. Propofol

B. Levodopa only

C. Levodopa plus carbidopa

D. Carbidopa

E. Flumazenil

F. *N*-Acetylcysteine

G. Lidocaine

H. Intravenous morphine

I. Ibuprofen

J. Nitrous oxide

Instruction: Match one of the options listed above to the statements given below.

1. To treat Parkinson's disease it is best to give

2. A patient is in serious respiratory depression following an excessive alcohol consumption while on a benzodiazepine. The most appropriate treatment would be

3. A young victim of assault makes an impulsive decision to take a paracetamol overdose but regrets it immediately and calls for help. On arrival at hospital she should be given

4. A local anaesthetic is required to allow excision of a small mole.

5. A road traffic accident victim, who was forced into the central reservation, is assessed by paramedics and found to have a patent airway and circulation but is in extreme pain.

4. Antibiotics and antivirals

A. Aciclovir

B. Penicillin

C. Fluconazole

D. Bleomycin

E. Chloroquine

F. Praziquantel

G. Ganciclovir

H. Rifampicin

I. Chloramphenicol

J. Trimethoprim

Instruction: Match one of the options listed above to the descriptions given below.

1. A bactericidal drug that prevents peptide cross-linking within the microbial cell wall is given to a 26-year-old woman presenting with an uncomplicated urinary tract infection to take for a course of 7 days.

2. A bacteriostatic drug was used to treat a respiratory tract infection in a 30-year-old man, who subsequently developed a hypersensitivity complex affecting the eyes, skin and mucous membranes. Treatment was immediately stopped.

3. A patient was put on a regimen of drugs to treat his tuberculosis. After his commencement he noted that his urine and tears had turned orange-red.

4. A 17-year-old student develops a red and tingling area of skin just above his lips. He is diagnosed as having a cold sore.

5. A patient who was on treatment for non-Hodgkin's lymphoma for many years developed shortness of breath resulting in reduced exercise capacity. Chest X-ray revealed lung fibrosis. It was thought to be caused by one of the cytotoxic antibiotic drugs he was taking, which worked by fragmenting DNA.

5. Cardiovascular system drugs

A. Quinidine

B. Lidocaine

C. Heparin

D. Glyceryl trinitrate

E. Erythropoietin

F. Amiodarone

G. Atorvastatin

H. Digoxin

I. Verapamil

J. Aspirin

Instruction: Match one of the options listed above to the descriptions given below.

1. An antianginal drug that involves the formation of nitric oxide, thereby dilating systemic veins.

2. An antiarrhythmic drug that blocks voltage-gated sodium channels, which slows phase 0 of the cardiac action potential and therefore increases the effective refractory period.

3. An antiarrhythmic drug that slows phases 0 and 3 of the cardiac action potential, prolonging the cardiac action potential duration and the effective refractory period.

4. An antiarrhythmic drug that shortens phase 2 of the cardiac action potential by calcium antagonism.

5. A cardiac glycoside with positive inotropic action that shifts the Frank–Starling ventricular function curve upwards.

6. Drug interactions

A. Moclobemide

B. Clozapine

C. Insulin

D. Diazepam

E. Ethanol

F. Phenytoin

G. Phenelzine

H. Aspirin

I. Vigabatrin

J. Hydrochlorothiazide

Instruction: Match one of the options listed above to the descriptions given below.

1. A French man who eats cheese and drinks wine daily is given medication for depression and becomes acutely ill with severely raised blood pressure. He is prescribed an irreversibly acting drug.

2. A young woman who has been taking epilepsy medication and has just started taking an oral contraceptive pill. Two months later, she finds that she is pregnant.

3. This drug was given to a student experiencing hallucinations, although it can cause potentially fatal neutropenia in 1% of the population. She drinks lots of high energy drinks, containing caffeine to study late. This is thought to inhibit metabolism of this drug (normally by cytochrome P450), resulting in an increase in serum levels and side effects.

4. A patient taking anxiolytic medication recently drank to excess while out one night. He was found on the street by paramedics who noted that he was not breathing.

5. A middle-aged man with bipolar affective disorder is found to have high serum levels of lithium. His general practitioner has recently started him on a diuretic to treat his hypertension.

---

7. Endocrine system drugs

A. Increase oral contraceptive

B. Isophane insulin

C. Glibenclamide

D. Insulin aspart and insulin zinc suspension

E. Take her off oral contraceptive

F. Prednisolone

G. Carbimazole

H. Levothyroxine

I. Beclometasone

J. Metformin

Instruction: Match one of the options listed above to the descriptions given below.

1. A 30-year-old woman presents to her general practitioner with increasing sweating, anxiety and weight loss despite an ever-increasing appetite. She is diagnosed with an endocrine condition and given medication.

2. A woman who is on the oral contraceptive pill and has asthma develops deep vein thrombosis. Appropriate management is required.

3. A young man requires modification to his insulin regimen for type 1 diabetes. His doctor thinks he needs to change only his intermediate-acting insulin from the protamine zinc insulin to a different one.

4. A 50-year-old man with heart failure has recently developed type 2 diabetes. He needs to take an oral antidiabetic drug.

5. A middle-aged man has been taking treatment for his rheumatoid arthritis. He now has increased central abdominal fat, a moon-shaped face, purple striae, thin arms and legs, and hypertension. A drug he is taking was thought to be responsible.

---

8. The kidney and urinary tract drugs

A. Mannitol

B. Amiloride

C. Aldosterone

D. Oxybutynin

E. Adrenaline

F. Methazolamide

G. Bumetanide

H. Doxazosin

I. Sildenafil

J. Bendroflumethiazide

Instruction: Match one of the options listed above to the descriptions given below.

1. A drug that inhibits the $Na^+/K^+/2Cl^-$ co-transporters in the luminal membrane of the loop of Henle.

2. A drug that acts by relaxing the detrusor smooth muscle of the bladder and is, therefore, used as a treatment for urge incontinence. This drug should not be given to patients with glaucoma.

3. A drug that blocks the sodium channels in the luminal membrane of the late distal convoluted tubule and collecting duct, thereby reducing potassium secretion into the lumen.

4. A drug to help maintain an erection through relaxation of penile smooth muscle that can be given to patients with multiple sclerosis. Relaxation of the smooth muscle happens through inhibition of phosphodiesterase-mediated degradation of cGMP.

5. A drug that inhibits the Na^+/Cl^- symporters in the luminal membrane of the early distal convoluted tubule.

---

9. Gastrointestinal system drugs

A. Domperidone
B. Aluminium hydroxide
C. Omeprazole
D. Prednisolone
E. Loperamide
F. Hyoscine
G. Senna
H. Lactulose
I. Mesalazine
J. Ursodeoxycholic acid

Instruction: Match one of the options listed above to the descriptions given below.

1. A 33-year-old banker visits her general practitioner with burning pain behind her sternum. A diagnosis of oesophageal reflux is made.

2. A 25-year-old patient with history of peptic ulcer disease is placed on aspirin following development of angina. Prophylactic treatment is indicated against ulcer reoccurrence and a drug which causes irreversible inhibition of H^+/K^+ ATPase is selected.

3. A 50-year-old patient who develops pain due to metastases is placed on opiate pain relief and subsequently develops constipation. She is put on a stimulant laxative to increase intestinal motility.

4. A 30-year-old woman, who suffers from motion sickness, needs to go on a business cruise. She is given an antiemetic which acts by competitive antagonism of muscarinic receptors.

5. A patient recently diagnosed with inflammatory bowel disease is placed on a maintenance drug.

---

10. Respiratory system drugs

A. Salbutamol
B. Salmeterol
C. Aminophylline
D. Naloxone
E. Dry mouth
F. Immunosuppression
G. Ephedrine
H. Coughing
I. Morphine
J. Oxygen

Instruction: Match one of the options listed above to the descriptions given below.

1. An example of physical defence mechanism.

2. An adverse effect associated with a drug used to treat chronic obstructive pulmonary disease (COPD).

3. A long-acting agonist used by asthmatic people for immediate relief of symptoms.

4. An intravenous xanthine given to treat a young adult, following admission to hospital with a life-threatening asthma attack.

5. A drug used as a respiratory stimulant in those with drug-induced respiratory depression.

BOF answers

Chapter 1 Introduction to pharmacology

1. E Up until phase 4, only a selected number of patients can be used. In preclinical phase, subjects are either animals or in vitro studies.

2. A Plasma pH in a healthy individual should be between 7.35–7.45. The average is 7.4.

3. B Generic names are given to government-approved drugs sold on prescription or over the counter. A and C are proprietary names. D and E are chemical names.

4. C A is an ion channel linked receptor. B and E are tyrosine linked receptors. D is a DNA linked receptor.

5. D The symbol for the dissociation constant is Kd. Ka is the association constant.

6. A The intravenous route is the most direct route of administering a drug as it avoids the need for absorption which is the rate limiting step.

7. C Corticosteroids can inhibit certain enzymes. The other drugs can induce certain enzymes, such as cytochrome p450.

Chapter 2 Cardiovascular system

1. A Phase 0 is depolarization. Partial repolarization occurs in phase 1, followed by a plateau in phase 2, then repolarization in phase 3. There is no phase 4.

2. D The resting membrane potential of nodal cells is −60 mv.

3. E Digoxin is a cardiac glycoside. Propanolol is a β-blocker. Hydralazine is a vasodilator used in hypertension. Milirinone is a PDE inhibitor.

4. C β-Adrenoceptor antagonists are a class II anti-arrhythmic. Class I block sodium channels. Class III block potassium channels. Class IV are calcium antagonists.

5. B ACE inhibitors are contraindicated in aortic stenosis, because they cause vasodilatation causing a reduced preload so that there blood pressure and cardiac output are not sufficient to overcome the stenosis.

6. A β-Blockers decrease heart rate. All of the others increase heart rate.

7. D The superior vena cava and inferior vena cava bring deoxygenated blood back to the heart from the body. Deoxygenated blood is pumped to the lungs through the pulmonary artery, where the blood becomes oxygenated and returns to the heart through the pulmonary vein. It then leaves the heart through the aorta.

Chapter 3 Respiratory system

1. A Asthma attack is a type 1 hypersensitivity reaction, which is immediate and IgE mediated.

2. E Long term oxygen therapy should not be given to patients until their COPD is severe enough to warrant it. Lifestyle changes such as stopping smoking should be promoted.

3. E The bronchioles are part of the lower respiratory tract.

4. B Glucocorticoids are anti-inflammatories used long term in asthmatics to try and prevent asthma attacks.

5. C Short acting, not long acting β_2-agonists are used first line in an asthma attack due to its quick acting bronchodilating action.

6. E 100% oxygen should be used in severe asthma attacks to get oxygen saturations up to above 92%.

7. A Tremor occurs with the use of β_2-agonists, alongside tachycardia and hypokalaemia after high doses.

Chapter 4 Peripheral nervous system

1. B Suxamethomium is the only depolarizing blocker used clinically. The others are non-depolarizing blockers and are used clinically, often in anaesthetics.

2. C Adrenaline should be used first line in anaphylaxis.

3. E Isoprenaline is an adrenoceptor agonist.

4. B M1 receptors are principally found in the CNS. M2 receptors are principally found in the heart. M3 receptors are principally found in smooth muscles and glands. M4 receptors are principally found in the eye. There is no M5 receptor.

5. D As aforementioned, M4 is the muscarinic receptor principally found in the eye.

6. E Atropine is a muscarinic antagonist used in bradycardia. It also reduces gastrointestinal motility and cardiac arrest.

7. A Ipratropium bromide is a muscarinic antagonist, but can also be used in an asthma attack as it is a bronchodilator.

Chapter 5 Central nervous system

1. B   The occipital lobe is responsible for processing vision.

2. D   Parkinson's disease is due to depletion of dopamine, which manifests in bradykinesia. Intention tremor is a sign of cerebellar pathology; resting tremor is a sign of Parkinson's disease.

3. E   Since Parkinson's disease is caused by a depletion in dopamine, dopamine antagonists would worsen symptoms. The other drugs act to increase dopamine or decrease its breakdown.

4. A   Citalopram is a common antidepressant and a SSRI. Amitriptyline is a TCA; Venlafaxine is a SNRI. Phenelzine is a MAOI; moclobemide is a RIMA.

5. C   TCAs are contraindicated in many conditions, but not asthma. Aditionally, it is contraindicated when taking lignocaine due to a potentially fatal drug interaction.

6. B   Haloperidol is an older drug, a typical antipsychotic. The other drugs are examples of atypical antibiotics.

7. C   Dopamine antagonists do not cause weight loss. However amenorrhoea, sedation, dystonia and parkinsonism can occur.

Chapter 6 Endocrine and reproductive systems

1. D   HRT is no longer recommended for general use in osteoporosis due to it increasing the risk of thromboembolism.

2. A   The COCP should not be used whilst breastfeeding as it contains oestrogen as well as progesterone.

3. E   Think of hyperthyroidism as the body working too quickly. Patients experience weight loss, not weight gain.

4. B   Fludrocortisone is a mineralcorticoid. The other drugs are glucocorticoids.

5. A   Subcutaneous insulin is used to control type 1 diabetes. Dietary control is also recommended at the same time, with regards to not eating high sugar foods.

6. C   Prolonged steroid use can cause hyperglycaemia not hypoglycaemia, leading to the chance of developing diabetes.

7. D   Salbutamol relaxes the uterus preventing contractions, hopefully postponing premature labour.

Chapter 7 Kidney and urinary system

1. E   The distal convoluted tubule is the main site of potassium secretion due to the negative potential difference that moves sodium into parietal cells and potassium out of the cells.

2. C   Furosemide is a loop diuretic. Other examples are bumetanide and torsemide. These act at the ascending segment of the loop of Henle.

3. B   Thiazide diuretics cause hypokalaemia, hyperuricaemia, hyponatraemia, hypermagnesaemia, and hypercalcaemia.

4. A   Sildenafil is used to treat erectile dysfunction. It is a selective PDEV inhibitor.

5. D   Acute urinary retention should be treated with urethral catheterization, providing there is no urethral damage. The cause should be investigated.

6. B   Oxybutinin is an antimuscarinic and therefore has anticholinergic side effects. Hypoglycaemia is not one of these.

7. E   99–100% of sodium is reabsorbed in the kidney.

Chapter 8 Gastrointestinal system

1. B   Parietal cells secrete hydrochloric acid. Peptic cells secrete digestive enzymes; G cells secrete gastrin.

2. D   *H. pylori* is present in most people and is believed to contribute to peptic ulcer formation in 75% of affected patients.

3. A   Ipecacuanha is a liquid which causes gastric irritation and causes emesis.

4. C   If a patient has bowel obstruction, laxatives that alter bowel movement tend to be contraindicated. Faecal softeners do not affect bowel movement and therefore are not contraindicated.

5. E   Before considering medication or surgery, patients should be persuaded to take up exercise and improve their diet.

6. B   Ursodeoxycholic acid should be given orally.

7. C   Trypsin, chymotrypsin and protease break down protein. Lipase breaks down fat. Starch is broken down by amylase.

Chapter 9 Pain and anaesthesia

1. A   Weaker opioids include codeine and pentazocine. Strong opioids include morphine, diamorphine and pethidine.

2. C   Opioids may be administered orally (e.g. Oramorph®), however its absorption is irregular and incomplete and therefore requires larger doses.

3. E   Naloxone is a short acting opioid antagonist used in opioid overdose.

4. B   Drugs such as carbamazepine and amitryptiline are used to treat neuralgic pain, such as post-herpetic neuralgia. Conventional analgesia does not usually work.

5. D   If migraines are frequent, serotonin antagonists such as pizotifen can be used to limit

pro-inflammatory and vascular changes that precede migraines. Serotonin agonists are used in acute attacks.

6. A Propofol is a white liquid used to induce general anaesthesia. The other drugs are gases used to maintain anaesthesia.

7. E Lignocaine is the quickest acting local anaesthetic. This is used, for example, to numb an area of skin before suturing.

Chapter 10 Inflammation, allergic diseases and immunosuppression

1. B Gastrin is not an anti-inflammatory mediator. It is secreted by G cells in the stomach in response to digestion.

2. C Paracetamol is an NSAID with no anti-inflammatory mediator.

3. D Chloroquine is an antimalarial, which is a DMARD used in rheumatoid arthritis.

4. A NSAIDs, such as indomethacin are most commonly used in acute gout. Colchicine may also be used, however this is second line after indomethacin.

5. C Allopurinol is used prophylactically, however it can induce an acute attack and should not be taken during an acute attack of gout.

6. B Hydrocortisone is the weakest of the topical steroids mentioned. Clobetasol propionate (Dermovate®) is considered very potent (Group 1).

7. E Ketokonazole is an antifungal and therefore not used in the treatment of psoriasis.

Chapter 11 Infectious diseases

1. E Polymyxins affect the bacterial cell membrane. Aminoglycosides and tetracyclines affect protein synthesis. Penicillin and cephalosporins affect cell wall synthesis.

2. C Tetracyclines are bacteriostatic. The others are bacteriocidal.

3. B Penicillin is used in the treatment of streptococcus.

4. A Tetracycline is not used in the treatment of TB.

5. D Herpes virus is a double stranded DNA virus. The others are single stranded RNA viruses except parvovirus which is a single stranded DNA virus.

6. C Aciclovir is used to treat cold sores, however it will not cure cold sores as the herpes virus remains dormant in the body. Ganciclovir is reserved for severe CMV infections.

7. B Clotrimazole is used to treat candidiasis, otherwise known as thrush.

Chapter 12 Cancer

1. B Cyclophosphamide is an alkylating agent used to treat leukaemia, lymphoma and some solid tumours.

2. B The G1 phase of the cell cycle is affected 40% of the time. S phase is affected by 39%; G2 phase 19% and M phase 2%. The G0 phase is not usually affected.

3. E Methotrexate, a folic acid antagonist, is an antimetabolite that affects the M phase of the cell cycle.

4. A Tamoxifen is a competitive oestrogen antagonist used in postmenopausal women with metastatic breast cancer.

5. C Trastuzumab is a monoclonal antibody used in HER2 breast cancer.

6. D Thrombocytopenia, not thrombocytophilia occurs with chemotherapy.

7. A 5-Fluorouracil is an anti-pyrimidine, an antimetabolite, which inhibits thymidylate synthetase which impairs DNA synthesis.

1. G-protein linked receptors

1. E   See Figure EMQ1.
2. B   Bradykinin initiates nitric oxide production in endothelial cells. Nitric oxide then acts as a second messenger to cause activation of guanylyl cyclase.
3. I   See Figure EMQ1.
4. H   See Figure EMQ1.
5. A   See Figure EMQ1.

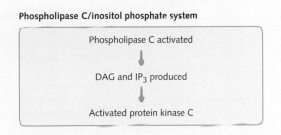

Phospholipase C/inositol phosphate system

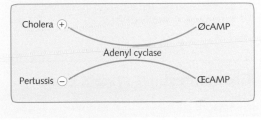

Activation/deactivation of adenyl cyclase

Fig. 1   E See Figure EMQ1.

2. Pharmacokinetics

1. G   Different routes of administration or an increase in dosage can be utilized to minimize the quantity of drug metabolized before reaching the target organ.
2. F   Phase 1 reactions usually result in the drug becoming more reactive.
3. E   Phase 2 reactions normally detoxify the metabolites of Phase 1 reactions.
4. B   An example of a Phase 1 reaction is reduction.
5. A   The distribution of a drug is dependent on the permeability between tissues; dependent on blood flow, perfusion rate and the ability of the drug to bind plasma proteins. Redistribution is an important factor in the termination of intravenous anaesthetics.

3. Emergency and nervous system drugs

1. C   Levodopa is a dopamine precursor used to treat Parkinson's disease and is usually given to replenish dopamine in the corpus striatum. To reduce the peripheral side-effects, by inhibiting extracerebral conversion of levodopa to dopamine, it is best given with carbidopa as co-careldopa.
2. E   Flumazenil is a benzodiazepine antagonist and so can reverse the overdose effect.
3. F   The antidote to paracetamol poisoning, *N*-acetylcysteine, is best given within 12 hours of overdose to provide the best protection against liver injury and renal failure.
4. G   Lidocaine can be given topically.
5. H   After vital signs have been checked it is important to administer pain relief. Trauma on the road is often severe and requiring strong pain relief as well as treatment of injuries sustained.

4. Antibiotics and antivirals

1. B   Penicillins, such as amoxicillin, are commonly given to treat urinary tract infections, which tend to occur more commonly in females due to the urethra being shorter than in males. They are bactericidal.
2. J   Stevens–Johnson syndrome is a rare but life-threatening condition which can be induced by certain drugs, such as the anti-folates. Trimethoprim is an antifolate and it is bacteriostatic.
3. H   Rifampicin dyes some body secretions, such as tears and urine, an orange-red colour.
4. A   Aciclovir inhibits herpes simplex virus DNA synthesis and viral DNA polymerase.
5. D   Bleomycin should be stopped immediately if there is suspicion of lung fibrosis, which occurs in a dose-related manner in patients who use it.

5. Cardiovascular system drugs

1. D   The dilatation of systemic veins decreases the preload of the heart and therefore decreases the oxygen demand of the myocardium. This makes organic nitrates very useful in acute angina attacks.
2. B   Class Ib drugs, such as lidocaine, are given for ventricular arrhythmias following myocardial

infarction. Adverse effects associated with these drugs include hypotension, bradycardia and drowsiness.

3. F Amiodarone blocks potassium, sodium and calcium channels and is a class III antiarrhythmic drug. However, it can cause dangerous torsades de pointes arrhythmias.

4. I Verapamil is a class IV drugs and so acts as a calcium antagonist. Class IV drugs are useful for supraventricular arrhythmias.

5. H Cardiac glycosides inhibit the membrane Na^+/K^+ ATPase of myocytes. Their positive inotropic effect means that they are useful in heart failure but they have a very narrow therapeutic index.

6. Drug interactions

1. G The answer is not moclobemide (which is a reversible MAOI) since the 'cheese reactions' usually occur with the older irreversible drugs of this class.

2. F Phenytoin induces the hepatic P450 system, therefore increasing the metabolism of several drugs, including oral contraceptives and anticoagulants. Therefore levels may be subtherapeutic, rendering them ineffective.

3. B Clozapine is an atypical antipsychotic drug and side-effects include hypersalivation, weight gain, tachycardia and neutropenia.

4. D Respiratory depression can occur when alcohol is combined with benzodiazepines.

5. J Thiazide diuretics cause a drug interaction with lithium by causing a rise in its plasma concentration, which can result in signs of lithium toxicity.

7. Endocrine system drugs

1. G Carbimazole and propylthiouracil inhibit thyroid peroxidase and therefore are treatments for hyperthyroidism.

2. E Oral contraceptives increase the risk of venous thromboembolism and must be stopped immediately if there is a suggestion of deep vein thrombosis.

3. B The correct answer is not insulin aspart and insulin zinc suspension as they are a short-acting insulin and intermediate-acting insulin, respectively. The only answer suitable is isophane insulin.

4. C Glibenclamide and metformin are oral antidiabetic drugs. Metformin is contraindicated in patients with heart failure.

5. F Prednisolone is a synthetic glucocorticoid used as an anti-inflammatory drug, an immunosuppressant or in physiological replacement therapy. Chronic use of such glucocorticoids can result in the development of Cushing's syndrome, as in this patient.

8. The kidney and urinary tract drugs

1. G This is a description of the action of loop diuretics. They are useful as a treatment for acute pulmonary oedema, oedema due to congestive heart failure, liver disease or nephrotic syndrome.

2. D Oxybutynin competitively antagonizes the muscarinic acetylcholine receptors in the smooth muscle of the bladder.

3. B This describes the potassium-sparing diuretics, amiloride and triamterene. Spironolactone is another member of this class of drug but it acts as an antagonist at aldosterone receptors in the cells of the distal tubule and collecting duct.

4. I Sildenafil is a selective inhibitor of phosphodiesterase type 5. Non-specific inhibition of phosphodiesterase type 6 in the retina is responsible for occasional disturbances in colour vision.

5. J Thiazide diuretics, such as bendroflumethiazide, have this action and are used in treating hypertension and oedema.

9. Gastrointestinal system drugs

1. B Antacids are used to treat gastro-oesophageal reflux disease. They work by raising the intraluminal pH of the stomach and therefore may neutralize acid and inhibit pepsin activity.

2. C There is an increased risk of gastrointestinal bleeding and peptic ulcer disease in patients taking aspirin. Omeprazole acts by irreversible inhibition of H^+/K^+ ATPase.

3. G Senna is a stimulant laxative, whereas lactulose is an osmotic laxative, working by increasing the water content of the bowel.

4. F Hyoscine is a muscarinic antagonist antiemetic; the other antiemetic, domperidone, acts via dopamine receptors in the chemoreceptor trigger zone.

5. I The aminosalicylate, mesalazine, is given for maintenance therapy, whereas prednisolone is used for acute exacerbations.

10. Respiratory system drugs

1. H   The respiratory system uses physical defence mechanisms, such as coughing or the mucociliary escalator, to protect itself from foreign bodies.

2. E   Anticholinergics are used in the treatment of COPD. Dry mouth may occur as a result of their antimuscarinic activity.

3. B β_2-Adrenoceptor agonists are used for immediate relief of symptoms in asthma. Salbutamol is an example of a short-acting drug and salmeterol is an example of a longer-acting drug.

4. C   Intravenous aminophylline is important for treatment of severe asthma attacks. However, care should be taken due to this drug's narrow therapeutic range and susceptibility to drug interactions.

5. D   Opiate (such as, heroin or morphine) overdose causes respiratory depression. Naloxone is the antagonist used as an antidote to reverse the respiratory depression.

Glossary

Aetiology The science of causation or origin of disease.

ACh (Acetylcholine) A neurotransmitter mainly used in parasympathetic neurotransmission.

Agonist A ligand that binds to receptors, thus activating the receptor and causing a response.

Agranulocytosis A serious condition in which white blood cells decrease to dangerously low numbers. Drugs which can cause this include antiepileptics, antithyroid drugs and some antipsychotics (such as clozapine).

Anaphylaxis An immediate and severe allergic reaction to a substance (e.g. certain foods or drugs). Symptoms of anaphylaxis include breathing difficulty loss of consciousness and a drop in blood pressure, or it could even be fatal.

Antagonist A ligand that binds to receptors and reduces the chance of an agonist binding, but which itself is unable to activate the receptor.

Ascites An abnormal collection of fluid in the abdominal cavity.

β-Blockers Drugs which antagonize β-adrenergic receptors.

BMI (Body mass index) is the weight (kg) of a person divided by the square of the height (m). Generally, normal is 20–25; below this is underweight and above is overweight.

cAMP (Cyclic adenosine monophosphate) A second messenger produced by conversion of adenosine triphosphate (ATP) by the enzyme adenyl cyclase.

Central nervous system Comprises the brain and the spinal cord

Congestive cardiac failure (CCF) Impaired ability of the heart to fill with or pump sufficient blood around the body, affecting both left and right sides of the heart.

CT (Computerized tomography) is a form of X-ray examination in which the X-ray source and detector rotate around the object to be scanned, to produce cross-sectional images.

Dementia A neurological condition characterized by a gradual, progressive decline in intellectual functioning as a result of damage or disease of the brain.

Dyskinesia Impaired ability to control movement with involuntary muscular activity.

Dyspnoea Shortness of breath.

ECG (Electrocardiogram) Record of the electric current produced by the contraction of the heart muscle.

Endogenous Produced within the body.

Exogenous Produced outside the body.

First-pass metabolism The phenomenon of a drug which taken orally is absorbed through the intestinal wall, goes directly to the liver through the portal vein system and gets metabolized there before reaching the target organ. This is avoided by giving the drugs by other routes (e.g. intramuscular, intravenous).

Fundoscopy Examining the back of the eye using an ophthalmoscope.

Half-life The time taken for the plasma concentration of a drug to fall by half after the administration of the drug is stopped.

Hepatomegaly An abnormally enlarged liver.

Hypersensitivity An exaggerated response by the immune system to a foreign substance.

Isoenzymes Enzymes that perform the same function but have different sets of amino acids. These enzymes may have different physical properties.

Jugular venous pressure The indirect, observed pressure measurement of the venous system. It helps by giving useful clues that may aid diagnosis of heart and lung diseases.

Ligand A small molecule that binds to a specific site on a protein.

Lipolysis The breakdown of fats.

M$_{1/2/3/4}$ Muscarinic receptor subtypes; they mediate parasympathetic neurotransmission.

MAO (Monoamine oxidase) is a neuronal enzyme that metabolizes monoamines (noradrenaline, serotonin and dopamine). It has two main isoforms: MAO$_A$ and MAO$_B$. Drugs may selectively target one isoenzyme or be non-selective.

Monoclonal antibodies Highly specific, purified antibodies that are derived from only one clone of cells and recognize only one antigen. They can be created to target a specific compound of interest and thus serve to detect specific characteristics of certain cells.

MRSA (Multiple drug resistant *Staphylococcus aureus*) is an increasingly dangerous bacterium that is resistant to many antibiotics.

Noradrenaline A neurotransmitter mediating sympathetic neurotransmission.

Na+/K+ATPase An energy dependent ion transporter.

Non-steroidal anti-inflammatory drug (NSAID) A drug used in the treatment of inflammation and mild pain.

Orthopnoea Breathlessness on lying flat.

Partial agonist A ligand that can activate a receptor, but cannot bring about a maximum response despite occupying all receptors.

Pathogenesis The cellular events, reactions and mechanisms resulting in the development of disease.

Peripheral nervous system (PNS) Comprises all nerves, with the exception of those in the brain and the spinal cord.

Pharmacodynamics The effects a drug will have on the body's organs and the relation between drug concentration and effect.

Pharmacokinetics The study of how compounds are absorbed, distributed, metabolized and eliminated by the body. In other words, the study of how the body acts on the drug.

Phosphorylation The addition of a phosphate group to a molecule, often causing activation, or sometimes deactivation, of proteins.

Receptor A molecule on the surface of a cell that serves as a recognition or binding site for antigens, antibodies, or other cellular or immunological components, resulting in a change in the activity of the cell.

Smoking pack years A measurement of a person's total cigarette smoking over a lifetime. It is calculated as the average number of packs smoked per day (where a pack is 20 cigarettes) multiplied by number of years. For example, somebody who smoked 10 cigarettes (half a pack) every day for 30 years would have a 15 pack year history: $0.5 \times 30 = 15$.

Systemic lupus erythematosus A chronic inflammatory connective tissue disease with features including skin rashes, joint pain and swelling, and inflammation of the kidneys and the fibrous tissue surrounding the heart (i.e. the pericardium).

Thrombocytopenia Reduced platelet numbers in the blood.

Torsades de pointes arrhythmia A potentially fatal form of ventricular tachycardia. On the electrocardiogram (ECG), it will present like ventricular tachycardia, but the QRS complexes will swing up and down around the baseline in a chaotic fashion.